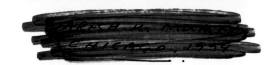

Cerebrovascular Occlusive Disease and Brain Ischemia

AANS Publications Committee
Issam A. Awad, MD, Editor

Neurosurgical Topics

American Association of
Neurological Surgeons

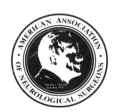

ISBN: 1-8792840-1-4

Neurosurgical Topics ISBN: 0-9624246-6-8

Robert H. Wilkins, MD, Chairman
AANS Publications Committee

Linda S. Miller, AANS Staff Editor

AANS1.3M792

Forthcoming Books in the *Neurosurgical Topics* Series

1992

Neurosurgery for the Third Millennium
   Edited by Michael L.J. Apuzzo, MD

Degenerative Disease of the Cervical Spine
   Edited by Paul R. Cooper, MD

1993

Surgery of the Cranial Nerves of the Posterior Fossa
   Edited by Daniel L. Barrow, MD

Current Management of Cerebral Aneurysms
   Edited by Issam Awad, MD

Spinal Instrumentation
   Edited by Edward C. Benzel, MD

Interactive Image-Guided Neurosurgery
   Edited by Robert Maciunas, MD

Dedication and Acknowledgments

This book is dedicated first and foremost to the memory of my father, whose premature death from complications of cerebrovascular occlusive disease heightened my awareness of and interest in this problem from a very early age. Since that time, my family has remained a great source of inspiration and support as I increasingly channeled my efforts to study the problem of brain ischemia in the laboratory and at the bedside. The pioneers in this field have prepared a solid foundation of scientific information, rational thinking, and conceptual analysis of brain ischemia. I am indebted to all of them for their vision, and most notably to my cerebrovascular mentors and teachers — Anthony J. Furlan, John R. Little, and Robert F. Spetzler. Each made a great effort in showing me their fascination with this problem, and in guiding me through the study and analysis of one or more facets of it.

The past decade has witnessed a revolution of scientific and clinical information related to cerebrovascular occlusive disease and brain ischemia. Based on this solid scientific foundation, there has been a renaissance of diagnostic and treatment approaches which have reached the bedside in a practical and beneficial way. There were landmark clinical studies confirming the usefulness of antiplatelet therapy and carotid endarterectomy in stroke prevention, and discrediting the widespread use of bypass revascularization procedures for brain ischemia.

Many advances have occurred in the classification of stroke types and in the tailoring of therapeutic measures to individual pathophysiologic scenarios. In this book, the contributors have attempted to synthesize some of this information in a practical way that would be of help to the practicing neurosurgeon, the resident in training, and other physicians who are not primary specialists in stroke. The book does not shy away from areas of controversy, but attempts to reach toward a consensus whenever possible. I am indebted to each of the contributors—true experts in their field—for simplifying, clarifying, and synthesizing a vast body of complex and controversial information. It has been a pleasure to work with each one of them, and I am particularly thankful for the timely and up-to-date compilations on their respective discussions on this topic.

I wish to acknowledge the expert secretarial assistance of Ms. Shirley McDaniel, who followed through the various stages of manuscript preparation with thoroughness and care. I am grateful to Ms. Linda Miller and Mr. Jeremy Longhurst, of the National Office of the American Association of Neurological Surgeons, for their expert and professional guidance through various phases of manuscript preparation and editing. Lastly, I wish to thank Dr. Robert Wilkins and all the members of the Publications Committee of the American Association of Neurological Surgeons for their inspiration, assistance, and support in the conceptualization and preparation of this work.

The Editor

Contents

CONTRIBUTORS   vii

PREFACE   ix

Chapter 1   Brain Metabolism, Blood Flow, and Ischemic Thresholds   1
             Fredric B. Meyer, MD

Chapter 2   Hemorheology of Cerebral Blood Flow and Ischemia   25
             Adam J. Davis, MD and Jafar J. Jafar, MD,

Chapter 3   Clinical Spectrum and Natural History of Cerebrovascular Occlusive Disease   59
             Marc I. Chimowitz, MB, ChB

Chapter 4   Diagnostic Evaluation of Ischemic Cerebrovascular Disease   73
             Joseph M. Zabramski, MD, and John A. Anson, MD

Chapter 5   Doppler Ultrasonography in Cerebrovascular Occlusive Disease   103
             Pierre B. Fayad, MD, and Lawrence M. Brass, MD

Chapter 6   Risk Factor Modification and Medical Therapy for Stroke Prevention   117
             Robert J. Dempsey, MD, and Robert W. Moore, PhD

Chapter 7   Medical Management of Acute Brain Ischemia   135
             Stephen Davis, MD

Chapter 8   Indications for Surgery in Extracranial Carotid Disease   155
             Christopher M. Loftus, MD, FACS

Chapter 9   Carotid Endarterectomy: Technical Aspects and Perioperative Management   167
             Daniel L. Barrow, MD, and Junichi Mizuno, MD

Chapter 10   Arterial Trauma and Dissection   187
             Cathy A. Sila, MD, and Issam A. Awad, MD, MS, FACS

Chapter 11   Vertebrobasilar Occlusive Disease   203
                  Fernando G. Diaz, MD, PhD

Chapter 12   Extracranial-Intracranial Bypass Surgery: Current Indications and Techniques   215
                  Issam A. Awad, MD, MS, FACS

Chapter 13   Endovascular Thrombolysis and Angioplasty   231
                  Bruce Mackay, MD

Chapter 14   Clinical Trials in Cerebrovascular Surgery   251
                  Marc R. Mayberg, MD

Chapter 15   Outcome and Rehabilitation in Ischemic Stroke   265
                  Bruce M. Coull, MD, and Dennis P. Briley, MD

Chapter 16   A Unified Concept of Cerebrovascular Occlusive Disease and Brain Ischemia   281
                  Issam A. Awad, MD, MS, FACS

INDEX   291

List of Contributors

John A. Anson, MD
Assistant Professor
Division of Neurosurgery
University of New Mexico
Albuquerque, New Mexico

Issam A. Awad, MD, MS, FACS
Head, Section of Cerebrovascular Surgery
Vice-Chairman, Department of Neurosurgery
The Cleveland Clinic Foundation
Cleveland, Ohio

Daniel L. Barrow, MD
Associate Professor of Neurosurgery
The Emory Clinic
Section of Neurological Surgery
Atlanta, Georgia

Lawrence M. Brass, MD
Associate Professor
Yale University School of Medicine
Department of Neurology
New Haven, Connecticut

Dennis P. Briley, MD
Chief, Neurology Section
Huntington VA Medical Center
Huntington, West Virginia

Marc I. Chimowitz, MB, ChB
Assistant Professor
Department of Neurology
University of Michigan Medical Center
Ann Arbor, Michigan

Bruce M. Coull, MD
Chief, Neurology Service
Portland VA Medical Center
Associate Professor of Neurology
Oregon Health Sciences University
Portland, Oregon

Adam J. Davis, MD
Fellow, Division of Neuroradiology
Department of Radiology
New York University Medical Center
New York, New York

Stephen Davis, MD
Head, Stroke Service
Royal Melbourne Hospital and
    University of Melbourne
Department of Neurology
Parkville, Victoria, Australia

Robert J. Dempsey, MD
Professor of Surgery
Division of Neurosurgery
University of Kentucky College of Medicine
Lexington, Kentucky

Fernando G. Diaz, MD, PhD
Professor and Chairman
Department of Neurological Surgery
Wayne State University of Medicine
Detroit, Michigan

Pierre B. Fayad, MD
Assistant Professor
Yale University School of Medicine
Department of Neurology
New Haven, Connecticut

Jafar J. Jafar, MD
Associate Professor
Department of Neurosurgery
New York University Medical Center
New York, New York

Christopher M. Loftus, MD, FACS
Associate Professor of Surgery
Division of Neurological Surgery
The University of Iowa College of Medicine
Iowa City, Iowa

Bruce C. Mackay, MD
Atlanta Neurologic Institute; and
Clinical Assistant Professor
The Emory Clinic
Section of Neurology
Atlanta, Georgia

Marc R. Mayberg, MD
Associate Professor of Neurosurgery
University of Washington School of Medicine
Department of Neurological Surgery
Seattle, Washington

Fredric B. Meyer, MD
Assistant Professor
Department of Neurosurgery
Mayo Clinic and Mayo
   Graduate School of Medicine
Rochester, Minnesota

Junichi Mizuno, MD
Research Fellow
The Emory Clinic
Section of Neurological Surgery
Atlanta, Georgia

Robert W. Moore, PhD
Senior Clinical Research Associate
Sanders-Brown Center on Aging, Stroke Program
University of Kentucky College of Medicine
Lexington, Kentucky

Cathy A. Sila, MD
Associate Medical Director
Cerebrovascular Center
Department of Neurology
The Cleveland Clinic Foundation
Cleveland, Ohio

Joseph M. Zabramski, MD
Assistant Professor of Surgery
University of Arizona
Head, Cerebrovascular Laboratory
Barrow Neurological Institute
Phoenix, Arizona

AANS Publications Committee

Preface

Stroke remains a major cause of death and disability and is gaining greater epidemiologic and socioeconomic prominence in the aging population of industrialized nations. In recent years, there have been major advances in the understanding of the pathophysiology of cerebrovascular occlusive disease and associated mechanisms of brain ischemia. Many therapeutic modalities have been accredited through a multitude of well-designed cooperative studies, while other treatment approaches have fallen out of favor. Traditional nihilistic attitudes about the diagnosis and treatment of stroke are being replaced rapidly by a rational diagnostic and treatment strategy based on pathophysiologic mechanisms.

Neurosurgeons have been at the forefront of advancing knowledge in this field, and continue to be called upon to assist in the diagnosis and treatment of this problem. Often, the decision whether to operate or withhold surgical treatment hinges upon the recommendation of a well-informed neurosurgeon with expertise and comprehensive understanding of brain ischemia. This book attempts to compile current knowledge on the pathophysiology and clinical presentation of cerebrovascular occlusive disease, prevention and medical management of brain ischemia, and the indications and surgical options for the treatment of extracranial and intracranial occlusive disease. A unified concept of cerebrovascular occlusive disease and brain ischemia encourages the adoption of therapeutic recommendations based on elucidation of pathophysiologic mechanisms operative in the individual case.

This book is aimed primarily at providing the practicing neurosurgeon and the resident in training with a useful and practical body of knowledge regarding this problem, including areas of consensus and of controversy. It is hoped that physicians of all specialties might use this book as a source of practical, readable, and accessible information about this complex topic.

Issam A. Awad, MD, MS, FACS
Cleveland, Ohio

CHAPTER 1

Brain Metabolism, Blood Flow, and Ischemic Thresholds*

Fredric B. Meyer, MD

Although the human brain accounts for only 2% of total body weight, it requires 15% of the resting cardiac output (approximately 750 ml per minute), 20% of the inspired oxygen at rest, and the liver's entire output of glucose in the fasting state. It is dependent on the oxidative phosphorylation of glucose for ATP production since it has no appreciable stores of glycogen.[58] The classic work of Kety and Schmidt established that resting cerebral blood flow (CBF) in man is approximately 50 ml/100 g of brain tissue/min.[27] This degree of blood flow reflects the brain's requirement of half of its own volume of blood flow per minute in the resting state. Total CBF remains relatively stable throughout fluctuations in body activity, cardiac output, and blood pressure. However, regional blood flow is closely coupled to metabolism and increases significantly with activation of a particular cortical region.[49]

This chapter reviews normal physiologic characteristics of brain metabolism and cerebral circulation and examines the mechanisms by which blood flow is coupled to cerebral metabolism. These concepts are applied to the pathophysiology of focal cerebral ischemia. Several significant differences exist between focal and global cerebral ischemia—patients with global ischemia have no col-

lateral flow during the ischemic insult. In focal ischemia the potential for low-level residual blood flow from collateral circulation results in a more complex biochemical picture, including the delivery of glucose under anaerobic conditions that may worsen brain acidosis. The residual perfusion in focal ischemia may provide sufficient substrate delivery to maintain a low level of metabolic activity; this will preserve membrane integrity, thereby retarding the evolution of irreversible injury. Global ischemia, as observed in patients suffering from cardiac arrest, rarely presents to a neurosurgeon for treatment. On the other hand, focal ischemia is frequently encountered in patients suffering from subarachnoid hemorrhage-induced vasospasm, embolic or hemodynamic stroke secondary to atherosclerotic occlusive disease, or temporary vessel occlusion during neurovascular operations.

Brain Metabolism: Basic Considerations

Oxygen Metabolism

The availability of oxygen, in sufficiently high concentrations to subserve the oxidative metabolism of glucose, is essential for brain function.[58] Normal atmospheric oxygen tensions of approximately 150 mm Hg result in alveolar tensions in the range of 100 mm Hg,

*Work performed in the author's laboratory was supported by NIH R01 25374.

which approximates arterial oxygen tensions (PaO_2). However, in clinical practice, PaO_2 usually varies between 80-90 mm Hg depending on patient age and pulmonary status. In chronic smokers who commonly have both pulmonary and cerebrovascular disease the PaO_2 is typically lower. Although the normal venous oxygen tension (PvO_2) is approximately 40 mm Hg, the complexity of the capillary network makes it difficult to determine a true average capillary oxygen tension by simply subtracting PvO_2 from PaO_2. In fact, the PaO_2 of the capillary bed is thought to be approximately 60 mm Hg.

The critical oxygen tension, defined as that tension below which oxygen consumption is reduced, varies considerably from species to species. In man, a PaO_2 of 30 mm Hg will result in loss of consciousness. Cortical grey matter oxygen tensions of approximately 25 mm Hg and white matter oxygen tensions of approximately 10 mm Hg have been reported. These tissue oxygen tensions are significantly lower than arterial oxygen tensions. Nonetheless, they are sufficient to subserve mitochondrial function, which requires intracellular oxygen tensions of approximately 1-2 mm Hg.

Energy Production

The energy requirement of the human brain, equivalent to the energy consumed by a 25-watt light bulb, is primarily provided by adenosinetriphosphate (ATP). The site of oxidative phosphorylation for energy production is the mitochondrial membrane. Its lipid membrane contains the enzymes necessary for oxidative phosphorylation, serves as a barrier that permits generation of electrochemical-proton gradients, and houses the proteins and coenzymes that transmit electrons from reduced nicotinamide adenine dinucleotide (NADH) to oxygen.

While oxygen enters mitochondria by simple diffusion, glucose delivery requires facilitated transport through the blood-brain barrier. Once within the mitochondrial cytoplasm, each molecule of glucose is split into two molecules of pyruvic acid by an anaerobic sequence of enzymatically activated reactions (glycolysis) that yields only two molecules of ATP for each molecule of glucose split. Pyruvic acid then enters mitochondria by way of a specific transporter and is oxidatively decarboxylated in the citric acid or Krebs cycle to CO_2 and hydrogen. Although the intricate details of these reactions are beyond the scope of this discussion, conceptualizing the events facilitates understanding the exquisite sensitivity of neuronal tissues to ischemia.[58]

Protons derived from pyruvic acid in the Krebs cycle are enzymatically added to NAD^+ to yield the reduced form of the dinucleotide (NADH). They are then transported as NADH to the mitochondrial membrane, where they are passed to the members of the respiratory chain. At this point, hydrogen ions are separated into electrons and protons (H+). During their passage down the electron transport chain to oxygen, the electrons generate more protons which are ejected from the mitochondria. Extrusion of protons leads to cytoplasmic acidification which is corrected by extrusion of H^+ into the extracellular space by the cytoplasmic membrane Na^+/H^+ pump. This local extracellular acidosis will lead to vasodilatation with increases in CBF, and is a mechanism by which blood flow is coupled to metabolism. The accumulation of protons in the extramitochondrial space will lead to an electric potential gradient of approximately 0.18 volts across the mitochondrial membrane.

In his chemosmotic theory, Mitchell proposed that the energy from both the proton and electron gradients could be combined with conformational changes in the mitochondrial membrane to drive ATP phosphorylation from adenosine diphosphate (ADP). The ATP then diffuses throughout the cytoplasm to provide energy in the form of high-energy phosphate bonds to drive various energy-dependent cellular functions such as membrane transport and ion pumps. It has been estimated that the brain oxidizes 90%

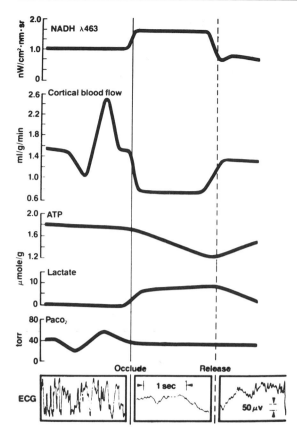

Figure 1. Correlation of cortical NADH fluorescence, cortical blood flow, and parenchymal ATP with lactic acid levels at various levels of $PaCO_2$ and during ischemia. Note that NADH remains at a constant level throughout a wide range of $PaCO_2$ and CBF but increases significantly during middle cerebral artery occlusion. Concordant with the increase in NADH is an increase in lactic acid and decline in ATP, also due to the ischemic injury. This failure of energy production is associated with EEG attenuation. (From Sundt TM Jr, Anderson RE, Sharbrough FW. Effects of hypocapnia, hypercapnia, and blood pressure on NADH fluorescence, electrical activity, and blood flow in normal and partially ischemic monkey cortex. J Neurochem. 1976; 27:1125-1133.)

Accordingly, there is an increase in the concentration of the reduced form of the membrane components (e.g. NADH) of the electron transport chain (Figure 1). The rise in NADH in the mitochondria coupled with the inability to process pyruvic acid in the Krebs cycle leads to a subsequent rise of pyruvic acid concentrations in the cytoplasm. With accumulation of NADH and pyruvic acid, cytoplasmic lactic dehydrogenase catalyzes the reduction of pyruvic acid in cytoplasm to lactic acid, which subsequently leads to a marked intracellular acidosis.

Cerebral Metabolic Rates

Cerebral metabolic rates are the product of the difference between the arterial and venous concentrations of metabolites such as oxygen or glucose multiplied by the CBF. The cerebral metabolic rate of glucose is 4.5-5.5 ml of glucose/100 g of brain tissue/min, or about 80 ml of glucose per minute for the entire brain.

The cerebral metabolic rate for oxygen is approximately 3.0-3.5 ml O_2/100 g brain tissue/min, which represents an oxygen consumption of approximately 50 ml per min for the total brain or approximately 20% of the body's total utilization of oxygen at rest. Since the respiratory quotient of the brain is roughly 1, oxygen consumption equals carbon dioxide production.

Finally, the cerebral metabolic rate of lactate is 2.3 μ mol/100 g brain tissue/min in nonpathologic states. As expected, it increases during ischemia or hypoxia.

Cerebral Blood Flow: Basic Considerations

Microanatomy

The cerebral circulation is a low-resistance bed composed of surface conducting vessels and penetrating arterioles. The penetrating or nutrient arterioles originate at right angles

to 100% of the glucose which it receives through facilitated transport.

In normal circumstances, there is sufficient oxygen to receive the electrons descending through the electron transport chain along the mitochondrial membrane. During ischemia the reduction in oxygen leads to a marked reduction in the flow of electrons.

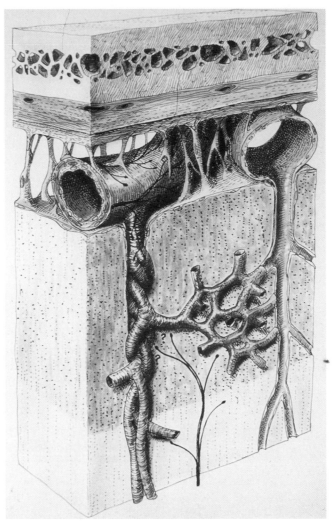

Figure 2. Depiction of surface conducting vessels and penetrating arterioles. The penetrating arterioles and precapillary sphincter are major sites of CBF regulation.

to the surface conducting vessels and penetrate the brain parenchyma. These penetrating vessels can be divided into a short arterial palisade that supplies the cortical capillary bed and a longer palisade that supplies white matter capillaries (Figure 2). There also appears to be a horizontal organization of capillary beds corresponding to cortical lamination. Of note is the probable existence of a precapillary sphincter which is thought to assist in local CBF regulation. Capillary beds appear to arise at right angles from the penetrating arterioles in a three-dimensional pyramid fashion with two to three capillary

loops being subserved by one precapillary sphincter.

The circumference of a typical brain capillary consists of a few endothelial cells making contact primarily with tight junctions. The endothelial cells are rich in mitochondria but have less vesicular structures (as observed in normal brain endothelium). On the abluminal surface, the endothelial cells are ensheathed by a basement membrane, which occasionally splits to enclose a pericyte. Beyond the basement membrane are investing end feet from glial cells. This combination of tight junction, basement membrane, and enveloping astrocytic processes is thought to be the anatomic substrate of the blood-brain barrier. In the penetrating arterioles and venules there is an intervening layer of smooth muscle cells between the basement membrane and glial foot processes.

Cerebral Blood Flow Regulation

Cerebral blood flow regulation has classically been defined as the ability of the brain to maintain a constant CBF despite changes in systemic arterial blood pressure. In non-hypertensive man, CBF will remain stable at an arterial blood pressure between 60 mm Hg and 160 mm Hg.[21] If arterial blood pressure rises above these parameters, CBF will either decline or increase accordingly. More recently, cerebral autoregulation has been redefined to describe the ability of the cerebral cortex to regulate and adjust CBF to satisfy its metabolic demands.[49] Many factors which contribute to CBF regulation can be conceptually divided into either intrinsic or extrinsic modulators.

Intrinsic Modulators

Balis Effect

The Balis effect is the intrinsic contractile response of smooth muscle cells in arteries and penetrating arterioles to an increase in intraluminal distending pressures. In all likelihood, the Balis effect is important for maintaining the overall tone of the vessel, but is not a major regulator of cerebral blood flow. It has been postulated that an increase in transluminal distending pressure leads to a release of intracellular calcium, which enhances myosin and actin filament crosslinking.

Extracellular pH

With increased metabolism, a local extracellular acidosis occurs due to an accumulation of H^+ and lactic acid. A longstanding theory holds that this extracellular acidosis induces a local vasodilatation that increases local CBF, thereby coupling blood flow with metabolic demand.[30] The mechanism by which a decline in extracellular pH (pH_e) induces vasodilatation has been thought to be due to altered membrane permeability or to changes in membrane receptor function. Profound extracellular acidosis induces a vasomotor paralysis in which CBF may depend directly on systemic arterial blood pressure.[29] Other evidence suggests that brain pH may not be the primary determinant of blood flow-metabolic coupling; for example, different anesthetics can cause differences in CBF despite similar intracellular pH (pH_i) changes. Moreover, there are differences in CBF between primary and secondary seizure foci despite essentially identical parenchymal brain pH_i.

Coupling Agents

Recent experimental data demonstrated that CBF regulation is a complex phenomenon that cannot be explained by one or two relatively simple mechanisms such as changes in extracellular pH. A large number of neuropeptides, including substance P and vasoactive intestinal peptide (VIP), have been shown to effect CBF. Certain neurotransmitters such as adenosine have been shown to modulate CBF, probably through a calcium antagonist effect.[28,75] Evidence now exists that endothelial cells can directly effect vascular tone through both endothelial-releasing factor (EDRF) and endothelin. Tables 1 and 2 list agents which may couple blood flow and metabolism.[17]

The fact that cerebral blood vessels receive a rich network of neurovascular nerve fibers containing monoamines, vasoactive peptides, and acetylcholine supports the contention that CBF regulation is complex. Although continued research is required to define the origin and function of these perivascular systems, there is definitive evidence for the existence of sympathetic innervation containing both norepinephrine and neuropeptide Y as neurotransmitters. These vasoconstrictive neurotransmitters likely have a physiologic role in preventing excessive cerebral vasodilatation due to systemic hypertension. The significance of serotonin-containing fibers origi-

TABLE 1
Potential Coupling Agents — Vasoconstrictors

Neurotransmitter	Origin	Role
Norepinephrine	Sympathetic ganglia	Dampens increases in CBF during severe hypertension
	Locus ceruleus	Modulates intracranial blood volume, BBB permeability
Neuropeptide Y	Sympathetic ganglia	Comparable to norepinephrine
Serotonin	Raphe nuclei	Unknown
Thromboxane A2	Blood vessel	Unknown
Endothelin	Endothelial cells	Unknown

TABLE 2
Possible Coupling Agents — Vasodilators

Neurotransmitter	Origin	Role
Acetylcholine	? 7th nerve sphenopalatine ganglia endothelial	Unknown
Substance P/ Neurokinin A	5th nerve	Prevents excessive vasoconstriction
Calcitonin-gene-related peptide	5th nerve	Unknown
Vasoactive intestinal peptide (VIP)/ Cholecystokinin (CCK)	Cortical neurons	Unknown
Prostacyclin	Blood vessel	? maintenance of basal tone
EDRF	Endothelial cells	Unknown
Adenosine	Cortical neurons	Blood pressure autoregulation coupling CBF to cortical activity

nating from the Raphe nucleus is unknown. The trigeminal ganglion, a source of perivascular fibers containing substance P, neurokinin A, and calcitonin gene-related peptide, may be responsible for preventing excessive vasoconstriction of circle of Willis arteries. The significance of perivascular nerve fibers originating from intracerebral neurons is unclear. Putative associated neurotransmitters include VIP, cholecystokinin (CCK), and adenosine. Finally, acetylcholine, an abundant perivascular neurotransmitter, is a vasodilator with functions in CBF regulation that remain largely unknown.

There is evidence indicating that prostaglandins and other derivatives of arachidonic acid play an important role in CBF regulation, in both physiologic and pathologic states.[47] Some eicosanoids such as thromboxane A_2 are potent vasoconstrictors, whereas others such as prostacyclin are potent vasodilators. Cerebral ischemia and other pathologic states effect a significant increase in the production of prostanoids and leukotrienes. The mechanism of action of the various eicosanoids on vascular smooth muscle are not well understood, but may be mediated by changes in adenylate cyclase. The release of vasoconstrictive prostanoids from platelets may be an important factor in reducing residual blood flow during an ischemic insult.

Extrinsic Modulators

Perfusion Pressure

Perfusion pressure is defined as the difference between cerebral arterial pressure and the cerebral venous pressure. In most circumstances the venous pressure is low except in cases of increased intracranial pressure. Cerebral autoregulatory mechanisms maintain CBF in a normal range over a wide range of perfusion pressures.[21] However, when arterial blood pressure declines below 60 mm Hg there will be a reduction in CBF. Alternatively, if systemic arterial blood pressure rises above 160 mm Hg, CBF will begin to increase. In hypertensive patients, compensatory autoregulatory mechanisms involve an increase in vascular tone to maintain CBF within a normal range with decreasing perfusion pressures. Variations in cardiac output do not significantly alter CBF if autoregulation is intact.

PaO_2 and $PaCO_2$ Tensions

Moderate changes in oxygen tensions do not significantly alter CBF. Hypoxia can be associated with an increase in CBF, presumably due to worsening of an extracellular acidosis with reflexive vasodilatation on that basis. Fluctuations in $PaCO_2$ will lead to significant changes in CBF. Carbon dioxide is a potent vasodilator of the cerebrovascular bed.

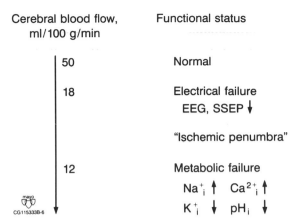

THRESHOLDS OF ISCHEMIA

Cerebral blood flow, ml/100 g/min	Functional status
50	Normal
18	Electrical failure EEG, SSEP ↓
	"Ischemic penumbra"
12	Metabolic failure Na^+_i ↑ Ca^{2+}_i ↑ K^+_i ↓ pH_i ↓

CG115333B-6

Figure 3. Schematic diagram of the thresholds of cerebral ischemia. Normal CBF in man is approximately 50 ml/100 g/min. When CBF declines to about 18 ml/100 g/min, there is loss of functional activity as evidenced by EEG attenuation. When CBF declines to approximately 12-10 ml/100 g/min, there is rapid alteration in extracellular ionic concentrations, representing depletion of ATP. This is ionic or membrane failure. Between these two thresholds of electrical failure and ionic failure, there is a circumscribed range of reduced CBF in which despite functional loss membrane activity is preserved, implying reversible ischemic neuronal damage.

An increase in $PaCO_2$ of 1 mm Hg will produce a 1-3 ml/100 g brain tissue/min increase in CBF. The mechanism by which $PaCO_2$ modulates CBF is thought to be due primarily to alterations in extracellular pH. Presumably the ineffectiveness of hypercapnia in increasing CBF in regions of ischemia is due to the pre-existing brain acidosis.

Ischemic Neuronal Injury
Thresholds of Cerebral Ischemia

Kety and Schmidt in 1948 first determined that CBF in man was approximately 50 ml/100 g brain tissue/min.[27] In 1973, in patients undergoing carotid endarterectomy with electroencephalography monitoring, it was shown that reductions in CBF to approximately 18 ml/100 g brain tissue/min caused attenuation in the electroencephalogram

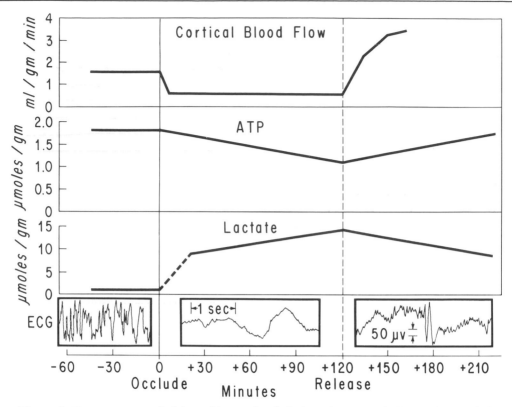

Figure 4. *Measurements of ATP and lactate levels before, during, and after occlusion of the middle cerebral artery in monkeys. Preocclusion ATP was 2 ± 0.11 $\mu mol/g$ and lactate was 2.32 ± 0.15 $\mu mol/g$. After vessel occlusion, ATP levels declined progressively to 25% of control values over 3 hours. Lactate levels increased rapidly during the first 30 minutes to about four times that of control values. Thereafter, lactate levels increased slowly to about seven times of that of control values after 2 hours. Despite acute EEG changes, residual collateral blood flow was sufficient to support limited metabolism for several hours. This study suggests that neuronal damage during focal ischemia after middle cerebral artery occlusion may be reversible. (From Michenfelder JD, Sundt TM Jr. Cerebral ATP and lactate levels in the squirrel monkey following occlusion of the middle cerebral artery. Stroke. 1971; 2:319-326.)*

(EEG).[56,71] Subsequent laboratory studies showed that reduction of CBF to 15 ml/100 g brain tissue/min suppressed somatosensory evoked potentials.[9] Accordingly, a threshold of electrical failure was quantitated at a critical CBF range of 18-15 ml/100 g brain tissue/min.

More recent investigations in a large number of experimental models showed that this threshold of electrical failure is reproducible, but may vary to a degree depending on the type and degree of anesthesia. In 1977, Astrup and colleagues demonstrated that a reduced blood flow of approximately 12-10 ml/100 g brain tissue/min led to significant alterations in extracellular ionic concentrations such as

K^+.[5] This was termed the threshold of ionic failure. Since neuronal tissue is critically dependent on a continuous delivery of oxygen and glucose for aerobic metabolism, declines in CBF to this approximate level of 12-10 ml/100 g brain tissue/min will cause a rapid depletion in ATP.[37] With depletion of ATP, there is failure of the Na^+/K^+ ATPase pump, which is essential for maintaining ionic gradients. Because of differences in the extracellular and intracellular concentration of these two ions, there is an efflux of potassium along with an influx of sodium into neurons, leading to membrane depolarization. In addition to these initial ionic fluxes, there is a rapid rise in intracellular lactic acid concentrations due to an anaerobic metabolic state.

During severe focal ischemia, lactic acid concentrations will increase four-fold during the first 30 minutes. With prolonged ischemia, lactic acid concentrations will climb to approximately 14 μmol/g of brain tissue (Figure 4). Although the tolerance of neuronal tissue for these reduced flows of approximately 10 ml/100 g/min is unknown, experimental evidence indicates that after 3-4 hours, irreversible neuronal injury may occur. Some brain regions are exquisitely susceptible to these low blood flow levels. For example, hippocampal CA1 neurons will demonstrate microscopic alterations after 3-5 minutes.

Between these two thresholds of electrical failure and ionic failure, there exists a small circumscribed range of CBF at which membrane homeostasis and structural integrity are maintained despite functional loss.[61] This circumscribed range of CBF has been termed "the ischemic penumbra."[4] It may explain why patients suffering from an acute focal ischemic event may have the potential for neuronal recovery, if there is sufficient collateral flow to satisfy basic energy requirements necessary for maintenance of membrane integrity.

The original intent of the term "ischemic penumbra" was to describe a zone of electrically silent but structurally intact parenchyma surrounding the core region of infarction during focal cerebral ischemia (Figure 5). Characterization of the ischemic penumbra relied primarily on electrophysiology, biochemistry, and histology during reduced cerebral blood flow.[23] There is now reasonable experimental evidence to confirm the probable existence of an ischemic penumbra. However, the question of ischemic penumbra stability remains unresolved. For example, CBF reductions to 18 ml/100 g/min in permanent middle cerebral artery (MCA) occlusion in the Macaca monkey leads to infarction, suggesting either deterioration in CBF or poor tolerance of neuronal tissue for prolonged reductions in blood flow. Variations in histological outcome following maintained CBF at the penumbra level led to categorization of the ischemic penumbra into two states.[68] Type 1 is charac-

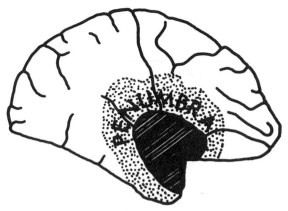

Figure 5. Schematic depiction of a core region of infarction surrounding a zone of reversibly injured tissue termed the "ischemic penumbra." (From Symon L. The relationship between CBF, evoked potentials, and the clinical features in cerebral ischemia. Acta Neurol Scand. 1980; 62 (Suppl 78):175-190.)

terized by EEG suppression, flow reduction, and neuronal structural preservation. Type 2 is defined by EEG attenuation, critical blood flow reduction, and repetitive transient increases in K^+_e. The Type 2 ischemic penumbra is associated with varying degrees of neuronal loss. The element of time also must be considered when analyzing the stability of the ischemic penumbra. Some experimental data indicates that a CBF of 18-23 ml/100 g/min may be tolerated for up to 2 weeks, while levels of 8-17 ml/100 g/min may result in infarction within 1-3 hours.

It is reasonable to assume that the ischemic penumbra is actually in a dynamic state that has the potential to decay over time. In fact, the source of decay may reflect a progressive decline in the residual collateral circulation due to either fatigue of collaterals or ischemic vasoconstriction. The clinical outcome following vessel occlusion reflects both the severity and duration of reduced CBF (Figure 6).[39]

Metabolic Events

The initial metabolic cascades which occur at a CBF of approximately 10 ml/100 g of brain tissue/min or less are complex and multifactorial. Some of these major events include brain acidosis, altered membrane

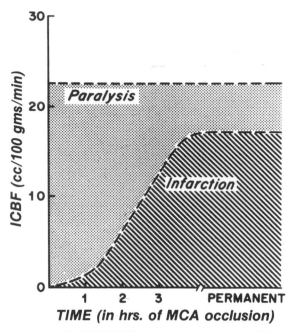

Figure 6. An analysis of ischemic thresholds relating time and severity of ischemia with morphologic injury. (From Jones TH, Morawetz RB, Crowell RM, et al. Threshold of focal cerebral ischemia in awake monkeys. J Neurosurg. *1981; 54:773-782.)*

Figure 7. Schematic depiction of relationship between energy failure and the major degradative metabolic pathways causing ischemic neuronal damage.

permeability to calcium and sodium, and release of sequestered intracellular calcium.

Conceptually, these events can all be related to energy failure (Figure 7). The release of excitatory amino acids, opening of membrane voltage-dependent calcium channels, and intracellular acidosis can all be linked to the failure of aerobic metabolism secondary to decreased glucose and oxygen delivery.

Calcium has a critical role in normal cellular events as secondary messenger, as metabolic regulator, and in effecting neurotransmitter release. Abnormal calcium accumulation can mediate anoxic death.[54] In 1977, Nicholson and colleagues demonstrated declines in extracellular calcium concentrations in hypoxic cerebellar cortex.[43] Subsequent observations that extracellular calcium declined in anoxia, status epilepticus, and hypoglycemic coma, led to an integrative hypothesis implicating calcium-related cell damage as the final common pathway for neuronal injury.[59] This theory postulated that calcium entered neurons through voltage-dependent calcium channels which opened following membrane depolarization. Under anaerobic conditions, the rapid depletion of ATP would result in failure of the Na^+/K^+ ATPase, which would lead to depolarization. Since intracellular calcium is largely sequestered in the endoplas-

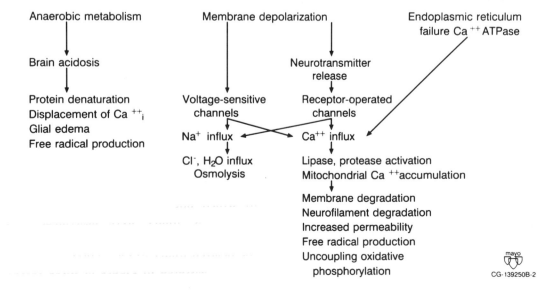

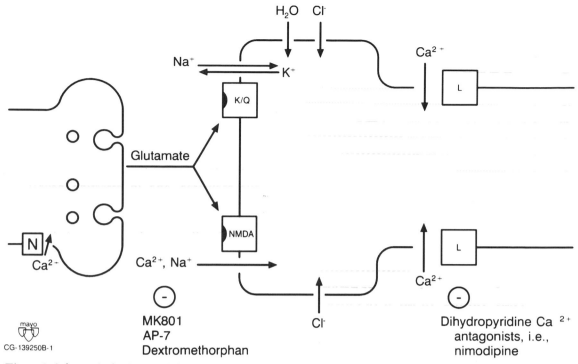

Figure 8. *Schematic depiction of the excitotoxic theory of ischemic neuronal injury. In this theory, early ischemic injury is due to Na^+ influx primarily through the kainate/quisquolate-operated channels. With this Na^+ influx, there is passive Cl^- and H_2O influx which leads to dendritic edema and subsequent osmolysis. The delayed ischemic injury is due to Ca^{2+} influx through the NMDA receptor. Note that presynaptically, Ca^{2+} influx through the N-type voltage-dependent calcium channel would lead to additional neurotransmitter release. In addition to NMDA receptor-operated channels, calcium could enter neurons through L-type voltage-dependent calcium channels. These L channels tend to be located closer to the cell soma. (Modified from Siesjö BK. Historial overview: calcium, ischemia, and death of brain cells.* Ann NY Acad Sci. *1988; 522:638-661.)*

mic reticulum by a Ca^{2+} ATPase, it was also suggested that energy failure would mediate release of intracellular calcium, which could contribute to neuronal injury independent from transmembrane calcium fluxes. Differences in vulnerability to ischemic injury between different neuronal populations was thought to be due to differences in the density of membrane calcium channels.

This original calcium hypothesis of cell injury was questioned by several observations: (1) in vitro studies demonstrated that neurons could die from a hypoxic insult in culture mediums devoid of calcium,[51] (2) there was a poor correlation between location of certain voltage-dependent calcium channels and ischemic vulnerability, and (3) the role of neurotransmitters such as glutamate in

hypoxic injury was demonstrated.[52]

Olney first suggested that excitatory amino acids such as glutamate and aspartate were cytotoxic, and if permitted to overexcite post-synaptic receptors could result in dendrosomatic injuries. This "excitotoxic hypothesis" has been implicated in both anoxic and hypoglycemic injury, which is concordant with the concept that overexcitation could involve either increased release or decreased reuptake of cytotoxic neurotransmitters. The mechanism of excitotoxic injury was elucidated by a series of eloquent tissue culture experiments in which both early and delayed forms of irreversible injury were described.[11,52] The early injury was ascribed to Na^+ influx and the delayed injury to Ca^{2+} entry.

As illustrated in Figure 8, three receptors

for these excitatory amino acids have been pharmacologically defined by analog binding: the N-methyl-D-aspartate (NMDA), kainic acid, and quisquolate receptors. The early injury has been attributed to Na^+ influx followed by obligatory Cl^- and H_2O entry with resultant cell swelling and osmolysis. The Na^+ influx is thought to occur primarily through channels gated by the kainic acid or quisquolate receptor. It can also be argued that Na^+ could enter cells by following its concentration gradient through membrane voltage channels independent from the receptor-operated channels. During ischemia with decreased ATP production, the Na^+/K^+ ATPase pump would fail. The delayed neuronal injury is considered to be secondary to calcium influx primarily through the NMDA receptor which gates a receptor-operated calcium channel. Similar to Na^+ influx, with energy failure and membrane depolarization, calcium may also enter the cell through voltage-dependent calcium channels independent from receptor-operated channels. Therefore, the concept of calcium related cell death in the excitotoxic hypothesis is similar to that proposed in the original calcium hypothesis.[60]

Several observations provide evidence that these excitotoxic mechanisms are important in ischemic injury: (1) the extracellular levels of glutamate and aspartate increase considerably during experimental anoxic insults; (2) both deafferentation of CA1 neurons by Schafferotomy (elimination of glutamatergic input) and local injection of a glutamate antagonist prevent decreases in extracellular calcium during ischemia; (3) competitive and noncompetitive glutamate receptor antagonists appear to ameliorate both in vitro and in vivo ischemic injury; and, (4) the excitotoxic theory may explain the phenomenon of selective vulnerability.[64] Brief periods of forebrain ischemia in the Wistar rat or gerbil result in injury limited to the subiculum, CA1 and CA4 regions of the hippocampus. With more prolonged ischemic insults, there is injury to hippocampal CA3, cortical pyramidal neurons, the caudate nucleus, and the putamen. Audiographic agonist binding stu-

dies have demonstrated that the NMDA receptor is concentrated in the Schaeffer collateral terminations of CA1 and CA4 while the kainic acid receptor is localized at the mossy fiber terminations on CA3, pyramidal neurons, caudate, and putamen. The distribution of the receptor sites for these excitatory amino acids corresponds well to regions with low ischemic tolerance.

Increases in intracellular free calcium are central to current theories on ischemic neuronal injury.[33] A wealth of information emerged over the last decade concerning the pivotal role of Ca^{2+} and neuronal function. Considering that extracellular calcium concentrations are approximately 10^{-3} versus an intracellular concentration of 10^{-7}, small alterations in calcium metabolism can have profound effects on neuronal function. Intracellular Ca^{2+} mediated events including excitation, contraction, and secretion are implemented by high-affinity processes which transpire at micromolar concentrations of ionized calcium. Inward calcium fluxes are driven by a high concentration gradient between extracellular and intracellular calcium through both voltage-dependent and receptor-operated calcium channels.

Currently, there are three recognized voltage-dependent membrane calcium channels: T, N, and L. The receptor-operated calcium channels refer to channels such as that regulated by the NMDA receptor for the excitatory acids. An increase in intracellular calcium concentrations from approximately 10^{-7} to 10^{-6} will give messenger status to ionized calcium. This is due to the tight control of intracellular calcium through a variety of mechanisms which act in unison to modulate intracellular calcium concentrations and mediate calcium dependent events. Some of the major regulators of Ca^{2+} metabolism include: (1) the Na^+/Ca^{2+} antiport pump which is electrogenic, with a ratio of approximately 3:1 in which the direction of calcium exchange can be either inward or outward depending on Na^+ gradients; (2) a Ca^{2+}-ATPase located both in the cytoplasmic and endoplasmic reticulum membranes; (3) mitochondria which can electrophoretically accumulate Ca^{2+} when intracellular free calcium rises; and, (4) intracellular calcium-binding proteins such as calmodulin.

Calcium influx during ischemia may contribute to neuronal injury by a number of mechanisms listed below.

1. Activation of degradative enzymes including lipases, proteases, and endonucleases which catabolize cellular membranes and neurofilaments. A loss of membrane phospholipids would increase the permeability of mitochondrial membranes, which would interfere with residual oxidative phosphorylation while injury to neurofilament structures would retard neuronal transport mechanisms. In addition, the accumulation of free fatty acids from membrane phospholipid degradation are thought to be oxidized through cyclo-oxygenase or lipo-oxygenase pathways during reperfusion. The net result of these pathways would be the production and release of prostaglandins, leukotrienes, and possibly free radicals. The prostaglandin thromboxane A^2 is a potent vasoconstrictor, leukotrienes alter membrane permeability and lead to vasoconstriction, and free radicals if present attack cellular membranes.

2. In an attempt to buffer rising intracellular free calcium concentrations, mitochondria would electrophoretically accumulate calcium. This in turn would uncouple residual oxidative phosphorylation at a time when ATP production was already limited due to anaerobic metabolism.

3. Receptor function would be altered.

4. Increased release of neurotransmitters such as glutamate or aspartate which would lead to a vicious repetition of this cycle.

5. A state of neuronal hyperexcitability could be potentially precipitated, since calcium influx appears to be critical for the initiation of epileptic activity.[34] If increased neuronal activity was induced through calcium influx at a time when

ATP reduction was already reduced, then there would be accelerated ATP depletion.

In addition to the above ionic disturbances with their associated detrimental effects, the primary importance of intracellular acidosis warrants emphasis.[48] Intracellular brain pH is approximately 7.01. Within 10 minutes of a severe focal ischemic event where CBF reductions are approximately 10-12 ml/100 g/min, there is a rapid deterioration in brain pH_i to approximately 6.65. This is a direct reflection of the four-fold increase in lactic acid concentrations.[37] With prolonged focal ischemia, intracellular brain pH continues to decline and reaches 6.10 over the next 4 hours. It is unclear at what level intracellular acidosis causes irreversible neuronal injury. However, intracellular acidosis has been demonstrated to have the following detrimental effects: (1) denaturing proteins with loss of enzymatic function, (2) increasing glial edema with the potential to compromise collateral flow thereby reducing residual CBF, (3) suppressing the cerebral metabolic rate for glucose, (4) suppressing the regeneration of NADH, (5) contributing to the increase in Ca^{2+}_i by H^+ competing for intracellular Ca^{2+} binding sites, and (6) creating an internal milieu that is favorable for free radical production.

Hyperglycemia worsens intracellular acidosis in core regions of ischemia and has a detrimental effect on survival in experimental studies.[32,40,73] Subsequent studies demonstrated that preischemic hyperglycemia impairs postischemic cerebral perfusion and ATP and phosphocreatine recovery, which results in tissue accumulation of lactic acid. Several researchers demonstrated that during ischemia the intracellular glial tissue pH may decrease to as low as 5.3, which may be responsible in part for the diffuse necrosis of cortical tissue during a severe ischemic insult.

Microcirculatory Alterations

Following vessel occlusion in core regions of ischemia, there occurs desaturation of the venous blood and a decrease in blood flow

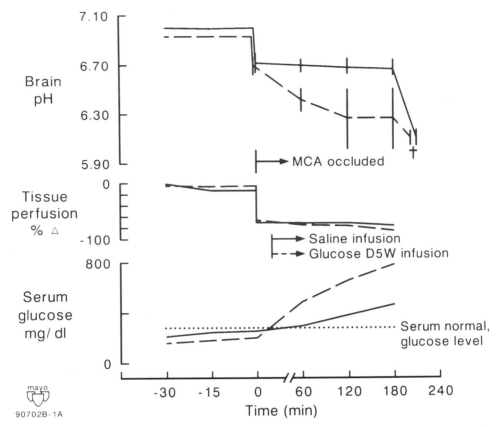

Figure 9. *Measurements of intracellular brain pH and percentage change in cortical blood flow in monkeys infused with either saline solution or D₅W. After occlusion of the MCA, an infusion of glucose caused a significant decrease in brain pH$_i$ when compared to controls. At 3 hours postocclusion, brain pH$_i$ was 6.66 ± 0.08 in controls vs. 6.27 ± 0.02 in glucose-infused animals. (From Marsh WR, Anderson RE, Sundt TM Jr. Effect of hyperglycemia on brain pH levels in areas of focal incomplete cerebral ischemia in monkeys.* J Neurosurg. *1986; 65:693-696.)*

through veins and venules. Shortly thereafter, in the surface conducting vessels and arterioles along the brain surface, sludging of the blood called "particulate flow" occurs. It is hypothesized that this particulate flow is due to a reduction in the shearing forces which tend to keep cellular blood components dispersed. Because of the sludging, blood viscosity increases and there is increased resistance to flow.

Experimental studies in which surface conducting blood vessels have been observed demonstrate an immediate slight increase in the vessel diameter, thought to be due to a local extracellular acidosis. During this time, there is vasomotor paralysis so that blood

flow through these dilated vessels directly reflects cerebral perfusion pressure. At a variable time after vessel occlusion, vasoconstriction of these same surface conducting vessels occurs. This vasoconstriction has been termed "ischemic vasoconstriction" or "secondary vasospasm" to distinguish it from subarachnoid hemorrhage-induced vasospasm.

Ischemia-induced vasoconstriction can be partially blocked by the use of dihydropyridine calcium antagonists which block voltage-dependent L channels (Figure 10). This supports the postulate that ischemic vasoconstriction is due to calcium influx into smooth muscle cells.[35] The decline in ATP presumably leads to smooth muscle cell depolarization,

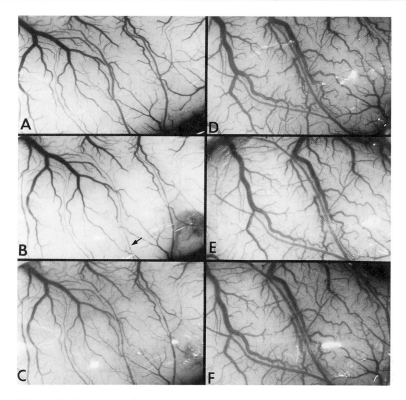

Figure 10. Intraoperative photographs of the cortical vasculature during temporary middle cerebral artery occlusion. The control animal was subjected to 45 minutes of MCA occlusion. *(A)* Cortical vasculature before MCA occlusion. *(B)* Within 15 minutes of MCA occlusion there is cortical pallor and severe ischemic vasoconstriction (arrow). *(C)* On reperfusion, there is cortical hyperemia with both red veins and vasodilatation. Severe cerebral edema and petechial hemorrhages developed in 8 of 10 animals during the 3 hours of reperfusion. *(D-F)* Comparison photographs of an animal treated with nimodipine 15 minutes before MCA occlusion. *(D)* Before MCA occlusion with the addition of nimodipine, vasodilatation and a dense pial network exist as compared to the control animal. *(E)* After 15 minutes of MCA occlusion cortical pallor is less severe and ischemic vasoconstriction is not present as compared to the control. *(F)* With reperfusion, mild cerebral edema developed in only three animals and in two cases the edema was associated with petechial hemorrhages. (From Meyer FB, Sundt TM Jr, Anderson RE, et al. Ischemic vasoconstriction and parenchymal brain pH. Ann NY Acad Sci. 1988; 522: 502-515.)

with calcium influx and subsequent actin and myosin crosslinking. Alternatively, this ischemic vasoconstriction may be due in part to an increase in extracellular potassium or to the release of endogenous vasoconstrictors such as norepinephrine or serotonin. If norepinephrine does play a critical component in ischemic vasoconstriction, the deactivation of

norepinephrine is energy dependent, since it must undergo reuptake at the presynaptic terminal. Ischemic vasoconstriction is important in that it reduces potential collateral flow.

A second microcirculatory change observed in focal ischemia is postischemic hypoperfusion.[14] Postischemic or delayed hypoperfusion following a focal ischemic insult is different

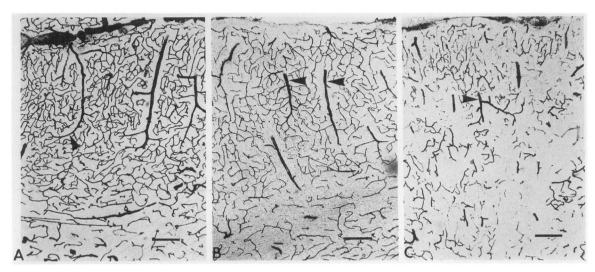

Figure 11. An example of the delayed hypoperfusion that occurs after MCA occlusion as demonstrated by carbon black perfusion. (A) Control nonischemic cortex. (B) Pale area of cortex after 3 hours of ischemia. Although penetrating arterioles (arrowheads) are well filled, many capillaries are narrowed and some failed to fill. (C) After 6 hours of ischemia, capillary filling is severely impaired. Capillaries appear to be obstructed at the origin from arterioles (arrowhead). Scale (lower right) equals 200 μm. (From Little JR, Kerr FWL, Sundt TM Jr. Microcirculatory obstruction in focal cerebral ischemia: relationship to neuronal alterations. Mayo Clin Proc. 1975; 50:264-270.)

than the original "no reflow phenomenon" as described in association with global ischemia[3,18] (Figure 11). In fact, the severity of postischemic hypoperfusion depends on the severity of the focal ischemic insult. If the ischemic insult is minimal, there will typically be no postischemic hypoperfusion.

In a severe focal ischemic event, on the other hand, the postischemic hypoperfusion following flow restoration can be profound. During postischemic hypoperfusion, there is an increase in both oxygen extraction and metabolism suggesting a mismatch between metabolic demand and substrate delivery. The perfusion derangement may secondarily injure surviving neurons in a delayed fashion after an ischemic insult. The pathophysiology of this hypoperfusion has been attributed to: (1) intravascular rheological factors including increased platelet aggregation or blood viscosity, or polymorphonuclear leukocyte injury to endothelium, (2) vascular wall alterations including smooth muscle contraction, micro-villi formation, and endothelial edema, and (3) extravascular edema, including glial tissue, causing mechanical capillary bed compression.[25,31]

Potential Therapeutic Interventions

Given the mechanisms of ischemic neuronal injury described above, therapeutic interventions can be conceptually identified as those which decrease neuronal energy requirements, increase CBF, or block degradative metabolic cascades. Interventions such as calcium antagonists may exert their therapeutic effect via more than one mechanism. No single therapeutic intervention will completely prevent neuronal injury during a focal ischemic event. The modalities subsequently discussed are those which have been shown in the experimental setting to be beneficial for the treatment of acute stroke or intraoperative ischemia.[72]

Decreasing Neuronal Energy Requirements

Barbiturates

Convincing experimental evidence indicates that barbiturates such as thiopental or pentobarbital limit ischemic neuronal damage. Michenfelder and Milde initially proposed that barbiturate protection was selective.[36] They suggested that cerebral metabolism could be divided into (1) a basal metabolic component, which consisted of the metabolism necessary to maintain membrane integrity, and (2) an activated metabolism component responsible for functional activity. They proposed that barbiturates selectively decreased the activated component of metabolism, thereby making a larger share of the energy charge available for basic cell function.[66] This required that barbiturates be delivered prior to the onset of focal ischemia to be effective. Other proposed mechanisms for barbiturate protection include free radical scavenging, decreasing cerebral edema, and enhancing microcirculatory flow.[63] Selman et al investigated the effects of timing of drug administration and duration of ischemia on effectiveness of barbiturates in focal ischemia.[55] Their research demonstrated that barbiturates must be administered within 1 hour after vessel occlusion to beneficially modulate ischemic injury. If flow was not restored, barbiturates had an adverse effect.

Unfortunately, clinical trials have not demonstrated beneficial effects of barbiturates in acute stroke, supporting Michenfelder's original hypothesis that barbiturates must be delivered before the onset of ischemia. In a double-blind prospective study, Yatsu and Coull administered phenobarbital (60 mg to 100 mg 3 times a day) in 26 patients within 24 hours of stroke onset.[77] The use of relatively low-dose phenobarbital in this study may have contributed to the lack of improved neurological outcome. In contrast, some beneficial effects of barbiturate pretreatment have been shown in patients undergoing open-heart surgery.[44] Complications reported with the use of barbiturates for acute stroke include respiratory depression and alterations in mental status.

In summary, experimental and clinical studies in which barbiturates were administered before the onset of ischemia demonstrated that barbiturates may have beneficial effects, whereas studies of barbiturate administration after the onset of ischemia showed a minimal effect. At our institution, thiopental at a dose of 3-5 mg/kg is administered in a controlled anesthetic setting prior to intraoperative temporary vessel occlusion. We do not administer barbiturates during routine carotid endarterectomy, in order to allow for complete intraoperative EEG monitoring.

Hypothermia

The original studies examining the effects of hypothermia during focal cerebral ischemia were reported by Rosomoff in 1957.[50] Subsequently, many laboratories examined the effects of both profound and mild hypothermia on brain metabolism, pathologic injury, and neurologic outcome. The original studies in which body temperature was reduced to 30°C suggested that hypothermia reduced the rate of brain energy depletion and ameliorated parenchymal brain acidosis. Yet, the clinical usefulness of profound hypothermia was limited by the adverse side effects associated with the severity and duration of hypothermia.[67]

There is evidence to suggest that low-grade hypothermia (1°C to 3°C reduction) preserves energy metabolites and attenuates intracellular acidosis, comparable to that observed during profound hypothermia >10°C, with minimal systemic side effects.[7,10,12] Some evidence demonstrates that mild hyperthermia increases brain acidosis and hastens high-energy phosphate depletion.[24] The precise mechanisms by which hypothermia exerts a beneficial modulatory effect are unknown. They may involve the many temperature-sensitive cerebral functions, including maintenance of blood-brain barrier integrity, calcium influx, CBF regulation, neurotransmitter release, and ionic homeostasis. Anecdotal reports of neurological deterioration in stroke patients with fever may justify aggressive treatment of high temperatures in patients who suffered an acute ischemic event.

Isoflurane

The halogenated anesthetic isoflurane has been shown to decrease both cerebral metabolic rate of oxygen consumption ($CMRO_2$) and CBF. The ability of isoflurane to reduce $CMRO_2$ outweighs its effects on cerebral perfusion, suggesting a protective effect on neuronal function.[42] In patients undergoing carotid endarterectomy, isoflurane anesthesia significantly reduces the threshold for electrical failure as compared to halothane. Accordingly, isoflurane is at present the anesthetic of choice for most neurosurgical procedures. In addition to the neuroprotective effect by decreasing $CMRO_2$, isoflurane effectively decreases intracranial pressure.

One advantage of isoflurane is that its inspired concentration can be easily titrated during the surgical procedure to provide protection when desired. It may prove to be more advantageous than medications such as barbiturates or etomidate which have a longer half-life.

Etomidate

Etomidate is a nonbarbiturate imidiazole compound that produces a dose-dependent decrease in EEG, $CMRO_2$, and cerebral blood flow.[6] The maximum depression in $CMRO_2$ obtainable with etomidate is approximately 46%, comparable to the effect of barbiturates. Despite these decreases in $CMRO_2$ and CBF, CO_2 reactivity of the cerebral vasculature remains intact. A potential advantage of etomidate over barbiturates is its fewer intraoperative systemic hemodynamic side effects. However, evidence suggests that etomidate may have the adverse effect of suppressing adrenal gland function, diminishing a patient's ability to respond to postoperative stress. Given the similar effects of etomidate and

barbiturates on $CMRO_2$, CBF, and EEG, cerebroprotective superiority of one agent over another has not been established. The dose of etomidate used is 0.4-0.5 mg/kg intravenous prior to vessel occlusion.

Modulation of CBF

Calcium Antagonists

There is general agreement that calcium antagonists, specifically those of the dihydropyridine class such as nimodipine or PN 200-110, increase CBF in both ischemic and nonischemic conditions.[22,38] In addition to increasing CBF during the ischemic insult, reasonable evidence indicates that these drugs attenuate postischemic hypoperfusion. Postulated mechanisms of improved CBF include the reversal of ischemic vasoconstriction, increase in pial collateral flow, or retardation of platelet aggregation causing reduced blood viscosity.[35,65] Unfortunately, recent metabolic and histologic studies in experimental focal ischemia have disappointingly failed to corroborate these blood flow data. One possible explanation is that calcium antagonists may increase the threshold of ionic failure, which would negate potential improvements in CBF.

Clinical experience with the use of calcium channel blockers for the treatment of acute focal ischemia is limited. In a double-blind study involving 186 patients at several medical centers, Gelmers et al found that administration of nimodipine in patients with acute stroke significantly reduced deaths only in males.[19] Patients receiving nimodipine had improved long-term functional outcome as measured by the Mathew scale assessing neurological deficit. Sherman et al, in a single-center randomized double-blind study, examined the usefulness of nimodipine given 30 mg every 4 hours for 20 days after stroke onset.[57] There was no difference in neurologic outcome between the two groups, and infarct size determined by CT scan was actually larger in the group receiving nimodipine. The small number of patients limits statistical significance, and these modest clinical results reflect the inconclusive nature of the experimental data.

The majority of experimental and clinical data are more promising regarding the use of nimodipine in subarachnoid hemorrhage. Although most clinical studies failed to demonstrate angiographic reduction in subarachnoid hemorrhage-induced vasospasm, there appears to be a consistent improvement in neurologic outcome.[2] This implies that nimodipine either increases microcirculatory flow not visualized on angiography or offers direct neuronal protection. This possible difference between the effects of nimodipine on acute stroke and subarachnoid hemorrhage-induced vasospasm may indicate that calcium antagonists have a potential therapeutic effect in progressive and moderate, but not acute, severe focal ischemia.

Hemorrheological Therapy

Based on the observation that there is an inverse relationship between blood viscosity and CBF, hemodilution has been proposed as a technique to increase CBF. Wood and colleagues conducted experimental studies examining this hypothesis: (1) hypervolemic hemodilution with autologous plasma increased CBF in both ischemic and non-ischemic regions, (2) intravascular volume expansion without hemodilution did not increase blood flow, and (3) animal studies using low-molecular-weight dextran revealed a reduction in infarct size by as much as 60% with a plasma volume increase.[76]

Hemodilution clinical trials have not been encouraging. The Scandinavian Stroke Study Group conducted a multicenter randomized trial involving 373 patients who were treated with either hemodilution or placebo.[53] Therapy began within 48 hours of stroke onset. The hemodilution protocol consisted of venesection of 250 to 1000 ml of whole blood during the first 2 days of treatment and daily infusions of 500 ml of low-molecular-weight dextran over the first 5 days of therapy. There was no benefit by hemodilution on either morbidity or mortality at 3 months.

The Italian Acute Stroke Study Group evaluated the use of isovolemic hemodilution consisting of venesection with dextran infusion commencing within 12 hours of stroke onset in 1,266 patients.[26] There was no significant improvement in morbidity in the treatment group, and additionally there was an increased mortality thought to be the result of an increase in cerebral edema.

Some experimental data indicate that induced hypertension with maximization of cardiac output may increase collateral flow.[69] Based on the clinical observation that this technique may be beneficial in reversing ischemic deficits caused by vasospasm following subarachnoid hemorrhage, the policy at our institution is to insure euvolemia in each patient suffering from a subarachnoid hemorrhage. This includes the daily administration of volume expanders. In patients demonstrating neurologic deterioration attributable to vasospasm, we use a protocol of induced hypertension with isoproterenol and central venous pressure monitoring. This technique can be effective in reversing ischemic neurologic deficits. Occasionally we use this technique in patients suffering from an acute stroke, although one must be wary of causing an increase in cerebral edema or hemorrhagic infarction.

Serotonin Antagonists

A novel calcium channel blocker of the phenylalkamine class (emopamil) has been reported to have potent S_2 antagonist activity.[41] When administered up to 1 hour after middle cerebral artery occlusion in Sprague-Dawley rats, emopamil significantly reduced cortical infarct volume by over 50%. However, it did not influence striatal ischemic damage. Although this and other experiments from a few laboratories demonstrated impressive therapeutic effects of emopamil in acute focal ischemia, the data are preliminary and further studies are necessary. Nonetheless, the use of such agents that may increase CBF through more than one mechanism is promising.

Thrombolysis

Some experimental data indicate that intravascular thrombolysis using intracarotid urokinase and intravenous tissue plasminogen activator (tPA) infusions may be beneficial in reducing infarct size and improving neurological outcome.[79] Zeumer demonstrated recanalization of either an occluded carotid or vertebrobasilar artery in 19 to 29 patients who received local intra-arterial urokinase infusion.[78] In the majority of patients in whom early reperfusion was obtained, there were minimal neurologic deficits. These clinicians also reported successful recanalization in 12 of 17 patients with acute middle cerebral artery thrombosis. Several other small series demonstrated successful recanalization following intra-arterial intravenous tPA therapy.

One of the major concerns with thrombolytic therapy is reperfusion-related hemorrhage.[15] The incidence of intracerebral hemorrhage in patients treated with streptokinase for noncerebral vascular occlusions is not insignificant, approximating 3%.[1] Clinical trials are currently evaluating the safety and efficacy of intravenous tPA in acute ischemic stroke.

Decreasing Degradative Metabolic Cascades

Excitatory Amino Acid Antagonists

Given the proposal of the excitotoxic theory, there has been tremendous interest in examining the effects of various competitive and noncompetitive antagonists to the amino acids, specifically the NMDA receptor.[13,74] Drugs investigated include AP-7, MK801, and dextromethorphan. Overall, it appears that these antagonists reduce neuronal damage during moderate but not severe ischemic insults.[45,46,62,70] Some investigators also suggest that the protective effects of these antagonists is actually due to mild hypothermia.[8] Several clinical trials are evaluating the use of excitatory amino acid antagonists in acute stroke.

Calcium Antagonists

As discussed previously, calcium antagonists may beneficially modulate ischemic neuronal damage by either increasing CBF or decreasing calcium entry into neuronal tissue. There is minimal evidence to suggest that calcium antagonists prevent calcium entry into ischemic neurons. A rise in intracellular free calcium during ischemia could occur through multiple avenues, including voltage-dependent calcium channels, receptor-operated calcium channels, and release from the endoplasmic reticulum.[33]

Within the subgroup of voltage-dependent calcium channels, there are actually three channels, with only one (L-channel) modulated by calcium antagonists. Therefore, it is unlikely that blockade of one channel would significantly attenuate the dramatic rise in intracellular free calcium during an ischemic insult. The only evidence to date supporting a direct modulating effect of calcium antagonists on neuronal activity is research demonstrating that some calcium antagonists are anticonvulsants.[34] Calcium antagonists such as nimodipine do appear to exert a beneficial effect in subarachnoid hemorrhage-induced vasospasm despite the lack of apparent angiographic evidence of cerebral vasodilatory effects.[2] Based on this finding, it has been suggested that calcium antagonists in the clinical setting reduce neurologic deficits through a direct neuronal effect.

Serum Glucose

Since the majority of data point to the deleterious effects of hyperglycemia during focal ischemia, serum glucose concentrations should be maintained within a normal range. Therefore, intravenous solutions for the patient suffering from acute ischemia should have minimal glucose; we infuse either Ringer's lactate solution or normal saline solution during neurovascular procedures.

Free Radical Scavengers

Some evidence suggests that oxygen free radical-mediated lipid perioxidation plays a detrimental role in focal ischemia. Research by Demopoulos et al and others showed that levels of endogenous antioxidants such as alpha-tocopherol, ascorbate, and glutathione decrease during focal cerebral ischemia.[16] Superoxide dismutase and alpha-tocopherol were effective in experimental focal cerebral ischemia followed by reperfusion. Hall and colleagues investigated the effects of a novel 21-amino acid steroid, a potent inhibitor of iron-dependent lipid perioxidation.[20] The limited number of experiments to date suggest that this drug decreases the size of infarction and improves neurologic outcome. As with any other free radical scavenger, this drug must be administered before the period of reperfusion, during peak free radical production. Mannitol has also been reported to be a free radical scavenger, and therefore beneficial in focal ischemia, leading some experienced neurosurgeons to routinely administer mannitol intraoperatively prior to vessel occlusion during aneurysm surgery.

Conclusion

Based on the mechanisms of ischemic neuronal injury thus far elucidated, some recommendations can be made regarding intraoperative protection. The author uses temporary vessel occlusion as opposed to the induction of significant hypotension when dissecting difficult vascular lesions. This maximizes potential collateral flow. The patient is anesthetized with isoflurane to provide an initial degree of brain protection.

Recently, we have been using intraoperative EEG monitoring to titrate the level of inhalation anesthetic (Figure 12). Prior to temporary occlusion, the concentration of inspired isoflurane is increased to obtain EEG isoelectricity. Following flow restoration, the concentration of inspired isoflurane is reduced under EEG guidance to allow awakening of the patient in the operating room, providing an immediate neurological examination. An alternative to the use of high concentrations of isoflurane is the traditional method of administering intravenous thiopental 3-5 mg/kg several minutes prior to

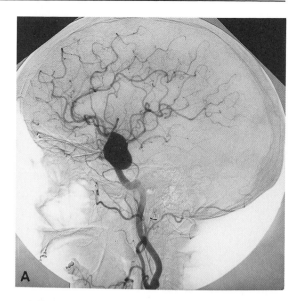

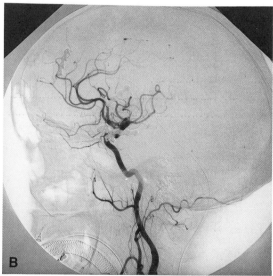

Figure 12. An example of the use of high concentrations of inspired isoflurane to provide intraoperative protection. *(A)* Obliteration of this aneurysm required temporary carotid occlusion for 28 minutes. Prior to vessel occlusion, the inspired concentration of isoflurane was increased to obtain EEG isoelectricity. Following successful repair, isoflurane was decreased to allow awakening of the patient in the operating room for an early examination. *(B)* Postoperative angiogram confirmed aneurysm obliteration.

vessel occlusion. Some surgeons prefer to use intravenous etomidate 0.4-0.5 mg/kg as opposed to barbiturates. In all three interventions, the effect is that of decreasing metabolic demand to a similar degree. Profound hypothermia is not proven to offer any greater degree of brain protection; the role of profound hypothermia may be limited to those unique circumstances in which it is thought necessary to induce severe reductions in blood pressure to decrease the size of the lesion.

New techniques to provide intraoperative protection will emerge, based on the principles of either increasing CBF or blocking metabolic cascades. It remains to be proven whether calcium antagonists, serotonin antagonists, or other novel interventions prove effective in increasing collateral flow over that which is now achievable by maintaining the patient euvolemic with occasional induced hypertension during the surgical procedure. Of perhaps greater interest is the rapid development of excitatory amino acid antagonists and free radical scavengers. Both of these classes of agents theoretically can decrease neuronal injury during and after the ischemic insult during reperfusion.

Recent advances in understanding the pathophysiology of ischemic injury have outpaced the development of protective interventions. Thus far, no single modality is a magic bullet. This reflects both the vulnerability and complexity of brain to ischemic injury. Future neuroprotective regimens will be a combination of agents with different mechanisms of action, acting in unison to provide ischemic brain protection.

References

1. Aldrich MS, Sherman SA, Greenberg HS. Cerebrovascular complications of streptokinase infusion. *JAMA.* 1985;253:1777-1779.
2. Allen GS, Ahns HS, Preziosi TJ, et al. Cerebral arterial spasm—a controlled trial of nimodipine in patients with subarachnoid hemorrhage. *N Engl J Med.* 1983;308:619-624.
3. Ames A III, Wright RL, Kowada M, et al. Cerebral ischemia, II: the no-reflow phenomenon. *Am J Pathol.* 1968;52:437-453.
4. Astrup J, Siesjö BK, Simon L. Thresholds in cerebral ischemia—the ischemic penumbra. *Stroke.* 1981; 12:723-725.
5. Astrup J, Symon L, Branston NM, et al. Cortical evoked potential in extracellular K^+/H^+ at critical levels of brain ischemia. *Stroke.* 1977;8:51-57.
6. Batjer HH, Frankfurt AI, Purdy PD, et al. Use of

7. etomidate, temporary arterial occlusion, and intraoperative angiography in surgical treatment of large and giant cerebral aneurysms. *J Neurosurg.* 1988; 68:234-240.
7. Berntman L, Welsh FA, Harp JR. Cerebral protective effect of low-grade hypothermia. *Anesthesiology.* 1981;55:495-498.
8. Block GA, Pulsinelli WA. Excitatory amino acid receptor antagonists: failure to prevent ischemic neuronal damage. *J Cereb Blood Flow Metab.* 1987;7:S149.
9. Bransten NM, Simon L, Crockard HA, et al. Relationship between the cortical evoked potential and local cortical blood flow following acute middle cerebral artery occlusion in the baboon. *Exp Neurol.* 1974;45:195-208.
10. Busto R, Dietrich WD, Gobus MY-T, et al. Small differences in intraischemic brain temperature critically determine the extent of ischemic neuronal injury. *J Cereb Blood Flow Metab.* 1987;7:729-738.
11. Choi DW. Glutamate neurotoxicity in cortical cell culture is calcium dependent. *Neurosci Lett.* 1985; 58:293-297.
12. Chopp M, Knight R, Tidwell CD, et al. The metabolic effects of mild hypothermia on global cerebral ischemia and recirculation in the cat: comparison to normothermia and hyperthermia. *J Cereb Blood Flow Metab.* 1989;9:141-148.
13. Croucher MJ, Collins JF, Meldrum BS. Anticonvulsant action of excitatory amino acid antagonists. *Science.* 1982;216:899-901.
14. Crowell RM, Olsson Y. Impaired microvascular filling after focal cerebral ischemia in monkeys. *J Neurosurg.* 1972;36:303-309.
15. Del Zoppo GJ, Zeumer H, Harker LA. Thrombolytic therapy in stroke: possibilities and hazards. *Stroke.* 1986;17:595-607.
16. Demopoulos HB, Flamm ES, Pietronigro DD, et al. The free radical pathology and the microcirculation in the major central nervous system disorders. *Acta Physiol Scan.* 1980 (suppl);492:91-119.
17. Edvinsson L, Mackenzie ET, McCulloch J, et al. Perivascular innovation and receptor mechanisms in cerebrovascular bed. In: Woods JH, ed. *Cerebral Blood Flow: Physiologic and Clinical Aspects.* New York, NY: McGraw-Hill Book Company; 1987: 145-172.
18. Fisher EG, Ames A III, Hedley-Whyte ET, et al. Reassessment of cerebral capillary changes in acute global ischemia and their relationship to the "no reflow phenomena". *Stroke.* 1977;8:36-39.
19. Gelmers HJ, Gorter K, de Weerdt CJ, et al. A controlled trial of nimodipine in acute stroke. *N Engl J Med.* 1988;318:203-207.
20. Hall ED, Yonkers PA. Attenuation of postischemic cerebral hypoperfusion by the 21-aminosteroid U74006F. *Stroke.* 1988;19:340-344.
21. Harper AM. Autoregulation of cerebral blood flow: influence of the arterial blood pressure on the blood flow through the cerebral cortex. *J Neurol Neurosurg Psychiatry.* 1966;29:398-403.
22. Harper AM, Craigen L, Kazda S. Effect of the calcium antagonist nimodipine on cerebral blood flow and metabolism in the primate. *J Cereb Blood Flow Metab.* 1981; 1:349-356.
23. Heiss W-D. Flow thresholds of functional and morphological damage of brain tissue. *Stroke.* 1983; 14:329-331.
24. Hindfelt B. The prognostic significance of subfebril-

ity and fever in ischemic cerebral infarction. *Acta Neurol Scand.* 1976;53:72-79.

25. Ianotti F, Hoff J. Ischemic brain edema with and without reperfusion: an experimental study in gerbils. *Stroke.* 1983;14:562-567.

26. Italian Acute Stroke Study Group. The Italian hemodilution trial on acute stroke. *Stroke.* 1988;19:145.

27. Kety SS, Schmidt CF. The nitrous oxide method for the quantitative determination of cerebral blood flow in man: theory, procedure, and normal values. *J Clin Invest.* 1948;27:476-483.

28. Ko KR, Ngai AC, Winn HR. Role of adenosine in regulation of regional cerebral blood flow in sensory cortex. *Am J Physiol.* 1990;259:H1703-H1708.

29. Lassen NA. The luxury-perfusion syndrome and its possible relation to acute metabolic acidosis localised within the brain. *Lancet.* 1966;2:1113-1115.

30. Lassen NA. Brain extracellular pH: the main factor controlling cerebral blood flow. *Scand J Clin Lab Invest.* 1968;22:247-251.

31. Little JR, Kerr FWL, Sundt TM Jr. Microcirculatory obstruction of focal cerebral ischemia: relationship to neuronal alterations. *Mayo Clin Proc.* 1975; 50:264-270.

32. Marsh WR, Anderson RE, Sundt TM Jr. Effect of hyperglycemia on brain pH levels in areas of focal incomplete cerebral ischemia in monkeys. *J Neurosurg.* 1986;65:693-696.

33. Meyer FB. Calcium, neuronal hyperexcitability and ischemic injury. *Brain Res Rev.* 1989;14:227-243.

34. Meyer FB, Anderson RE, Sundt TM Jr, et al. Selective central nervous system calcium channel blockers— a new class of anticonvulsant agents. *Mayo Clin Proc.* 1986;61:239-247.

35. Meyer FB, Sundt TM Jr, Anderson RE, et al. Ischemic vasoconstriction and parenchymal brain pH. *Ann NY Acad Sci.* 1988;522:502-515.

36. Michenfelder JD, Milde JH. Influence of anesthetics on metabolic, functional and pathological responses to regional cerebral ischemia. *Stroke.* 1975;6:405-410.

37. Michenfelder JD, Sundt TM Jr. Cerebral ATP and lactate levels in the squirrel monkey following occlusion of the middle cerebral artery. *Stroke.* 1971; 2:319-326.

38. Mohammed AA, Mendelow AD, Teasdale GM, et al. Effect of the calcium antagonist nimodipine on local cerebral blood flow and metabolic coupling. *J Cereb Blood Flow Metab.* 1985;5:26-33.

39. Morawetz RB, Crowell RH, DeGirolami U, et al. Regional cerebral blood flow thresholds during cerebral ischemia. *Fed Proc.* 1979;38:2493-2494.

40. Myers RE. Lactic acid accumulation as cause of brain edema and cerebral necrosis resulting from oxygen deprivation. In: Korobkin R, Guilleminault C, eds. *Advances in Perinatal Neurology.* New York, NY: SP Medical & Scientific Books; 1979;1:85-114.

41. Nakayama H, Ginsberg MD, Dietrich WD. (s) Emopamil, a novel calcium channel blocker and serotonin S$_2$ antagonist, markedly reduces infarct size following middle cerebral artery occlusion in the rat. *Neurology.* 1988;38:1667-1673.

42. Newberg LA, Michenfelder JD. Cerebral protection by isoflurane during hypoxemia or ischemia. *Anesthesiology.* 1983;59:29-35.

43. Nicholson C, Bruggencate GT, Steinberg R, et al. Calcium modulation in brain extracellular microenvironment demonstrated with ion-selective micropipette. *Proc Natl Acad Sci USA.* 1977;

74:1287-1290.

44. Nussmeier NA, Arlund C, Slogoff S. Neuropsychiatric complications after cardiopulmonary bypass: cerebral protection by a barbiturate. *Anesthesiology.* 1986;64:165-170.

45. Ozyurt E, Graham DI, Woodruff GN, et al. Protective effect of glutamate antagonist MK-801 in focal cerebral ischemia in the cat. *J Cereb Blood Flow Metab.* 1988;8:138-143.

46. Park CK, Nehls DG, Graham DI, et al. Focal cerebral ischemia in the cat: treatment with the glutamate antagonist MK-801 after induction of ischemia. *J Cereb Blood Flow Metab.* 1988;8:757-762.

47. Pickard JD. Role of prostaglandins and arachidonic acid derivatives in the coupling of cerebral blood flow to cerebral metabolism. *J Cereb Blood Flow Metab.* 1981;1:361-384.

48. Plum F. What causes infarction in ischemic brain?: the Robert Wartenberg lecture. *Neurology.* 1985; 33:222-233.

49. Raichle ME, Grubb RL Jr, Mokhtar HG, et al. Correlation between regional cerebral blood flow and oxidative metabolism: in vitro studies in man. *Arch Neurol.* 1976;33:523-526.

50. Rosomoff HL. Hypothermia and cerebrovascular lesions, II: experimental interruption followed by induction of hypothermia. *Arch Neurol Psychol.* 1957;78:454-464.

51. Rothman SM. The neurotoxicity of excitatory amino acids is produced by passive chloride influx. *J Neurosci.* 1985;5:1483-1489.

52. Rothman SM, Olney JW. Glutamate in the pathophysiology of hypoxic-ischemic brain damage. *Ann Neurol.* 1986;19:105-111.

53. Scandinavian Stroke Study Group. Multicenter trial of hemodilution in acute ischemic stroke, I: results in the total patient population. *Stroke.* 1987;18: 691-699.

54. Schanne FAX, Kane AB, Young EE, et al. Calcium dependence of toxic cell death: a final common pathway. *Science.* 1979;206:700-702.

55. Selman WR, Spetzler RF, Roessmann UR, et al. Barbiturate-induced coma therapy for focal cerebral ischemia: effect after temporary and permanent MCA occlusion. *J Neurosurg.* 1981;55:220-226.

56. Sharbrough FW, Messick JM Jr, Sundt TM Jr. Correlation of continuous electroencephalograms with cerebral blood flow measurements during carotid endarterectomy. *Stroke.* 1973;4:674-683.

57. Sherman DG, Easton JD, Hart RG, et al. Nimodipine in acute cerebral infarction. A double blind study of safety and efficacy. In: Battistini N, Fiorani P, Courbier R, et al, eds. *Acute Brain Ischemia. Medical and Surgical Therapy.* New York, NY: Raven Press; 1986:257-261

58. Siesjö BK. *Brain Energy Metabolism.* New York, NY: John Wiley and Sons; 1978.

59. Siesjö BK. Cell damage in the brain: a speculative synthesis. *J Cereb Blood Flow Metab.* 1981;1:155-185.

60. Siesjö BK, Bengtsson F. Calcium fluxes, calcium antagonists, and calcium related pathology in brain ischemia, hypoglycemia, and spreading depression: a unifying hypothesis. *J Cereb Blood Flow Metab.* 1989;9:127-140.

61. Simon L, Bransten NM, Strong AJ, et al. The concepts of thresholds of ischemia in relation to brain structure and function. *J Clin Pathol.* 1977;30 (suppl 11):149-154.

62. Simon RP, Swan JH, Griffith T, et al. Blockade of

N-methyl-d-aspartate receptors may protect against ischemic damage in the brain. *Science.* 1984; 226:850-852.

63. Smith AL, Hoff JT, Nielsen SL, et al. Barbiturate protection in acute focal cerebral ischemia. *Stroke.* 1974;5:1-7.

64. Smith M-L, Auer RN, Siesjö BK. The density and distribution of ischemic brain injury in the rat following 2-10 min of forebrain ischemia. *Acta Neuropathol.* 1984;64:319-332.

65. Smith M-L, Kagström E, Rosén I, et al. Effect of the calcium antagonist nimodipine on the delayed hypoperfusion following incomplete ischemia in the rat. *J Cereb Blood Flow Metab.* 1983;3:543-546.

66. Steen PA, Michenfelder JD. Mechanisms of barbiturate protection. *Anesthesiology.* 1980;53:183-185.

67. Steen PA, Soule EH, Michenfelder JD. Detrimental effect of prolonged hypothermia in cats and monkeys with and without regional cerebral ischemia. *Stroke.* 1979;10:522-529.

68. Strong AJ, Venables GS, Gibson G. The cortical ischemic penumbra associated with occlusion of the middle cerebral artery in the cat, 1: topography of changes in blood flow, potassium ion activity, and EEG. *J Cereb Blood Flow Metab.* 1983;3:86-96.

69. Sundt TM Jr, Onofrio BM, Merideth J. Treatment of cerebral vasospasm from subarachnoid hemorrhage with isoproterenol and lidocaine hydrochloride. *J Neurosurg.* 1973;38:557-560.

70. Swan JH, Evans MC, Meldrum BS. Long-term development of selective neuronal loss and the mechanism of protection by 2-amino-7-phosphonoheptanoate in a rat model of incomplete forebrain ischemia. *J Cereb Blood Flow Metab.* 1988;8:64-78.

71. Trojaborg W, Boysen G. Relation between EEG, regional cerebral blood flow and internal carotid artery pressure during carotid endarterectomy. *Electroencephalogr Clin Neurophysiol.* 1973;34:61-69.

72. Weinstein PR, Faden AL. *Protection of the Brain from Ischemia.* Baltimore, MD: Williams & Wilkins; 1990.

73. Welch FA, Ginsberg MD, Rieder W, et al. Deleterious effect of glucose pretreatment on recovery from diffuse cerebral ischemia in the cat, II: Regional metabolite levels. *Stroke.* 1980;11:355-363.

74. Wieloch T. Hypoglycemia-induced neuronal damage prevented by an N-methyl-d-aspartate antagonist. *Science.* 1985;230:681-683.

75. Winn HR, Rubio GR, Berne RM. The role of adenosine in the regulation of cerebral blood flow. *J Cereb Blood Flow Metab.* 1981;1:239-244.

76. Wood JH, Simeone FA, Fink EA, et al. Correlative aspects of hypervolemic hemodilution: low molecular-weight dextran infusions after experimental cerebral artery occlusion. *Neurology.* 1984; 34:24-34.

77. Yatsu FM, Coull BM. Barbiturate therapy in stroke. In: Fisher M, ed. *Medical Therapy of Acute Stroke.* New York, NY: Marcel Dekker Inc.; 1989:109-115.

78. Zeumer H. Survey of progress: Vascular recanalizing techniques and interventional neuroradiology. *Neurology.* 1985;231:287-294.

79. Zivin JA, Fisher M, DeGirolami U, et al. Tissue plasminogen activator reduces neurological damage after cerebral embolism. *Science.* 1985;230: 1289-1292.

CHAPTER 2

Hemorheology of Cerebral Blood Flow and Ischemia

Adam J. Davis, MD and Jafar J. Jafar, MD

Rheology is the study of the deformation and flow of matter. *Biorheology* was a phrase first coined 50 years ago by Alfred Copley[28] in response to the growing interest in the rheologic study of biologic organisms. Inherent in the study of biorheology is the observation of how and why biologic materials flow and deform in response to the internal and external physical and chemical stresses placed on the living organism.[30] Hemorheology is concerned with the deformation and flow of the cells and plasma of the blood on a macroscopic and microscopic basis, as well as the rheologic properties of the vessel with which the blood comes into contact.[29] Hemorheology was the earliest of the biorheologic sciences to be studied and still generates the most interest. The past two decades have produced a great amount of information concerning the basic rheologic properties of cerebral blood flow, in part secondary to the knowledge gained in general hemorheology. This information has led to an understanding of the importance of the physical properties of cerebral blood flow in both normal and pathophysiologic states. Progress in cerebral hemorheology has encouraged clinicians to manipulate the rheologic properties of blood in order to treat cerebrovascular disease. The study of hemorheology allows a greater understanding of the cellular and fluid properties of blood, and provides a rationale for further therapy of cerebral ischemia.

General Principles of Hemorheology

Viscosity and Shear

The relative importance of the rheologic principles of blood flow for the cerebrovascular circulation is largely determined by the size of the vessel that the blood is coursing through. The rheologic properties of blood that are significant for determining blood flow within the microcirculation of the brain (vessels less than 70-100 μm in diameter that penetrate the parenchyma) are different from those for the macrocirculation (conductance vessels greater than 100-300 μm in diameter).

The viscosity, or fluidity, of blood is a major determinant of blood flow. Viscosity is defined as the internal friction of liquids. It may be understood best by imagining a perfect liquid, such as water, placed between two plates. As one plate is moved and the other remains stationary, the layer of water closest to the moving plate travels in the same direction. Each successive layer of water will also travel in the same direction, though at a somewhat slower velocity due to the loss of energy from friction between the molecules of the adjacent fluid layers. Each fluid layer farther away from the moving plate tends to hold back the faster-moving adjacent layer.

One can imagine another similar situation,

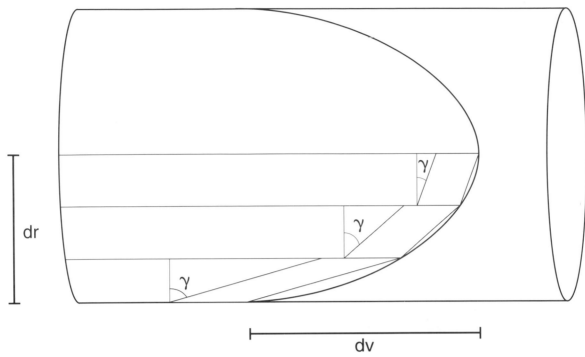

Figure 1. *Axial laminar flow. The velocity of the central layer is greater than that of the peripheral layers, defining a parabolic velocity profile. The* change *in velocity is greater at the periphery than near the center of the vessel. This is demonstrated by the greater angulation of the rhomboid representing the deformation of each layer. Angle Y reflects the change in velocity for a given length of radius and is termed the* shear angle. *The change in the shear angle over time is the* shear rate. *The shear rate is greatest at the periphery.*

in which a liquid is flowing through a hollow cylinder due to a pressure gradient across the length of the tube. In this case the layer with the least velocity will be adjacent to the immobile outer wall owing to friction between the stationary wall and the fluid molecules. The fastest flowing layer will be within the center of the flowing fluid column. Each concentric layer from the center moving outward will be flowing at a slightly slower velocity due to the internal friction, or viscosity, of the fluid. This is axial flow, and for perfect fluids has a parabolic velocity profile. As seen in Figure 1, each moving fluid layer will be deformed by the the adjacent layer. This is conceptually represented as a rhomboid segment within each layer with an angle γ. This is termed the *shear angle γ*. The amount of deformation is defined by the amount of shear angle g over time and is called the *shear rate γ*.

Shear rate within a given vessel is determined by the change of velocity over the change in radius over time. If vessel size is constant, then the shear rate will be directly proportional to the velocity of the fluid. Conversely, for a given velocity, the shear rate in small vessels is greater than that of large vessels; however, this is a simplification. As schematically demonstrated in Figure 1, shear rates vary within a vessel even with constant average fluid flow because the velocity of the fluid is not uniform across the vessel. Flow velocity is parabolic such that the magnitude of velocity is exponentially greater at the center of the vessel than at the periphery. Therefore, the *change* in velocity, or shear rate, is greatest near the vessel wall and becomes progressively smaller toward the center. For a newtonian fluid, the average shear rate of a vessel is ⅛ of the wall shear rate. Change in shear rate has an important influence on flow resistance and the axial distribution of cells within the microcirculation, as will be discussed later in this chapter.

The force propelling the fluid within the

cylinder, causing each layer to deform to shear angle γ, is called the *shear stress*. The shear stress is related to the shear rate by viscosity.[113]

shear stress = viscosity × shear rate
shear rate = shear stress ÷ viscosity

Since shear rate is the deformability of a fluid, the second equation informs us that as the viscosity of a liquid increases, the amount of shear stress required to maintain that deformity also increases. Thus higher viscosity requires greater forces to generate axial laminar flow.

Hagen-Poiseuille Equation

The preceding situation pertains to perfect liquids only and follows the principles of newtonian physics. Plasma is similar to (but not identical to!) a perfect liquid whose flow behavior may be closely approximated by using the newtonian equations given here. The Hagen-Poiseuille equation describes the flow of newtonian fluids as follows:

$$Q = \frac{\Delta P \ \pi r^4}{8ln}$$

(where Q is the flow, ΔP is the pressure gradient, r is the radius, l is the length of the vessel, and n is the viscosity.)

Flow is inversely proportional to the viscosity of the fluid. One will note, however, that the greatest contribution to this equation is the r^4 component. Thus in large vessels, such as those in the macrocirculation, with diameters 100 μm or greater, the viscosity plays a much less significant role than in the microcirculation where capillary and arteriole diameters range from 4-40 μm. Even in the precapillary arterioles, one can see how flow is more significantly affected by changes in the vessel diameter, such as those brought about by autoregulatory mechanisms, than by viscosity.

When the driving pressure and vessel diameter are fixed, the Hagen-Poiseuille equation suggests that viscosity becomes the predominant determinant of flow. This relationship is the basis for the concept that viscosity becomes a relatively more important determinant of cerebral blood flow during ischemic conditions; however, blood is not a perfect newtonian fluid, and this relationship is not strictly true, particularly within the microcirculation.

The equations for flow dynamics presented are intended only for fluids that display newtonian physical properties. By definition, biorheology is the study of non-newtonian flow and deformation, though for simplicity, newtonian physics is often employed. Blood is a complex liquid, a suspension, and displays non-newtonian behavior. Blood viscosity is a result of many influences, the most important of which include but are not limited to velocity; shear rate; shear stress; hematocrit; aggregating properties of red blood cells and platelets; red blood cell deformability; plasma viscosity and proteins; and the intrinsic rheologic properties of white blood cells and platelets. Furthermore, each of these contributing variables is influenced by its own intrinsic properties and external influences. The apparent viscosity of blood is constantly changing as the internal and external influences change. Accordingly, the flow of blood cannot be precisely defined by the Hagen-Poiseuille equation.

Thixotropy

Thixotropy is the property of certain gels and suspensions to become less viscous when shaken or subject to shearing forces. Thixotropy is characterized by the isothermal structural change of a system when a mechanical force is applied, which then returns to its original structure after the disturbance is removed.[73]

Blood is a thixotropic fluid. A common example of a thixotropic fluid that is analogous to blood is ketchup. One is familiar with the seemingly endless wait for the flow of ketchup to begin when the bottle is first inverted. At first it flows extremely slowly and is very thick, acting more like a paste than a fluid. As velocity increases the ketchup seems to become thinner and the column of flow appears to be more like that of a flowing

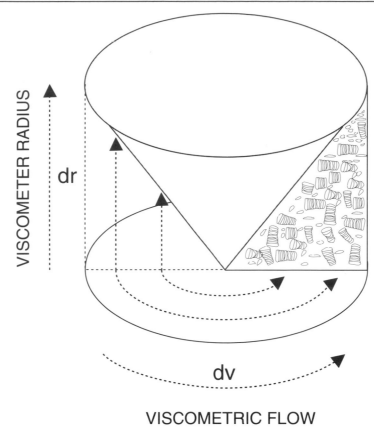

VISCOMETRIC FLOW

Figure 2. Rotational viscometer (schematic). This common method for determining whole blood viscosity is more representative of the macrocirculation than the microcirculation. The dimensions of the container are many orders of magnitude larger than the size of the circulating erythrocytes. Note that both the velocity and radius are greater at the periphery of the device. Modified from Gaehtgens and Marx.[53]

fluid. This is secondary to the decrease in viscosity as the ketchup suspension encounters greater shear forces (e.g. the force of gravity or banging on the bottle).

Thixotropy and the Apparent Viscosity of Blood Within the Macrocirculation Versus the Microcirculation

The viscosity of blood cannot be measured directly. It is often calculated by measuring blood flow, or the energy (shear stress) needed to maintain blood flow, under controlled in vivo or in vitro conditions and then determined by using the Hagen-Poiseuille or viscosity/shear stress equation. This is the *apparent* viscosity of blood. The most common laboratory method for measuring whole blood viscosity was for many years the rotational coaxial viscometer (Figure 2). This method provides reliable information concerning the bulk flow of whole blood at a variety of shear rates as determined by the physiochemical and mechanical properties of the cellular and fluid components.[53] Using this method, the thixotropic properties of blood have been studied by numerous investigators. In accordance with the known physical properties of thixotropic fluids, the prevailing opinion for many years was that within the circulation, as shear rate decreased, the apparent viscosity of blood increased

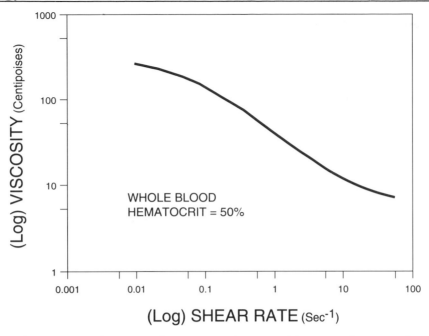

Figure 3. *Viscosity versus shear rate. As determined by a coaxial rotational viscometer, viscosity increases exponentially as shear rate decreases from high (100 sec⁻¹) to low (1 sec⁻¹) values that are commonly encountered in the circulation. At extremely high or low shear rates, the viscosity plateaus. This is representative of the macrocirculation only. Modified from Chien et al.[27]*

exponentially and then plateaued (Figure 3).[21,27,95,97,124,159] This was felt to be due to the aggregation and decreased deformability of red blood cells at low shear rates.[12,20,25-27,84,125]

It is now known that the principle of increasing viscosity with decreasing shear rate within the physiologic range applies only to the macrocirculation. An exponential increase in viscosity as shear rate declined was demonstrated in the rotational viscometer, and thought to be confirmed by studies conducted within both large tubes and small horizontal capillary tubes.[6,96] More recent studies conducted within narrow *vertical* capillary tubes failed to demonstrate this relationship within the physiologic and anatomic range of the microcirculation.[11,57,105,111,112] These newer studies demonstrate that the results from previous studies conducted within narrow *horizontal* tubes, which were felt to confirm the principles demonstrated within the rotational viscometers, were complicated by an artifact (red blood cell sedimentation), which is discussed later in this chapter.

Therefore, the basic rheologic principles demonstrated by the rotational viscometer are only applicable to whole blood flow within large vessels and do not reflect the actual state of flow within small tubes or the cerebral microcirculation. The large dimensions and inappropriate geometry of the rotational viscometer are more representative of the macrocirculation, especially vessels greater than 300 μm, where the size of the lumen is significantly larger than the size of the cellular constituent. The large distances between the inner and outer container walls of the rotational viscometer (see Figure 2), in comparison to the cellular components, make the device insensitive to events occurring at the fluid-wall interface. This interface is an important determinant of apparent viscosity within the microcirculation. The rotational viscometer fails to mimic the laminar configuration of flow and the central aggregation of blood cells that occurs within narrow tubes and is accentuated at decreasing shear rates. These characteristics are responsible for the decrease in apparent viscosity during flow through small tubes (Fahraeus-Lindqvist effect), and the maintenance of low viscosity as shear rates decrease.

In summary, within the macrocirculation only, as shear rate decreases, red cell aggregation increases, red cell deformability decreases, and the apparent viscosity of the blood increases. Within the microcirculation certain rheologic properties prevent this increase in viscosity from occurring and will be discussed below.

Red Blood Cell Aggregation and Deformability

It is well known that under certain conditions, red blood cells form aggregates termed *rouleaux.* Rouleau formation depends on three phases: transport of the red blood cell to another cell so that they physically interact; activation of the red blood cell; and aggregation (adhesion).[138] For erythrocyte aggregation to occur, macromolecules such as fibrinogen or globulins (both contained within plasma) or high molecular weight dextran (HMWD) must be present within the medium.[21-23,83,132] Aggregation of red blood cells does not occur to any significant degree within a saline or serum medium. Aggregation results from macromolecular bridging between erythrocyte membranes and may have either nonspecific binding, as in the case of fibrinogen or HMWD, or specific binding, as occurs during antigen-antibody reactions.[132] Fibrinogen and dextran act at different binding sites; there is no competitive binding.[132] Albumin interferes with the aggregating properties of fibrinogen, presumably secondary to competition at the adsorbing sites on the erythrocyte membrane.[83] Whereas HMWD increases red cell aggregation,[100] low molecular weight dextran (LMWD), often used for hemodilutional purposes, has been shown[54] to cause *disaggregation* of erythrocytes, and will be discussed later in this chapter.

Aggregation is a reversible process and is the result of the sum of the adhesive versus the antiaggregating forces. Surface electrostatic charges, as well as increased mechanical stress from the enlarged and deformed erythrocyte membrane surface area, tend to promote disaggregation[132]; however, the overwhelming energy that promotes dissociation is the mechanical force of shear stress. Multiple experimental studies have shown that at increasing shear rates, there is increasing disaggregation of rouleaux into individual red blood cells.[12,20,21,23,27,31,132] The size of the rouleaux also decrease with increasing shear as larger rouleaux break up into smaller ones.[99] Depending on the experimental method,[31,127] in the moderate to high shear rate range of 50-100 sec[-1], commonly encountered within the cerebral circulation, rouleaux are entirely dispersed into individual erythrocytes. In a steady state condition, a dynamic equilibrium exists between the applied shear rate and the formation and size of rouleaux.[99] When albumin is added to red blood cell suspensions with fibrinogen, disaggregation occurs at lower shear rates.

The deformation of red blood cells plays an important role in their ability to aggregate and is an important factor in whole blood rheology. The deformability of red blood cells depends on both external shear stress and on the intrinsic rheologic properties of the cell. The basic rheologic parameters[37,133] that determine deformability are the following:

1. The shape of the cell; when biconcave it provides a large surface-volume ratio.
2. The internal viscosity of the cell, which is affected by changes in the hemoglobin content and concentration, external osmolality, pH, oxygen pressure, as well as by abnormal types of hemoglobin.
3. The membrane viscoelasticity (membrane flexibility), which is determined by the degree of polymerization (cross linking) between the spectrin and actin molecules that constitute the cytoskeleton.
4. The membrane fluidity, which is a

result of the translational and rotational mobility of the lipids and proteins within the cell membrane and is affected by numerous factors such as temperature, lipid/protein/ion interactions, and cholesterol-phospholipid ratios.

5. The "tank tread" motion of the membrane (the rotation of the membrane around the cytoplasm), which allows for transmission of the shear stresses within the cell and makes cell transfer and adhesion easier.

Red blood cell deformability and red blood cell aggregation are directly related. The flexibility of the erythrocyte membrane facilitates the formation of macromolecular bridging and allows for the maximum attached surface area.[22] With increased cross linking of the membrane proteins (spectrin cytoskeleton), flexibility is decreased and the rate of aggregation is consequently decreased.[89] pH has a profound effect on erythrocyte shape and membrane flexibility. At alkaline pH there is an increase of the surface-volume ratio due to erythrocyte flattening, which maximizes the surface area available for macromolecular bridging between cells. Hence, at a higher pH, the rate of aggregation increases and the rouleaux formed are more stable at higher shear rates.[91] A decrease in membrane flexibility has been documented at low pH, which may contribute to the decreased aggregation in an acidic (i.e. ischemic) environment.[90]

At higher shear rates, there is an increased deformation of the red blood cell to improve alignment with the local flow profile.[21] This is believed to be the reason for the apparent decrease in viscosity at high shear rates demonstrated within rotational viscometers, large tubes, and the macrocirculation. This decrease in viscosity at moderate to high shear rates (greater than 10 sec[-1]) may be blunted by rigidification of the red blood cells.

As discussed earlier, studies utilizing rotational viscometers concluded that the increase in apparent viscosity associated with a decrease in shear rate is secondary to enhanced erythrocyte aggregation.[12,20,25-27,73,83,124] This results in an increased erythrocyte concentration for

a given volume of blood. This relationship is intensified by the addition of HMWDs, which further enhance erythrocyte aggregation.[93] Fibrinogen and globulins have a similar effect and may play an important role in increased whole blood viscosity and cerebral ischemia as discussed later within this chapter. Conversely, experimentally abolishing the membrane deformability and aggregating tendencies of red blood cells, by using a saline or serum medium, was found to reduce the relationship between increasing viscosity and decreasing shear rate for the macrocirculation. These results coincide with the findings of nonbiologic, polymer rheology in which suspensions of long-chain molecules have a higher viscosity than those of short-chain molecules for a given weight fraction.

The effect of red cell aggregation on the rheologic properties of blood in small tubes is more complex than its effect on bulk flow as measured in a rotational viscometer. As noted earlier, the aggregation of erythrocytes in the microcirculation results in a significantly different effect on viscosity than in the macrocirculation. Red blood cell aggregation and the central axial flow of red blood cells cause a *decrease* in the apparent viscosity of whole blood flow in the microcirculation and are discussed below.

Fahraeus-Lindqvist Effect and Axial Cellular Flow

In 1931 Fahraeus and Lindqvist[47] published their classic work that demonstrated that within tubes of less than 300 μm in diameter, the apparent viscosity of blood flow decreased as the lumen of the tube narrowed (Figure 4). This finding has been substantiated by multiple in vitro and in vivo studies and has been termed the *Fahraeus-Lindqvist effect*. The decrease in relative viscosity has been attributed to two effects:

1. The central (axial) migration and aggregation of the cellular constituent.
2. A reduction in the "dynamic" hemato-

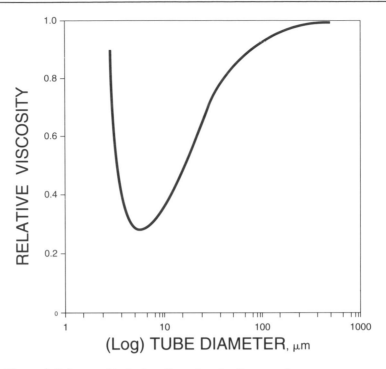

Figure 4. *Fahraeus-Lindqvist effect. As tube diameter decreases, apparent viscosity of whole blood also decreases for a given shear rate. The effect is maximal at a lumen diameter of approximately 5 μ m. Viscosity then increases again as the flow characteristics become less optimal and the lumen diameter approaches the size at which erythrocytes can no longer pass. Modified from Gaehtgens.[51]*

crit within tubes of narrow diameter (Fahraeus effect).

Within the circulation, flow characteristics, including variations in flow velocity and shear rate, lead to an axial distribution of the cellular constituents (Figure 5) so that they migrate to and aggregate within the center of the vessel lumen.[8,53,56] This phenomenon is most pronounced with the erythrocytes, which make up the great majority of the blood cells. At the vessel wall, where shear rates are greatest, the red blood cells tend to remain dissociated, while within the center of the vessel, where shear rates are lowest, aggregation occurs and rouleaux are formed. This central migration and aggregation create an outer marginal zone of decreased cellular concentration consisting mainly of plasma. Between the inner axial core of red blood cell rouleaux and the plasma margin lies a dy-

namic transitional zone of cells that are constantly aggregating and dissociating.

Within rotational viscometers and the macrocirculation, where the wall dimensions are infinitely large compared with the size of the blood cells, the cell free plasma outer margin constitutes a small percentage of the lumen cross section and makes an insignificant contribution to the overall flow properties; however, within smaller tubes and in the microcirculation, the peripheral plasma margin constitutes a greater percentage of the lumen diameter. This "wall exclusion" effect increases as the tube diameter decreases and has been measured directly.[111,112] Depletion of red blood cells from the periphery, where shear rates are greatest, is very significant as it leads to a reduction in the frictional energy loss that occurs during blood flow.[53,111,112] As lumen size decreases, this reduction in friction becomes proportionately larger and plays

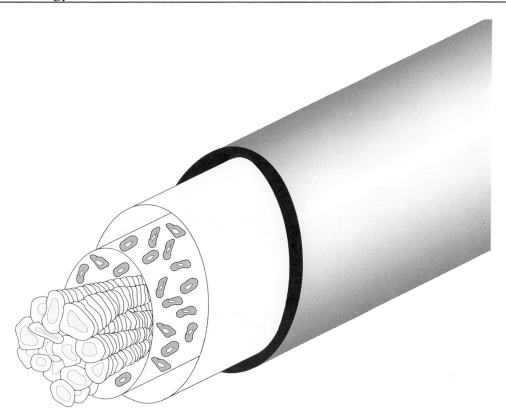

Figure 5. *Axial distribution of the cellular constituents of the blood within the microcirculation. In the center is a core of aggregated, stacked erythrocytes (rouleau), surrounded by a transitional zone of aggregating and dissociating red blood cells. At the periphery is a relatively cell free laminar zone consisting of plasma that interfaces with the vessel wall.*

a critical role in reducing the resistance to flow and the apparent viscosity of the blood within the microcirculation.

An increase in the concentration of red blood cells increases the viscosity of the blood; hence, it follows that the high central concentration of aggregated erythrocytes decreases the fluidity of the local axial flow. This causes a blunting of the velocity profile, so that the central laminar flow velocity is decreased. Although this situation causes an increase in energy loss as compared to newtonian liquids, this detrimental effect is far outweighed by the significant reduction in frictional energy loss due to the lubricating effect of the cell free outer margin.[111,125] In fact, the reduction in friction at the plasma-endothelium interface leads to an enhancement of the net forward displacement of the

entire content of the vessel for a given pressure gradient.[125]

The importance of aggregation on the size of the cell free margin is seen in Figure 6. These graphs demonstrate the ratio of the diameter of the central aggregated cell column to the overall vessel diameter, at varying shear rates, within small-diameter capillary tubes. When the ratio is high, the erythrocyte column constitutes a large portion of the vessel lumen, and the outer cell free margin is correspondingly small. When the ratio approaches zero, the erythrocyte column constitutes a smaller portion of the lumen and the cell free zone is larger. Notice that within the saline medium, where red blood cell aggregation is severely reduced, the cell free margin remains small for all shear rates in both the smaller and larger tubes. Of inter-

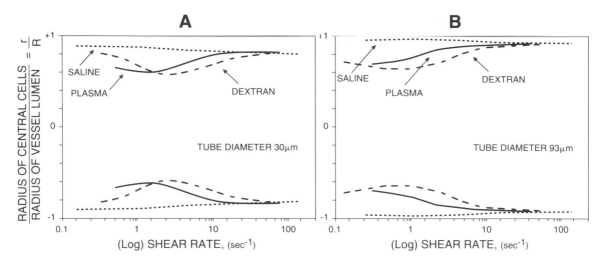

Figure 6. *Ratio of the red blood cell core to the vessel lumen diameter within microcirculation-sized tubes. As the ratio approaches 1, the red blood cells constitute a larger portion of the cross-sectional area of the vessel lumen. Conversely, the smaller the ratio, the more compact the central red blood cell core and the larger the peripheral cell free plasma margin are. The graph lines are presented in a "mirror image," which gives a rough visual approximation of the change in the central red blood cell core. The red blood cells within the saline medium show only a minimal change as the shear rate decreases, while in the plasma medium and HMVP medium, which promotes red blood cell aggregation, there are more tightly packed cores as the shear rate decreases below 10⁻¹. Note that at extremely low shear rates, the ratio begins to increase again. This is more pronounced in the smaller tube and especially within the dextran medium. Modified from Reinke et al.[111]*

est, the ratio of the cell free margin is slightly greater within the 30-μm tube as compared to the 93-μm tube, as predicted by the Fahraeus-Lindqvist effect. Within the plasma medium, which promotes red blood cell aggregation and allows for more efficient packing of erythrocytes within the central axial flow, there is a wide cell free outer margin that increases as the shear rate is reduced and aggregation increases. The addition of HMWD, which enhances aggregation, further increases the size of the cell free plasma margin for a given shear rate.

The impact of axial flow and aggregation on the relative viscosity of flow in small tubes is summarized in Figure 7. Within the serum medium, there is minimal red blood cell aggregation and the compact central core of rouleaux fails to form (Figure 7A). As the shear rate diminishes, the cell-cell interactions increase, the cells become less dispersed, and they lose the favorable shape produced by high shear deformation. The viscosity

climbs exponentially as very low shear rates are encountered. Within the plasma medium, direct observation confirmed the presence of red cell aggregates (Figure 7B). As shear rate decreases, the relative viscosity remains nearly constant and even decreases slightly as low shear is encountered. The effect is enhanced with the addition of HMWD, which promotes increased cell aggregation and plasma margination (Figure 7C). It is interesting to note that within the dextran medium at low shear rates, the maximum reduction in viscosity is attained within all tubes, since the enhanced red blood cell aggregation results in the most densely concentrated rouleaux column possible, regardless of tube size, and consequently the greatest possible reduction in friction.

There is an additional interesting phenomenon. As shown in Figure 4, once the maximal peripheral plasma margin size is reached, the margin begins to decrease again as the shear rate continues to decline. This effect is

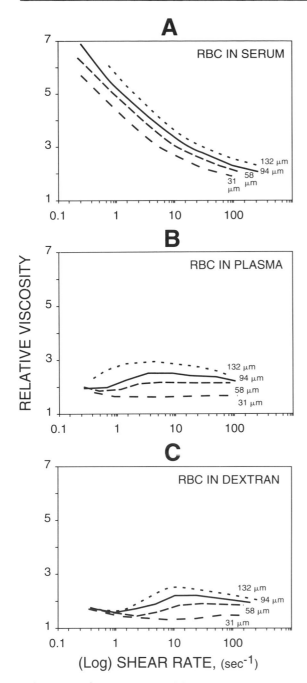

Figure 7. *Relative viscosity of different red blood cell suspensions. See text for explanation. Modified from Reinke et al.[111]*

Figures 7B and C. Within the smallest capillary tube in the plasma medium, and within all the tubes containing the plasma plus HMWD medium, viscosity is increased at very low shear rates. Once the maximum concentration of the central red blood cell column is reached, further decreases in flow cause the long continuous column of rouleaux to contract longitudinally and break up into fragments. This leads to a radial expansion of the red blood cell rouleaux, and therefore a proportionately larger cross-sectional volume for the central cellular core, which increases frictional losses.[111]

This phenomenon is related to the inversion phenomenon of the Fahraeus-Lindqvist effect, demonstrated by Dintenfass[36] and depicted in Figure 4. One notes that as the size of the tube diameter decreases, the relative viscosity decreases until approximately 5 μm, when the viscosity begins to exponentially increase. This is due to the diameter of the tube approaching the resting size of the erythrocyte, which must now undergo extreme deformation to pass through the vessel. As this diameter is approached, the central rouleaux core is disrupted, the plasma margin becomes less optimal, and the frictional forces begin to increase.

As the size of the tube diameter decreases, the shear rate that produces the maximal cell free outer margin is shifted to a higher value (Figure 6). This indicates that as flow decreases within the smallest vessels of the microcirculation, optimal axial flow characteristics occur earlier than in the larger vessels. Therefore, at very low shear rates, the viscosity within the smallest of the microvessels may begin to increase before the rest of the circulation. One may conclude that erythrocyte aggregation, due to variations in vessel size, shear rate, or aggregation strength, is a two-edged sword with regard to viscosity.

Hematocrit

The hematocrit is a major determinant of blood viscosity. For almost 90 years[35] the

more pronounced in tubes of smaller diameter and with increased erythrocyte aggregation tendencies (HMWD medium). The decrease in size of the peripheral plasma margin at very low shear rates is reflected in

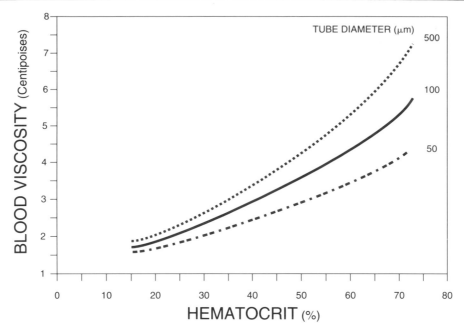

Figure 8. Effect of hematocrit on apparent blood viscosity. As hematocrit increases, apparent viscosity increases for all tube sizes. The influence of hematocrit is more profound within larger-diameter tubes, and at higher hematocrit values. Modified from Stadler et al.[131]

relationship between increased concentration of erythrocytes and decreased fluidity of blood flow has been studied. Laboratory studies using both human and nonhuman blood within both rotational viscometers[27,134,140] and capillary tubes[10,112,131] as well as indirect yield shear stress methods[61] repeatedly confirm the strong influence of hematocrit on viscosity. At a given shear rate, the effect of hematocrit on viscosity is more pronounced within large tubes representative of the macrocirculation than in small capillary tubes (Figure 8); however, it must be emphasized that even within the smallest capillary tubes, hematocrit still remains a major determinant of apparent viscosity. The impact of hematocrit on viscosity is more profound at high hematocrit values. This principle applies to the macrocirculation (Figure 8) as well as the microcirculation (see Figure 10) but is more significant within the macrocirculation.

In the macrocirculation, shear rate modifies the influence of hematocrit on viscosity. Within the rotational viscometer, the effect of hematocrit on viscosity is more profound at low shear rates and becomes progressively less significant as the shear rate increases. Erythrocyte aggregation is a contributing factor, since impaired rouleaux formation decreases viscosity for a given hematocrit and is most significant at low shear rates (Figure 9). Within small vertical tubes representative of the microcirculation, shear rate has less influence on the relationship between hematocrit and viscosity (Figure 10).

Fahraeus Effect, Exclusion Effects, and the Reduction of Hematocrit Within the Microcirculation

Experimental and clinical studies demonstrate that hematocrit is not constant within the circulation. As blood flows through tubes of decreasing diameter, there is a reduction in the measured hematocrit. This phenomenon was first postulated by Fahraeus[46] and hence bears his name. It was later demonstrated in vitro[5,11,51] and in vivo[52,123] by multiple investigators. The migration of cellular blood components perpendicular to the direction of flow, due to shear effects, leads to a segregated axial distribution of cells and plasma. Red blood cells migrate inward, platelets and leukocytes marginate outward, and the plasma margin is most peripheral. Other influences (e.g. gravity, vessel branching points, vessel size) further complicate this arrangement. As a result, different blood components are segregated within separate lamina with different flow velocities. Within the microcirculation, the erythrocytes occupy the central, fastest-flowing lamina and have a higher average velocity than the average velocity of the combined contents of the vessel. The erythrocytes have a shorter "residence time"[125] within the vessel than does the slower-moving peripheral plasma. This leads to a reduction in the dynamic hematocrit of the vessel relative to the arterial source or receiving veins. The reduced hematocrit contributes to the decrease in apparent

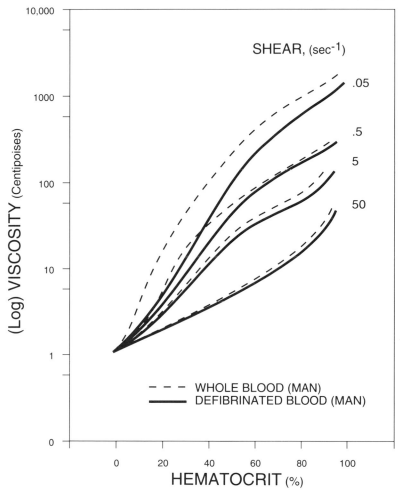

Figure 9. Effect of hematocrit on apparent blood viscosity at different shear rates (macrocirculation). Within a rotational viscometer, reflecting the rheologic characteristics of the macrocirculation, as hematocrit increases, apparent viscosity increases; however, the influence of hematocrit on viscosity is more profound at low shear rates (0.05 sec⁻¹) than at high shear rates (50 sec⁻¹). When the aggregation of erythrocytes is impaired (defibrinated blood), the influence of the hematocrit at low shear rates is attenuated. Modified from Chien et al.[27]

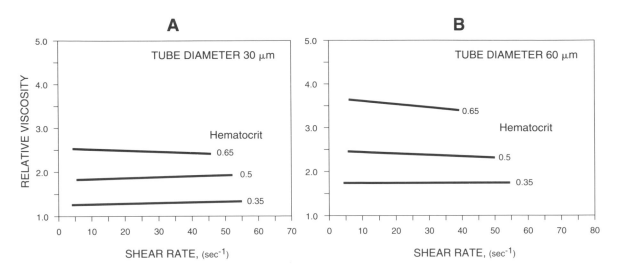

Figure 10. *Effect of hematocrit on apparent blood viscosity at different shear rates (microcirculation). Change in shear rate from a moderate to low value within small vertical capillary tubes has little impact on the influence of hematocrit on apparent viscosity. Of note, for a given hematocrit, as tube diameter decreases, apparent viscosity decreases, as predicted by the Fahraeus-Lindqvist effect. Modified from Reinke et al.[112]*

viscosity within the microcirculation.

The Fahraeus effect may be represented schematically by considering the cerebral circulation to be composed of three different hematocrits: the feed hematocrit (H_F), or hematocrit of the reservoir supplying a vessel; the tube hematocrit (H_T), or hematocrit of the vessel under consideration; and the discharge hematocrit (H_D), or hematocrit of the reservoir filled by a vessel. Although this is an in vitro laboratory paradigm, it is easily applied to the real circulation. Within the microcirculation, the precapillary arterioles and capillaries are the "study tubes" and the small arteries and veins are the reservoirs. Since the erythrocytes are traveling faster than the peripheral plasma, the H_T/H_D is less than 1 and the blood has a lower apparent viscosity secondary to a lower relative hematocrit. As depicted in Figure 11, the relative hematocrit decreases as the diameter narrows, due to a progressively smaller and more compact red cell volume traveling faster than the peripheral plasma lamina. Once the tube diameter reaches approximately 15 μm, the hematocrit begins to rise again, as the flow effects become less optimal, and the

maximum benefit from rouleau formation and erythrocyte deformation has been surpassed. As the "critical diameter" is approached (the point at which red cells can no longer flow despite deformation), the hematocrit exponentially rises.[51]

Other rheologic and flow mechanisms reduce the cellular concentration within the microcirculation by restricting the delivery of cells to the microvessels. These are termed *exclusion effects*.[51] Three different mechanisms have been identified:

1. Size limitation—when the diameter of the capillary approaches the critical diameter (2.7 μm) and erythrocytes have difficulty entering the lumen.
2. Plasma skimming—when the feeding vessel has an segregated axial cellular distribution and the branching capillary is fed primarily by the cell-depleted outer plasma margin.
3. Screening effect—when flow properties at branch points cause streamlines that prevent cells from entering the capillary orifice.

Animal and human studies indicate that

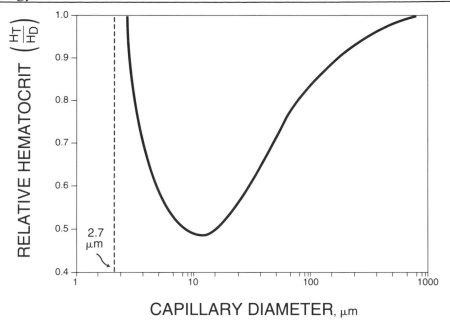

Figure 11. *Fahraeus effect. Relative hematocrit is expressed as the ratio of the tube hematocrit to the discharge hematocrit (H_T/H_D). As capillary diameter narrows, the relative hematocrit decreases, reaching its nadir at approximately 10 μm. The reduction in hematocrit is secondary to the faster rate of flow of the central red blood cell rouleaux relative to the peripheral plasma margin. The relative hematocrit increases again as the critical diameter is approached; the flow characteristics are less optimal and the red blood cells have difficulty passing through the capillary tube. Modified from Gaehtgens.[51]*

the true body hematocrit is less than the large-vessel hematocrit, presumably secondary to the Fahraeus effect and exclusion effects. Direct microscopic observation of the microcirculation[52,123] indicates that hematocrit is reduced to approximately 75% of its macrocirculation value. Studies using positron emission tomography[84,114] reveal that the cerebral hematocrit/large-vessel hematocrit ratio in humans ranges from 69% to 76%.

Human experimental studies[114] support the theoretic basis of the Fahraeus effect. During systemic hemodilution, single photon emission computed tomography demonstrates an increase in the ratio of the cerebral hematocrit to peripheral hematocrit. Meanwhile, there is a simultaneous decrease in the cerebral blood mean transit time, which is characterized by a reduction in the red blood cell velocity relative to the plasma velocity. As

the Fahraeus effect predicts, this leads to an increased dynamic hematocrit.

Sedimentation

Experimental work on blood flow conducted within horizontal tubes demonstrates the important effect of gravity on the distribution of cells and apparent viscosity. At high shear rates, there is dispersion of the blood cells. The flow is characterized as a more or less homogenous plasma and blood cell mixture with an axisymmetric velocity profile. As the shear rate decreases, aggregation and central cellular migration become more pronounced and the symmetric, peripheral, cell free plasma margin develops and enlarges; however, as the shear forces decrease, the pull of gravity on the cellular elements is more pronounced, and sedimentation occurs. The erythrocytes then settle to the dependent portion of the vessel. A cell free plasma zone develops in the superior aspect of the vessel. This cell free zone enlarges until a steady state is reached. A steady state of sedimentation occurs faster in small vessels and at higher shear rates. The *size* of the cell free plasma zone is larger at low shear rates compared to high shear rates, since there is less of a force to counteract the downward pull of gravity. The influence of shear on the extent of sedimentation varies depending on the vessel size, but overall, for a given tube size, the greatest determinant of sedimentation is low shear rate.[1]

As new erythrocytes enter a vessel in which sedimentation is occurring, the red blood cell sediment enlarges and coalesces and the velocity profile of the vessel becomes skewed. The velocity of the sedimented red blood cells becomes progressively slower while the velocity of the superior cell free plasma layer is maintained or increases. Therefore, the residence time of the erythrocyte component is greatly increased, and the relative hematocrit increases. This has been termed *Fahraeus effect reversal.*[125] The combination of a blunted velocity profile, increased apparent hematocrit, and loss of the lubricating plasma sleeve leads to a higher relative viscosity, which continues to increase as sedimentation enlarges. It is postulated[1] that a positive feedback develops in which flow retardation causes an increase in tube hematocrit, resulting in lower conductance and further flow retardation. Eventually there is complete rheologic occlusion as the vessel is packed by sedimented red blood cells. This is termed *compaction stasis.*[125]

Within vessels positioned in series, the pressure head built up by red cell blockage leads to increased shear forces that then disperse the aggregating cells and layered sediment so that a new equilibrium is reached. When compaction stasis occurs within vessels positioned in parallel, such as the capillaries and venules, there is no compensatory increase in shear forces because increases in pressure are dispersed by the parallel conductance vessels. These vessels remain partially

or entirely occluded when a cycle of sedimentation is initiated and reflect what is commonly known clinically; during slow flow, venules are the preferential site of stasis and occlusion.[1]

Leukocyte Rheology

The white blood cells have been implicated as a potentially important factor in the rheology of cerebral blood flow and ischemia. Rheologic studies indicate that their significance is manifest predominantly within the microcirculation, especially under pathologic low-flow conditions. Their special morphologic, rheologic, and chemoimmunologic properties make them prime targets for stroke therapy, and they are currently the subject of intense experimental and clinical investigations.

Granulocytes and lymphocytes constitute approximately 60% and 30% of the circulating leukocytes, respectively. Granulocytes contain three subpopulations of cells: neutrophils, eosinophils, and basophils. The majority of granulocytes are neutrophils, but for the purpose of rheologic description, all subpopulations will simply be considered together.

Leukocyte morphology and deformability are distinctly different from those of erythrocytes. Granulocytes are approximately 10 μm, and lymphocytes 8 μm, in diameter; lymphocytes are slightly larger than erythrocytes.[64,152] Granulocytes contain prominent, highly lobulated or bilobed nuclei; lymphocytes contain large, darkly stained nuclei that may occupy more than 40% of the cellular volume. Their membranes have numerous fine folds demonstrated by scanning electron microscopy. In the quiescent state, leukocytes maintain a spherical shape; when chemotactically activated, they project cytoplasmic pseudopods. Leukocytes demonstrate viscoelastic properties under stress, with granulocytes being more deformable than lymphocytes.[82,121] Both are considerably more rigid than erythrocytes.[117] In the activated state, leukocytes assume stiffer elastic properties with reduced "creep" movement along the vessel surface.[119]

Leukocytes are responsible for impeding the flow of erythrocytes within the microcirculation. The meager deformability of the leukocytes, and their large rigid nuclei, slow their entrance into the small channels of the microcirculation. Entry time into capillary-sized tubes may be many seconds, whereas that of erythrocytes is only milliseconds,[50,82,117] a three order of magnitude difference. Erythrocyte entry into capillaries may be delayed or prevented. The velocity of leukocytes is less than that of red blood cells[122] and erythrocyte trains may be observed to follow behind slower-moving leukocytes in the microcirculation.[102]

Experimental evidence suggests that the rigidity and decreased deformability of leukocytes may be only a minor factor in their interference with erythrocyte movement and microcirculation flow.[50,82] Blood flow resistance increases linearly with an increase in the number of leukocytes only up to 1000 cells/mm³, after which resistance plateaus. Thus, variation within the normal physiologic range of leukocyte concentration (4-10 x 103 cells/mm³) will have little additional effect on blood flow. Under normal flow conditions, leukocytes are diverted into the larger, faster-flowing channels,[24,92,120] which may attenuate their rheologic influence; however, under conditions of low shear stress within the microcirculation, the importance of leukocyte rigidity, deformability, and size becomes pronounced.

In normal flow, the radial distribution of the leukocytes is affected by fast-moving streamlines and interactions with erythrocytes. During fast, homogenous flow, the passing red cells impact the leukocytes and cause random radial displacements.[117] When red cell aggregation occurs, the leukocytes are displaced radially. As blood moves from the capillaries to the venules, the leukocytes assume a more radial position secondary to flow divergence.[121] All of these phenomena tend to increase leukocyte interaction with the vessel endothelium. Under normal conditions, there is very little adhesion within the arterioles or venules. In the nonactivated state in vitro, granulocytes detach from the endothelium at shear forces commonly found in the capillaries and venules,[82] in accordance with in vivo observations.[122] Leukocyte capillary occlusion secondary to the "tight fit" and relative rigidity is only transient during normal flow states. In the activated state however, or during low shear stress, leukocyte-endothelium interaction leads to pathologic consequences.

It is believed that the most important rheologic factor for the leukocyte impedance of blood flow is endothelial adhesion and capillary plugging. This is most prominent under conditions of low shear stress or when leukocytes are chemoimmunologically activated. Under low-flow conditions, leukocytes are unable to deform sufficiently to pass through capillaries, and plugging occurs within the lumen or at the entry site.[117] A common contact area between the leukocyte and the endothelium is formed. The adhesion strength is influenced by the production of adhesion complexes or local inflammatory injury, in part produced by the release of lysosomes, leukotrienes, and prostaglandins or by the production of oxygen free radicals.[118] Once entrapped, all flow within the vessel is obstructed. Shear forces required to dislodge the cells are about the same order of magnitude as the pressure gradient across unobstructed capillaries[117] and may be significantly higher if the leukocyte is activated. In a fluid dynamic system in parallel, such as the cortical capillaries, the high perfusion force needed to dislodge trapped leukocytes is difficult to attain since patent capillaries in parallel provide an alternative "pressure sink." Therefore, postischemia reperfusion may be insufficient to completely restore microcirculation flow. It has been suggested[7] that leukocyte plugging is responsible for the "no reflow" phenomenon described by Ames[2] and has been observed within capillaries of the cat cerebral cortex following hemorrhagic shock.[161] Within the venules, leukocytes may adhere to the endothelium but rarely cause obstruction.[72] Vascular resistance is, however, increased.

A decrease in the total number of leukocytes has been observed during the initial phase of hypotension, the so-called flight of leukocytes.[129] Presumably leukocytes that would normally be diverted from small capillary lumens become wedged within the capillaries during the low-flow state secondary to maximum vessel dilatation and decreased cell deformability. Increased cell activation from the hemorrhagic insult potentiates adhesion. Prolonged or irreversible capillary flow obstruction results.

The importance of leukocyte plugging *during* the period of low shear force has considerable experimental support. During hemorrhagic shock, individual peripheral muscle capillary obstruction occurs from a single leukocyte; rarely is there more than one cell within the lumen.[4] Unobstructed neighboring capillaries are leukocyte free. Mortality from short-term hemorrhagic shock in animals is most accurately predicted by the number of activated neutrophils prior to the hemodynamic insult.[118] Neutrophils that are already activated are most capable of becoming quickly and irreversibly lodged within the microcirculation during a transient hypotensive state, and they play a decisive role in ultimate organ perfusion. The prehemorrhage activated neutrophil count is a more sensitive predictor of outcome than the total number of neutrophils, the hematocrit, or traditional hemodynamic parameters. In a rat transient ischemia model, pretreatment with antineutrophil serum, which decreases neutrophil count, substantially improves postischemic reperfusion.[60] Treatment after the onset of ischemia provides no benefit. If hemorrhagic shock is prolonged, the greater the activated neutrophil count the lower the chance for animal survival.[118] Hence, prolonged or irreversible leukocyte plugging secondary to a low-flow state or chemoimmunologic activation is a principal aspect of the hemorheology of vessel occlusion and flow resistance.

Viscosity of Blood Flow in the Macrocirculation and Microcirculation—A Caveat

As is obvious from the preceding sections, the viscosity and blood flow through the circulation are products of multiple and complex rheologic properties, involving multiple cellular components, which vary significantly depending on the specific conditions present within any given vessel. Generalizations and simplifications of rheologic principles (e.g. "red cell aggregation increases viscosity," "low shear increases viscosity," "small lumen size increases viscosity") are frequently untrue and misleading when applied to the entire spectrum of the cerebral vasculature. The rheologic determinants of blood flow have meaning only when discussed in a specific situation, when other parameters are controlled. Otherwise, their exact influence on cerebral blood flow can, at best, only be guessed at. With this in mind, the figures presented in the preceding sections only serve to broadly summarize the major rheologic trends applicable to cerebral blood flow. They do, however, give the reader a gestalt for the patterns and changes of flow and viscosity encountered within the cerebral circulation. Keeping in mind the detailed and interrelated concepts of hemodynamics and cellular rheology discussed in the preceding sections gives the reader an appreciation for the pearls and pitfalls contained within the results and conclusions of animal rheologic experiments and human clinical trials.

Clinical Hemorheology

The clinical importance of hemorheology has undergone considerable study and debate. Clinical research demonstrates a strong correlation between hemorheologic abnormalities and the incidence and severity of cerebral ischemia. Unfortunately, there is no consensus as to which factors are of paramount importance; nor are the hemorheologic mechanisms resolved. A central issue continues to be the relationship between hematocrit, whole blood viscosity, and cerebral blood flow during both normal and pathologic states. The influence of plasma viscosity and plasma proteins on cerebral blood flow has long been recognized and has become the focus of increased attention following the disappointing results of the large multicenter hemodilutional trials. Most recently, leukocyte rheology and capillary plugging have been implicated as important occurrences during the acute phase of cerebral ischemia. The hemorheologic mechanisms underlying cerebral blood flow and ischemia will be discussed within the following sections. Whenever possible, the theoretic and experimental concepts will be related to the clinical manifestations. Although definitive conclusions are often difficult, broad rheologic concepts emerge that provide the foundation for the prevention and treatment of stroke.

Platelet rheology appears to play a significant role in ischemic pathology and is intimately involved with the chemical mediators of endothelial and parenchymal injury during stroke. For the sake of brevity, and in order not to do injustice to this important subject, it has been omitted from the following discussion. The reader is referred to other references.[33,38,39,66,126,142,145]

This chapter is primarily concerned with the rheologic principles of cerebral blood flow and ischemia. Therapeutic practices are considered briefly and only when they serve to illustrate or clarify a particular issue. The one exception is hemodilutional therapy for cerebral ischemia, which, because of its widespread interest within the neuroscience community and its direct relevance to the subject of clinical hemorheology, is discussed in detail from a rheologic point of view.

Hematocrit, Viscosity, and Cerebral Ischemia

Experimental and Clinical Studies

It has long been recognized that hemorheologic alterations are associated with cerebrovascular disease. Early studies focused on the role of hemoglobin concentration and packed cell volume. It was suggested that an elevated hematocrit correlated with a decreased cerebral blood flow and an increased incidence and severity of cerebral ischemia. Polycythemia vera and relative polycythemia (increased hematocrit secondary to a decreased plasma volume) are associated with a higher

incidence of cerebrovascular accidents and decreased cerebral blood flow.[17,75,81,101,107,139] The incidence of cerebrovascular accidents is directly proportional to the packed cell volume in patients with polycythemia rubra vera.[107] Conversely, patients with anemia are noted to have increased cerebral blood flow.[70] It was felt that variations in blood viscosity secondary to an abnormally low or high hematocrit accounted for these findings.

Population studies provided conflicting results regarding the impact of hematocrit on cerebrovascular disease. The Framingham study[77] suggested that a higher than average hemoglobin concentration was a risk factor for cerebral infarction, although multivariate analysis indicated that the relationship was probably secondary to other factors such as blood pressure and tobacco smoking. None the less, the authors concluded that the impact of hemoglobin may be mediated by its effect on blood pressure or that hemoglobin may mediate the effect of smoking. A Japanese autopsy study[142] demonstrated that the incidence of cerebral infarction increased dramatically as hematocrit increased above 0.45. The relationship was independent of age, blood pressure, and degree of cerebral atherosclerosis, but notably, tobacco smoking was unaccounted for. This finding was felt to confirm the uncertain conclusion of the Framingham study; however, a large prospective population study[80] failed to find any correlation between elevated hematocrit and cerebral infarction and even suggested that in women a low hematocrit was deleterious.

Overall, population studies fail to offer any decisive conclusion regarding the issues of hematocrit, viscosity, and infarction, but the suggestion of a causal relationship between hematocrit and cerebral infarction prompted numerous human studies concerning cerebral blood flow and abnormal blood viscosity. Since hematocrit is a major determinant of in vitro blood viscosity as measured by the capillary and rotational viscometer,[10,95,134] it was proposed that cerebral blood flow was inversely proportional to whole blood viscosity. Initial studies suggested a strong correlation. Venesection in patients with polycythemia decreased blood viscosity measured at a low shear rate by 30% and increased cerebral blood flow an average of 70%.[139] A high *normal* hematocrit was also associated with decreased cerebral circulation,[75,140] as was suggested by the population studies. In patients without polycythemia, both with and without cerebrovascular disease, those patients with a hematocrit greater than 0.46 had a significantly decreased cerebral blood flow as compared with matched controls with a lower hematocrit.[75,140] Following venesection, whole blood viscosity in the high hematocrit patients decreased and cerebral blood flow increased between 30% to 50%. A strong correlation between hematocrit and cerebral blood flow was demonstrated. In all studies, treated patients had subjective clinical improvement as well.

The theory that hematocrit determined cerebral blood flow by virtue of its influence on viscosity was significantly challenged by studies examining the relationship between oxygen delivery and cerebral blood flow. Paulson, Henriksen, and others suggested that changes in cerebral blood flow in patients with a normal[105] or high hematocrit[68] depended on both oxygen-binding capacity and changes in hematocrit, but they were unable to satisfactorily distinguish their individual influence. They did demonstrate that blood flow increased to compensate for decreased oxygen content and, more importantly, that oxygen delivery remained constant after the hematocrit was decreased. This contradicted earlier studies[149] that claimed an increase in cerebral oxygen delivery secondary to the improved hemorheologic state resulting from decreased blood viscosity following venesection.

Further studies demonstrated that the relationship between hematocrit and cerebral blood flow was mediated by oxygen delivery and not viscosity. It was known[150,151] that patients with polycythemia secondary to hypoxic lung disease or patients with high oxygen affinity hemoglobin have normal, or greater than normal, cerebral blood flow despite increased hematocrit and whole blood

viscosity. Brown and Marshall[13,14] demonstrated that in patients with paraproteinemia or leukemia with elevated whole blood viscosity, the cerebral blood flow was determined by arterial oxygen content and was independent of blood viscosity. Furthermore, following plasma exchange that results in a significant decrease in whole blood viscosity but no change in oxygen content, there was no change in cerebral blood flow. In patients with either anemia or polycythemia, multivariate analysis revealed that any correlation between cerebral blood flow and viscosity or hematocrit was secondary to changes in oxygen content.[15] It became apparent that cerebral blood flow was tightly coupled to the cerebral metabolic rate and the regulation of cerebral oxygen delivery. The importance of hematocrit as a determinant of cerebral blood flow by virtue of its effect on viscosity was almost discounted.

However, there is still a strong suggestion within the literature that the effect of hematocrit on cerebral blood flow is not entirely mediated by changes in the oxygen-carrying capacity of blood. One study[76] demonstrated that in anemic patients with and without paraproteinemia and matched for hematocrit, increased whole blood viscosity resulted in diminished cerebral blood flow, emphasizing the importance of viscosity as an independent variable. Improved cerebral blood flow after venesection in patients with polycythemia or a moderately elevated hematocrit is not completely accounted for by the change in oxygen delivery.[15,75,138,140,149] Increased oxygen delivery to the brain was demonstrated after venesection in patients with polycythemia[149] and in some hemodilutional studies,[124] reflecting an increase in cerebral blood flow that was more than compensatory to a reduction in oxygen content. This was attributed to enhanced flow properties resulting from decreased blood viscosity. In a well-controlled animal study, up to 50% of blood flow within an intact cerebral circulation was found to be directly related to changes in red blood cell concentration, independent of changes in blood oxygen content, hemoglobin oxygen affinity, or cerebral metabolic rate.[74]

In conclusion, experimental results strongly suggest that viscosity does contribute to the correlation between hematocrit and blood flow but is overshadowed by the significantly larger influence from oxygen delivery regulation. How the importance of each of these determinants changes during ischemic conditions is uncertain.

Some studies suggest that the influence of an elevated hematocrit or whole blood viscosity may be more prominent in patients with a compromised cerebral blood flow. The relationship between hematocrit and cerebral infarction in the Japanese necropsy study[142] was most striking in the patients with the most advanced cerebral atherosclerosis. This important finding was supported by a study[65] that revealed that the severity of cerebral infarction in patients with significant carotid occlusion was directly proportional to the hematocrit. A strong correlation between cerebral blood flow and viscosity as measured by yield shear stress was demonstrated only for patients with cerebrovascular disease and diminished cerebral blood flow[61]; patients with average or elevated cerebral blood flow had a significantly *smaller* correlation with viscosity.

Hemodilutional Therapy for Cerebral Ischemia

Animal Research

The relationship between hematocrit, viscosity, cerebral blood flow, and oxygen transport prompted researchers and clinicians to speculate whether variations in hematocrit could be exploited for the treatment of ischemic stroke. Experimental animal studies were undertaken that examined the impact of both isovolemic and hypervolemic hemodilutional therapy on cerebral blood flow following focal arterial occlusion. Wood et al[156] demonstrated that hemodilutional therapy with LMWD significantly increased cerebral blood flow within the region of cerebral ischemia following focal arterial occlusion. The increase in blood flow inversely correlated with the reduction in hematocrit, although the role of oxygen delivery was not studied. Intravascular volume expansion without hemodilution was found to have no effect on cerebral blood flow in regions of low blood flow.[159] These same authors[157] demonstrated that hypervolemic hemodilution increased cerebral blood flow preferentially within ischemic regions; nonischemic regions had no change in cerebral blood flow. These studies demonstrated a significant reduction in the size of cerebral infarction following hemodilution but failed to reach statistical significance. A later study[144] demonstrated that in both the acute and subacute period following arterial occlusion, the size of the cerebral infarction was dramatically and significantly reduced by isovolemic hemodilution with venesection and LMWD infusion. It was concluded that a reduction in hematocrit produces a beneficial increase in blood flow following focal cerebral ischemia.

Several important objections should be considered with regard to this conclusion. These same studies[144,157] produced conflicting reports on whether blood flow was preferentially increased in nonischemic regions as compared to normal parenchyma. This casts doubt on the theory that within maximally dilated arterioles, changes in whole blood viscosity resulting from changes in hematocrit preferentially influence cerebral blood flow. Decreased oxygen content resulting from hemodilution may not be beneficial for ischemic brain already subject to low blood flow and high oxygen extraction. Regional cortical oxygen transport did not change in either ischemic or nonischemic regions, suggesting that hemodilution did not improve overall oxygen delivery despite the increase in blood flow. A recent study[148] demonstrated a decrease in oxygen transport to the cerebral parenchyma following hemodilutional therapy and hypotensive hypoxia. The authors demonstrated that the reduction in arterial oxygen content was not compensated for by the increase in cerebral blood flow, further supporting the finding that within maximally dilated arterioles, whole blood viscosity reduction does not enhance oxygen delivery. In conclusion, animal research produced suggestive, but not compelling, evidence that hemodilutional therapy is advantageous in the setting of focal cerebral ischemia. Furthermore, disturbing evidence arguing against the theoretic and practical benefit of hemodilution was raised.

Hemodilutional Therapy for Cerebral Ischemia

Clinical Trials

The results from large population studies and clinical experiments suggesting that hematocrit correlates with cerebral blood flow and ischemia, as well as evidence from experimental studies indicating that hemodilution attenuates infarction severity, prompted numerous human clinical studies evaluating hemodilution therapy for ischemic stroke. An initial uncontrolled, retrospective study[58] suggested that treatment of acute cerebral ischemia with LMWD decreased mortality and neurologic morbidity as compared to therapy with vasodilating agents. An uncontrolled study conducted by Wood et al[154] with small numbers of patients showed marked neurologic improvement during and immediately following therapy with hypervolemic hemodilution. These same authors also demonstrated that isovolemic hemodilution produced a small but statistically significant reduction in slow-wave electroencephalogram (EEG) activity within the region of ischemia during the acute phase of stroke.[155] An impressive 20% reduction in hematocrit and an 18% increase in cerebral blood flow were documented. Unfortunately no clinical correlation was made and long-term EEG changes were not presented; however, this study did suggest at least temporary functional improvement of ischemic cerebral parenchyma resulting from hemodilution. An early randomized study[55] of 100 patients claimed that

treatment with LMWD decreased mortality and improved neurologic function.

Studies clearly demonstrating no benefit to hemodilution therapy were also appearing in the literature. A randomized, controlled trial of hypervolemic hemodilution with LMWD within 24 hours of onset of symptoms of acute cerebral ischemia demonstrated no difference in neurologic condition among survivors in the control or treatment groups at 3 weeks.[130] Unfortunately, no information regarding the reduction in hematocrit was presented, and the effectiveness of the hemodilution cannot be evaluated. A randomized, controlled, and blinded study[91] also demonstrated no neurologic or functional benefit following hypervolemic hemodilution with LMWD versus 5% dextrose at 3 weeks and 6 months; however, acute mortality in patients with the most severe infarctions was significantly lower in the treatment group, although these patients remained severely disabled and made no meaningful recovery. The authors postulated that the decrease in mortality in the most severe stroke group was a result of the osmotic action of dextran on the cerebral edema. This finding is in keeping with previous studies[55,130] in which mentation and level of consciousness in treated patients improved, but neurologic status did not. It was concluded that LMWD therapy did not reduce the size or severity of cerebral infarction.

Overall, no convincing argument for hemodilution therapy had been made in the literature until 1984 when a prospective, randomized, controlled Scandinavian study[135] demonstrated that isovolemic hemodilution accomplished with venesection and infusion of LMWD improved neurologic function at 10 days and functional outcome at 3 months. Mortality was unaffected. Hematocrit decreased approximately 14% in treated patients with a concomitant decrease in whole blood viscosity measured at both low and high shear rates. The beneficial effect was attributed to the reduction in hematocrit, although the authors could not discount the possibility that the disaggregating effect of LMWD on platelets and erythrocytes, or its ability to decrease platelet adhesiveness, played a role in improving outcome.

Enthusiasm over the initial results of the Scandinavian stroke study were short-lived. Within 3 years, a large, prospective, randomized, and controlled multicenter trial conducted within both university and nonuniversity hospitals by the Scandinavian Stroke Study Group[3,115,116] demonstrated that isovolemic hemodilution accomplished by venesection and infusion of LMWD produced no benefit regarding mortality, neurologic status, or functional outcome at 3 months. All patients were treated within 48 hours of the onset of symptoms and most within 24 hours. The hematocrit was reduced 16% over a 5-day period; the average reduction within the first 24 hours was 9%. An extensive follow-up study demonstrated that hemodilution produced no beneficial effect in any subset of patients including those with the most rapid or pronounced reduction of hematocrit or those most quickly entered into the study after the onset of symptoms. Notably hemodilution even failed to help those patients with the highest initial hematocrits on entry into the trial (47%-50%).

One year later, a second large randomized and controlled multicenter trial conducted by the Italian Acute Stroke Study Group[63] demonstrated that patients treated with isovolemic hemodilution accomplished by venesection and LMWD infusion were no different from control patients with regard to mortality, neurologic state, or functional status at the time of discharge from the hospital or at 6 month follow-up. All patients were treated within 12 hours of the onset of symptoms, and the mean reduction of hematocrit was 13% at 48 hours. Patients treated within 6 hours, or those with the highest hematocrit or most rapid hemodilution, also showed no benefit.

The results of these two studies convincingly demonstrated that current hemodilutional practice does not provide measurable benefit for ischemic stroke. Critics[67,81] argued that these studies were faulted by the long

period between the onset of symptoms and entrance into the study, the mild reductions in hematocrit achieved, and the long length of time required to achieve the hemodilutional goal. It was argued that the "optimal" hematocrit for oxygen delivery (0.30-0.35) was not achieved in either of these two studies. These arguments are not persuasive. Both studies clearly demonstrated that subsets of patients treated most rapidly, within less than 6 hours of the onset of symptoms in the Italian multicenter trial, had no additional benefit. It is evident that hemodilution was only mild in both of these studies (13%-16% over 2-5 days)—far less than the approximate 20% baseline hematocrit reduction required to achieve an "optimal" hematocrit of less than 0.35. However, both studies did produce a 10% hematocrit reduction within 24 hours in the majority of patients; a 15% reduction was accomplished within 48 hours in a large number of patients in the Scandinavian trial. Neither of these groups showed any benefit. Furthermore, those patients with the highest hematocrits (more than 0.45) showed no benefit either. Hematocrit reductions may have been less than those advocated for optimal hemodilution, but it may be argued that if any benefit were to be gained from this therapy, clinical trials with such large numbers of subjects (over 1600 for both studies combined) would at least show a statistical trend toward improvement in the most aggressively treated subgroups.

Two studies attempted to correct the faults of the large multicenter trials by accomplishing a more rapid and profound hemodilution in patients with acute ischemic stroke. One study[67] was unable to provide sufficient pentastarch hemodilution to satisfy protocol guidelines despite intensive care monitoring with a Swan-Ganz catheter. The study did suggest that the few patients with a greater than 15% hematocrit reduction treated within less than 12 hours had marked improvement over controls, but did not reach statistical significance. The other study,[81] a prospective, randomized, blinded trial of hypervolemic hemodilution accomplished with venesection and LMWD, achieved an impressive 30% reduction in hematocrit within 9 hours of the initiation of therapy. Hematocrit was reduced to less than 0.35 in 84% of the patients. Treated patients demonstrated significantly improved neurologic status and fine motor skills at 8 days, 3 weeks, and 3 months. Mortality was not different among groups. This well-controlled study provides the only statistically significant and compelling evidence for the benefit of rapid and aggressive hemodilution therapy. Until other supporting studies are published, the benefit of hemodilutional therapy as currently practiced for acute cerebral ischemia remains questionable.

Optimal Hematocrit

The hematocrit that results in the maximal oxygen delivery to the brain parenchyma has been a subject of considerable discussion and debate. Optimal hematocrit is defined as that value that produces the maximal ratio of hemoglobin content to viscosity, hence the most efficient transfer of oxygen. It has frequently been stated in the stroke literature that oxygen transport increases during hemodilution secondary to the augmentation in cerebral blood flow, maximizing at a hematocrit between 0.30 to 0.35.[79,159,160] This is based on both animal and clinical research[34,49,58,71,98] and is a foundation for the theoretic basis of hemodilution therapy.

Numerous basic science, experimental, and clinical evidence argues against this premise. Oxygen delivery within the microcirculation may not be maximal when the large-vessel hematocrit is reduced to such low levels. The Fahraeus-Lindqvist effect (the decrase in apparent viscosity as blood flows through narrow-diameter tubes) suggests that for a given feed hematocrit, red blood cell transport efficiency will be greater in vessels of decreasing diameter. This was supported by Stadler et al[131] who demonstrated that in vitro optimal hematocrit increased as tube diameter decreased. Within 50- and 100-μm diameter tubes, optimal feed hematocrit occurred at

0.51 and 0.44, respectively, and then plateaued. Within 500 μm-tubes, more representative of the macrocirulation, optimal feed hematocrit was 0.38. The authors stated that other studies[108,134] demonstrate varying optimal hematocrits that are directly proportional to the diameter of the needle or tube viscometer used to measure viscosity. Gaehtgens and Marx,[52] pooling cerebral blood flow data from several studies, demonstrated that maximal cerebral oxygen delivery occurs at a packed cell volume of 0.42, and postulated that during periods of ischemia, optimal hematocrit may be shifted even higher.

The Fahraeus effect (decrease in apparent hematocrit as blood flows through narrow-diameter tubes) also suggests that large-vessel hematocrit reductions may not be beneficial. Since microcirculation or whole body hematocrit is approximately 70% of that of the large vessel hematocrit[52,84,114,123] when large-vessel hematocrit is 0.45-0.50, then microcirculation dynamic hematocrit is approximately 0.31-0.35. Hence, a normal physiologic hematocrit provides the same optimal feed hematocrit for the microcirculation as demonstrated by in vitro studies using microcirculation-sized tubes (50-100 μm). This idea is supported by two large clinical studies. In a Japanese necropsy study,[142] patients with hematocrits between 0.36 and 0.45 had a *lower* incidence of cerebral infarction than patients with an average hematocrit between 0.31 and 0.35. Similarly, the Scandinavian Multicenter Stroke trial[135] found the lowest incidence of mortality in patients whose hematocrits at the time of admission ranged between 0.44 and 0.47. As the hematocrit decreased or increased from these values, mortality increased.

It may be concluded that optimal oxygen delivery may not necessarily occur at a reduced hematocrit. Within the intact circulation, normal rheologic mechanisms ensure the most efficient transport of red blood cells and oxygen. It must be cautioned that during abnormal flow states resulting from hyperviscosity syndromes or polycythemia, favorable changes in whole blood viscosity resulting from hemodilution may provide increased oxygen delivery; however, during low-flow states secondary to cerebrovascular occlusive disease, therapy involving a severe hematocrit reduction is theoretically suspect, may not provide an optimal hematocrit, and should be approached with caution.

Hematocrit, Viscosity, Cerebral Blood Flow, and Ischemia

Conclusions

Popular hemorheologic theories describing a direct relationship between whole blood viscosity or hematocrit and cerebral blood flow are inadequate to explain the complex relationship characterized by experimental and clinical studies. Hematocrit and whole blood viscosity are certainly important determinants of cerebral blood flow, but their influence remains secondary to that of oxygen delivery in the intact, and probably also the impaired, cerebral circulation.

The clinical effect of hematocrit reduction on cerebral blood flow is probably mediated within the macrocirculation. Packed cell volume is more important to whole blood viscosity within the macrocirculation than the microcirculation. Rheologic studies demonstrate that an exponential increase in whole blood viscosity secondary to an elevation in hematocrit beyond the normal physiologic range occurs predominantly within larger tubes.[10,27,131,134] The Fahraeus-Lindqvist and Fahraeus effects maintain decreased viscosity within the microcirculation. Furthermore, within the macrocirculation, reductions in shear rate more profoundly influence viscosity at a high hematocrit than a low hematocrit; this preferential effect is much less pronounced within the microcirculation.

These findings suggest that the relationship between an elevated hematocrit and ischemic stroke is a large-vessel phenomenon. Clinically this is documented by studies[142] showing that a high hematocrit has a greater association with stroke when associated with atherosclerotic cerebrovascular disease, which involves the large vessels more so than the microcirculation.[18] It is also consistent with the association between a high hematocrit and increased infarction severity resulting from carotid stenosis.[66] Although there is no firm conclusion regarding the clinical importance of a normal or low hematocrit, several studies identify an abnormally elevated hematocrit as a determinant of decreased cerebral blood flow[76,139,140] and a risk factor for stroke.[66,138,142] Consequently, the conclusion that a significantly increased hematocrit (greater than 0.46) worsens infarction severity when secondary to a large-vessel occlusion or atherosclerosis appears to be in agreement with both the clinical findings and the known rheologic principles as applied to the macrocirculation.

It is frequently stated that during periods of cerebral ischemia, whole blood viscosity plays a significant role in determining cerebral blood flow as predicted by the Hagen-Poiseuille equation. It is hypothesized that during an episode of occlusive cerebrovascular ischemia, when maximal arteriolar dilatation has been achieved and an increase in the pressure gradient is no longer feasible secondary to a proximal occlusion, whole blood viscosity becomes the sole determinant of direct and collateral cerebral blood flow; however, this often-quoted generalization is not strictly true. The Hagen-Poiseuille equation reflects a purely newtonian fluid phenomenon. At best it may only be applied to the macrocirculation under high shear rate conditions, when blood achieves its most "newtonian" character. Studies indicate that within regions of cerebral hypoxia, when arteriolar (microcirculation) dilatation is presumed to be maximal, whole blood viscosity does not influence cerebral blood flow more preferentially than in nonischemic regions.[144,148]

Many of the hemodilutional trials were based on the assumption that hematocrit is the major determinant of blood viscosity and hence is a major determinant of blood flow during cerebral ischemia; however, this is a predominantly macrocirculation phenomenon and is not applicable to the entire cerebral circulation. Hematocrit is a relatively less important determinant of viscosity in the microcirculation than it is within the large vessels. Within the normal physiologic range of 0.35-0.50 there is only moderate variation in viscosity as hematocrit changes in small capillary tubes less than 50 μm (Figures 8 and 10). As described earlier, it is not so much the concentration of red blood cells, but their axial distribution, aggregation, deformation, and axial flow pattern that critically influence the apparent viscosity of blood within the microcirculation. This is especially true at low shear rates (less than 10 sec^{-1}), suggesting an even smaller role for hematocrit within the microcirculation during periods of cerebral ischemia.

Studies suggest that erythrocytes enhance initial platelet adhesion and aggregation.[66,126,145] However, erythrocytes also inhibit the growth and sedimentation of already established platelet aggregates[87] that have been implicated in the pathogenesis of stroke.[33,38,39,141] Hematocrit reduction from 0.50 to 0.30 results in increased platelet aggregation in vitro.[88] Thomas,[138] reviewing clinical trials involving antiplatelet drugs, remarked on the significance of erythrocyte/platelet interaction and the use of aspirin as an adjunct to hemodilution "in order for the potential benefits not to be lost." Hematocrit reduction may have a deleterious effect on platelet aggregation, releasing secondary mechanisms of cerebral injury.

Therapeutic paradigms based on hematocrit as the single important determinant of viscosity and cerebral blood flow should be approached with caution. They ignore the role of small-vessel disease and the abnormal flow conditions present within the capillaries and arterioles when proximal feeding arteries are compromised. They disregard other important determinants of microcirculation viscosity such as erythrocyte aggregation and plasma protein concentration. They do not take into account the role of other blood components or their interaction with ery-

throcytes. Furthermore, the presumption that hemodilution produces the optimal hematocrit for maximal oxygen delivery may be invalid. Regardless of the therapy employed, improvement in large-vessel flow will not significantly increase oxygen delivery or collateral blood supply unless the numerous and interrelated microcirculation rheologic mechanisms are optimized to enhance microcirculation flow.

Rheologic Characteristics of Cerebral Ischemia

Plasma Viscosity and Plasma Proteins

Increased blood viscosity has been frequently associated with cerebrovascular disease and acute stroke. Although partially due to increased values of hematocrit, a significant contribution is made by increases in plasma viscosity and plasma protein concentrations.[32,40,85,104] Several studies[32,48,85] demonstrate increased plasma viscosity following stroke as compared with controls, but whether this finding represents a consequence of stroke or a pathogenetic mechanism is debated. Increased plasma viscosity immediately following stroke was shown to return to normal 6 months following the event,[85] suggesting a reactive phenomenon; however, several recent studies clearly demonstrate that plasma viscosity is increased not only in patients post stroke, but also in those patients with risk factors for stroke or transient ischemic attacks (TIAs).[32,44,48] This strongly argues for an etiologic mechanism. Schneider et al[128] demonstrated increased plasma viscosity with subcortical arteriolsclerotic encephalopathy (Binswanger's disease) as compared with patients with lacunar infarctions; other parameters (hematocrit, red cell deformity, and aggregation) were not different. The implication of increased plasma viscosity mediating microvascular disease is complemented by in vitro experiments demonstrating the importance of the peripheral plasma sleeve in reducing frictional forces within capillary tubes. Animal experiments demonstrate that cerebral blood flow varies inversely with plasma viscosity when hematocrit is controlled for,[143] a finding confirmed within the peripheral vasculature as well.[62]

Plasma viscosity per se may not be the only or most significant factor involved in the studies described above. Some animal studies[16,19] demonstrate only a minor effect of plasma fluidity on cerebral blood flow. Although clinical evidence strongly supports an association between increased plasma viscosity and the risk of stroke, there is no compelling evidence that decreased fluidity is the significant etiologic mechanism. As noted earlier, plasma exchange studies demonstrated that the increased plasma viscosity associated with paraproteinemia was not an important determinant of decreased blood flow.[13,14] How may these divergent clinical findings be reconciled? The answer may be that increased plasma viscosity, while perhaps contributing to the pathogenesis of cerebrovascular disease due to decreased plasma fluidity, also acts as a marker for changes in plasma proteins. It is these proteins that may be intimately involved in the mechanisms of stroke.

Although hematocrit is the overwhelming determinant of whole blood viscosity, fibrinogen makes a smaller but significant contribution to whole blood viscosity[10,40] and is an important determinant of plasma viscosity.[32] Fibrinogen has been found to be closely associated with cerebral ischemia. Increased serum levels are found not only postcerebral infarction,[40,85] but also in patients at risk for stroke.[32,48] Similarly a decreased albumin-globulin ratio was found in patients post stroke and at risk for stroke.[32] In a prospective population study[153] using multivariate analysis, fibrinogen was found to be an independent and significant risk factor for the incidence of stroke. Furthermore, the incidence of stroke appeared to be "dose dependent," increasing with the fibrinogen level.

Fibrinogen is clearly related to cerebrovascular disease. Although the mechanisms of action are still speculative, there is strong evidence that it is mediated through the rheologic properties of erythrocytes. Animal studies demonstrate enhanced red blood cell aggregation following focal cerebral ischemia.[103] Red blood cell aggregation has been demonstrated to be increased during the acute and chronic phase of cerebral ischemia[136] and also in patients with TIAs.[44] Deep subcortical infarction, presumably due to microvascular terminal arterioles, has been associated with a higher degree of erythrocyte aggregation than cortical infarction.[139] It is proposed that fibrinogen plays a role in enhanced erythrocyte aggregation. Fibrinogen[23,83,95,132] and plasma globulins[23] are known to induce aggregation of red blood cells, which increases blood viscosity within the macrocirculation at low shear rates, as discussed earlier within this chapter. Albumin may interfere with red blood cell aggregation.[83] Increased fibrinogen correlates inversely with cerebral blood flow and is even more significant when hematocrit is considered.[60] Several stroke studies demonstrate that increased erythrocyte aggregation correlates significantly with increasing levels of fibrinogen[136,137] and a decreased albumin-globulin ratio.[136]

In conclusion, there is strong evidence that fibrinogen and serum globulins are etiologic factors in the pathogenesis of cerebral infarction. The mechanism may be enhanced erythrocyte aggregation, which increases viscosity within rotational and large-tube viscometers, particularly at low shear rates. This would be a deleterious factor in large-vessel flow, especially at stenotic regions with decreased flow rates. Within the microcirculation the situation is more complex. Erythrocyte aggregation *decreases* apparent viscosity by maximizing the peripheral cell free margin at mid and low shear rates; however, at extremely low shear rates (less than 1 sec[-1]) encountered during ischemic conditions, viscosity may increase again (see Figure 7B). Enhanced aggregation shifts the curve to the right (see Figure 7C), allowing the increase in microcirculation viscosity to begin at higher shear rates (1-10 sec[-1]), resulting in an earlier and greater impediment to blood flow as shear rate declines. In conclusion, experimental and clinical evidence indicates that during periods of cerebral ischemia with extremely slow flow, plasma fibrinogen and globulins may enhance aggregation, increase viscosity, and further impede cerebral blood flow in both the micro- and macrocirculation, contributing to the pathogenesis of stroke.

Rheologic Characteristics of Cerebral Ischemia

Leukocytes

The rheologic characteristics of leukocytes are an important determinant of cerebral ischemia. Epidemiologic data strongly suggest that white blood cell counts, especially neutrophils, correlate with the risk of coronary[43] and cerebral[110] ischemia. Over a 2-year period, subjects with neutrophil counts greater than 5000/mm[3] have a relative risk of ischemic stroke 1.5 times that of patients with neutrophil counts less than 2500/mm[3]. Patients with white blood cell counts greater than 10,000/mm[3] have a relative risk of 2.5 as compared with those with counts of 4000/mm[3]. Increased white blood cell counts on admission have been demonstrated to correlate with increased mortality following stroke.[86]

The etiology of this leukocyte-associated cerebral ischemia is undoubtedly multifactorial, being secondary to both toxic chemoimmunologic mechanisms as well as pathologic rheologic mechanisms. Altered leukocyte rheology in association with human cerebral ischemia has been firmly established. Diminished whole blood filterability following stroke, initially attributed to decreased erythrocyte deformability, is in fact partly or wholly due to rheologic changes in the leukocyte population.[45,94,109,146] Decreased leukocyte filterability has been demonstrated in acute and subacute ischemic stroke[45,94] and in patients with chronic cerebrovascular disease.[146] It appears certain that white blood cells are an important determinant of decreased whole blood filterability. The rheologic mechanisms by which low-flow states create leukocyte-induced

microvasculature occlusion was detailed earlier in this review.

Whether increased leukocyte counts or increased leukocyte activation is a contributing mechanism to the development of cerebral ischemia, a marker of other concomitant disease processes, or a postischemic reactant is still undetermined. Epidemiologic evidence demonstrates that elevated white blood cell counts are present prior to the onset of stroke and are predictive for the event. Correlations between altered rheology and stroke are suspect as they occur after the event. There are some clinical studies indicating a causal role for leukocytes in the development of cerebral ischemia. A statistically significant increase in leukocyte counts was demonstrated in patients with stroke, TIAs, as well as those with high risk factors (and no history of cerebrovascular accident) as compared with controls.[32] Unfortunately, leukocyte rheology was not specifically investigated. Blood filterability, which is highly dependent on leukocyte rheology, has been shown to be decreased in patients with TIAs as compared with matched controls.[44] This complements the previously noted studies that demonstrate altered leukocyte filterability in patients with a history of stroke.[45,94,146]

Experimental work also supports a causal role, since therapies directed at reducing circulating neutrophils appear to be effective when given prior to the ischemic event in the intestinal,[69] coronary,[41,42] and cerebral[9,60] microvasculature. Neutropenia induced prior to transient ischemia improves postischemic cerebral reperfusion[9,60] and reduces infarction size significantly.[9] Neutropenia induced after the onset of ischemia is ineffective.[60] This is in keeping with the rheologic evidence for early plugging of leukocytes during the period of ischemia. Preischemic neutropenia may be attenuating or preventing the "no reflow" phenomenon. One conflicting study demonstrated increased leukocyte activation in patients with ischemic and hemorrhagic stroke as compared with healthy controls, but it failed to show this same increase in patients with TIAs, who would be expected to share the same leukocyte characteristics as patients with completed strokes.[147] In summary, epidemiologic, laboratory, and clinical evidence strongly implicates altered leukocyte rheology as a factor in the genesis of cerebral infarction; however, firm conclusions regarding the relative contribution of rheologic mechanisms, as opposed to toxic chemoimmunologic mechanisms, await prospective, randomized clinical studies.

Promises of Hemorheology

What is Going Wrong?

The reader possibly has an obvious question. If hemorheology is an important determinant of cerebral blood flow, and a large body of information concerning the rheologic properties of blood is available, and pharmaceuticals exist today that are known to profoundly change the rheologic character of plasma and blood cells, then why is there still no clearly beneficial rheologic therapy available for the treatment of cerebral ischemia? As described earlier, part of the reason may be an inappropriate application of theoretic or basic science knowledge to clinical problems; however, part of the answer may lie in the dynamics of treatment and monitoring.

Cerebral blood flow is a dynamic phenomenon and critically depends on cerebral perfusion pressure, cardiac output, and blood rheology that changes from minute to minute. Unfortunately, treatment of stroke is based on a paradigm that is static. After the acute event, medications are given according to predetermined protocols. The cerebral blood flow or neurologic/pathologic endpoints are then measured later as a means of evaluating the effect of therapy, usually at predetermined times and often at long intervals. Compare this treatment with that of patients in a cardiac critical care unit. In this setting intravenous fluids, pressors, antihypertensive, or antiarrhythmic medications may be administered and altered in a moment to moment fashion based on continuous information

gained from dynamic monitoring. Electrocardiogram monitoring, Swan-Ganz catheterization, or arteriovenous oxygen differences provide the physician with instantaneous information regarding the patient's physiologic condition. It is obvious that if various cardiac therapies were applied immediately and indiscriminately following surgery or an acute cardiac event and not closely watched for their impact on cardiovascular physiology, few patients would survive. Yet, this is precisely how acute cerebrovascular ischemia is currently managed. Hemodilution may improve cerebral blood flow and oxygen delivery following a thrombotic or embolic event, but it is doubtful that it does so in all cases or even within the same patient over time, given the large number of constantly changing rheologic, vascular, and metabolic parameters. As the cerebrovascular armamentarium increases, its use must be selective and directed.

In order for hemorheologic therapy of acute cerebral ischemia to prove beneficial, continuous and dynamic monitoring of cerebrovascular and physiologic function is required. Many of the current methods are limited by either expense, lack of portability, or the need for specialized personnel. Until practical and reliable cerebrovascular monitoring is developed, hemorheology may remain a promise unrealized.

Epilogue

The large body of experimental and clinical data demonstrating the importance of rheologic factors on cerebral blood flow in the intact and compromised circulation generates enthusiasm regarding the future of hemorheologic therapy in the prevention and treatment of cerebral ischemia. The complexity of the issue and the disappointing results of the neuroscience community's first large effort using hemodilution therapy generate a humble and cautious attitude. The lack of adequate dynamic monitoring must be corrected. The significant theoretic, basic science, and clinical knowledge regarding hemorheologic mechanisms, and the ability to capitalize on them, provide great promise that therapy for cerebral ischemia is not only possible, but may be imminent.

Editorial Comment: Hemorheology and Practical Clinical Management

The preceding chapter clearly illustrates the complexity of factors and mechanisms affecting the hemorheology of cerebral blood flow and brain ischemia. There appears to be agreement that blood viscosity is of utmost importance in the pathophysiology of brain ischemia. Yet, there is no consensus over the "optimal hematocrit level," which maximizes oxygen and substrate delivery in the ischemic brain. Factors affecting viscosity and the optimal hematocrit level may be different at various levels of the cerebral circulation and may change over time during evolving ischemia.

Clinical implications must be guarded and sweeping conclusions cannot be supported by available scientific evidence. Although Davis and Jafar make many arguments against the clinical practice of hemodilution in brain ischemia, most of their discussion is based on theoretic considerations and contradictory empiric data. Many clinical trials on hemodilution in brain ischemia have been uniformly criticized on design or execution or both. Others instituted therapy quite late after the ischemic insult, and many did not ensure therapeutic objectives were in fact accomplished. All such clinical trials to date have not distinguished subclasses of ischemic stroke (thromboembolism, hemodynamic compromise, small-vessel disease, and so forth) likely to respond differently to hemodilution therapy, nor have they stratified patients according to stroke severity or infarction size. These methodologic factors may be as much to blame for the apparent "therapeutic failure" as the theoretic factors invoked by Davis and Jafar.

Clinicians would be safe to conclude, from numerous basic and clinical lines of evidence, that an elevated hematocrit (above 0.40) is probably harmful in brain ischemia and should be avoided. To what extent the converse, i.e. hemodilution, is helpful remains controversial. Anemia is certainly not helpful either, with hematocrit below 0.33 probably impairing oxygen delivery. Avoiding either extreme is strongly recommended in the setting of acute evolving ischemia.

Hypervolemia and hypertension are clearly helpful in situations of brain ischemia secondary to hemodynamic insufficiency, as in clinical vasospasm following subarachnoid hemorrhage. These measures are most likely effective in the absence (i.e. prior to the development) of significant parenchymal infarction. These measures are likely to worsen cerebral edema across a disrupted blood-brain barrier in established brain infarction. They will certainly not reverse tissue damage in brain infarction and may be harmful by worsening focal edema and further microcirculatory compromise.

Clinicians should be aware of complex interactions affecting the hemorheology of brain ischemia. They should avoid therapeutic extremes in the management of brain ischemia. In certain clinical scenarios, hyperviscosity or anemia may accentuate ischemic damage and should be judiciously corrected. Much research is needed to clarify additional aspects of hemorheology that may affect the pathophysiology and clinical management of brain ischemia.

Issam A. Awad, MD, MS, FACS

References

1. Alonso C, Pries AR, Gaehtgens P. Time-dependent rheological behaviour of blood flow at low shear in narrow horizontal tubes. *Biorheology.* 1989;26:229-246.
2. Ames A, Wright RL, Kowade M, et al. Cerebral ischemia, II: the no-reflow phenomenon. *Am J Pathol.* 1968;52:437-447.
3. Asplund K. Randomized clinical trials of hemodilution in acute ischemic stroke. *Acta Neurol Scand.* 1989;127(suppl):22-30.
4. Bagge U, Amundson B, Lauritzen C. White blood cell deformability and plugging of skeletal muscle capillaries in hemorrhagic shock. *Acta Physiol Scand.* 1980;108:159-163.

5. Barbee JH, Cokelet GR. The Fahraeus effect. *Microvasc Res.* 1971;3:6-16.

6. Barbee JH, Cokelet GR. Prediction of blood flow in tubes with diameters as small as 29 μm. *Microvasc Res.* 1971;3:17-21.

7. Barroso-Aranda J, Schmid-Schönbein GW, Zweifach BW, et al. Granulocytes and the no-reflow phenomenon in irreversible hemorrhagic shock. *Circ Res.* 1988;63:437-447.

8. Bayliss LE. The axial drift of the red cells when blood flows in a narrow tube. *J Physiol (Lond).* 1959; 149:593-613.

9. Bednar M, Raymond S, McAuliffe T, et al. The role of neutrophils and platelets in a rabbit model of thromboembolic stroke. *Stroke.* 1991;22:44-50.

10. Begg TB, Hearns JB. Components in blood viscosity: the relative contribution of haematocrit, plasma fibrinogen and other proteins. *Clin Sci.* 1966;31:87-93.

11. Braasch D. The missing negative effect of red cell aggregation upon blood flow in small capillaries at low shear forces. *Biorheology.* 1984;1(suppl):227-230.

12. Brooks DE, Goodwin JW, Seaman GVF. Interactions among erythrocytes under shear. *J Appl Physiol.* 1970;28:172-177.

13. Brown MM, Marshall J. Effect of plasma exchange on blood viscosity and cerebral blood flow. *Br Med J.* 1982;284:1733-1736.

14. Brown MM, Marshall J. Regulation of cerebral blood flow in response to changes in blood viscosity. *Lancet.* 1985;1:604-609.

15. Brown MM, Wade JPH, Marshall J. Fundamental importance of arterial oxygen content in the regulation of cerebral blood flow in man. *Brain.* 1985;108:81-93.

16. Brückner UB, Messmer K. Blood rheology and systemic oxygen transport. *Biorheology.* 1990;27:903-912.

17. Burge PS, Johnson WS, Prankerd TAJ. Morbidity and mortality in pseudopolycythaemia. *Lancet.* 1975; 1:1266-1269.

18. Caplan L, Stein R. Basic pathology, anatomy and pathophysiology of stroke. In: *Stroke: A Clinical Approach.* Stoneham, Ma: Butterworth Publishers Inc.;1986;27-50.

19. Chen RYZ, Carlin RD, Simchon S, et al. Effects of dextran-induced hyperviscosity on regional blood flow and hemodynamics in dogs. *Am J Physiol.* 1989;256: H898-H905.

20. Chien S. Shear dependence of effective cell volume as a determinant of blood viscosity. *Science.* 1970; 168:977-978.

21. Chien S. Biophysical behavior of red cells in suspensions. In: *The Red Blood Cell.* 2nd ed. Surgenor D Mac N eds. New York, NY: Academic Press Inc. 1975;1031-1133.

22. Chien S, Jan KM Ultrastructural basis of the mechanism of rouleaux formation. *Microvasc Res.* 1973;5:155-166.

23. Chien S, Sung LA. Physiochemical basis and clinical implications of red cell aggregation. *Clin Hermorh.* 1987;7:71-91.

24. Chien S, Tvetenstrand CD, Farrell Epstein MA, et al. Model studies on distribution of blood cells at microvascular bifurcations. *Am J Physiol.* 1985;248: H568-H576.

25. Chien S, Usami S, Dellenback RJ, et al. Blood viscosity: influence of erythrocyte deformation. *Science.* 1967;157:827-829.

26. Chien S, Usami S, Dellenback RJ, et al. Blood viscosity: influence of erythrocyte aggregation. *Science.* 1967;157:829-831.

27. Chien S, Usami S, Taylor HM, et al. Effects of hematocrit and plasma proteins on human blood rheology at low shear rates. *J Appl Physiol.* 1966;21:81-87.

28. Copley AL. Rheological Problems in Biology. In: Burgess JM, et al, eds. *Proceedings of the International Congress on Rheology, Holland 1948.* Amsterdam, Netherlands, North-Holland Publishing Co; 1949;I-47-I-61, III-8-III-11.

29. Copley AL. The rheology of blood: a survey. *J Coll I Sci.* 1952;7:323-333.

30. Copley AL. Fluid mechanics and biorheology. *Thromb Res.* 1990;57:315-331.

31. Copley AL, King RG, Chien S, et al. Microscopic observations of viscoelasticity of human blood in steady and oscillatory shear. *Biorheology.* 1975; 12:257-263.

32. Coull BM, Beamer N, deGarmo P, et al. Chronic blood hyperviscosity in subjects with acute stroke, transient ischemic attack, and risk factors for stroke. *Stroke.* 1991;22:162-168.

33. Crouch JR, Hassanein RS. Platelet aggregation, stroke, and transient ischemic attack in middle-aged and elderly patients. *Neurology.* 1976;26:888-895.

34. Czer LSC, Shoemaker WC. Optimal hematocrit value in critically ill postoperative patients. *Surg Gynecol Obstet.* 1978;147:363-368.

35. Denning ADP, Watson JH. The viscosity of blood. *Proc R Soc Lond (Biol)* 1906;78:328-358.

36. Dintenfass L. Inversion of the Fahraeus-Linqvist phenomenon in blood flow through capillaries of diminishing radius. *Nature.* 1967;215:1099-1100.

37. Dormandy JA. Red cell deformability. *Eur Neurol.* 1983;22(suppl 1):23-29.

38. Dougherty H Jr, Levy DEB, Weksler B. Platelet activation in acute cerebral ischaemia: serial measurements of platelet function in cerebrovascular disease. *Lancet.* 1977; 1:821-824.

39. Dougherty JH, Levy DE, Weksler BB. Experimental cerebral ischemia produces platelet aggregates. *Neurology.* 1979;29:1460-1465.

40. Eisenberg S. Blood viscosity and fibrinogen concentration following cerebral infarction. *Circulation.* 1966;33(suppl 2):10-14.

41. Engler RL, Dahlgren MD, Morris DD, et al. Role of leukocytes in response to acute myocardial ischemia and reflow in dogs. *Am J Physiol.* 1986;251: H314-H322.

42. Engler RL, Schmid-Schönbein WG, Pavelec RS. Leukocyte capillary plugging in myocardial ischemia and reperfusion in the dog. *Am J Pathol.* 1983;111: 98-111.

43. Ernst E, Hammerschmidt DE, Bagge U, et al. Leukocytes and the risk of ischemic diseases. *JAMA.* 1987; 257:2318-2324.

44. Ernst E, Matrai A, Marshall M. Blood rheology in patients with transient ischemic attacks. *Stroke.* 1988;19:634-636.

45. Ernst E, Matrai A, Paulsen F. Leukocyte rheology in recent stroke. *Stroke.* 1987;18:59-62.

46. Fåhraeus R. The suspension stability of the blood. *Physiol Rev.* 1929;9:241-274.

47. Fåhraeus R, Lindqvist T. The viscosity of the blood in narrow capillary tubes. *Amer J Physiol.* 1931;96: 562-568.

48. Falke P, Lindgarde R, Stavenow L. Differences in blood viscosity, glycosylated hemoglobin and platelet

count between male patients with carotid territory transient ischemic attacks and minor strokes. *Clin Hemorh.* 1991;11:35-40.

49. Fein J, commentator. *Neurosurgery.* 1984;14:722-723. Comment on: Wood JH, Simeone FA, Kron RE, et al. Experimental hypervolemic hemodilution: physiological correlations of cortical blood flow, cardiac output, and intracranial pressure with fresh blood viscosity and plasma volume.

50. Fenton BM, Wilson DW, Cokelet GR. Analysis of the effects of measured white blood cell entrance times on hemodynamics in a computer model of a microvascular bed. *Pflugers Arch.* 1985;403:396-401.

51 Gaehtgens P. Flow of blood through narrow capillaries: rheological mechanisms determining capillary hematocrit and apparent viscosity. *Biorheology.* 1980;17:183-189.

52. Gaehtgens P. Distribution of flow and red cell flux in the microcirculation. *Scan J Clin Lab Invest.* 1981; 41(suppl 156):83-87.

53. Gaehtgens P, Marx P. Hemorheological aspects of the pathophysiology of cerebral ischemia. *J Cereb Blood Flow Metab.* 1987;7:259-265.

54. Gelin L-E, Ingelman B. Rheomacrodex—a new dextran solution for rheological treatment of impaired capillary flow. *Acta Chir Scand.* 1961;122:294-302.

55. Gilroy J, Barnhart MI, Meyer JS. Treatment of acute stroke with dextran 40. *JAMA.* 1969;210:293-298.

56. Goldsmith HL. The microrheology of red blood cell suspensions. *J Gen Physiol.* July 1968;52(special issue):5S-28S.

57. Goldsmith HL, Cokelet GR. Decreased resistance in the two-phase flow of blood through small tubes at low shear rates. *Biorheology.* 1986;23:279. Abstract.

58. Gottstein U. Normovolemic and hypervolemic hemodilution in cerebrovascular ischemia. *Bibl Haematol.* 1981;47:127-138.

59. Gottstein U, Sedlmeyer I, Heuss A. Behandlung der akuten zerebralen Mangeldurchblutung mit niedermolekularem Dextran [Treatment of acute cerebral ischaemia with low-molecular dextran: results of a retrospective study]. *Dtsch Med Wochenschr.* 1976; 7:223-227. English Abstract.

60. Grøgaard B, Schürer L, Gerdin B, et al. Delayed hypoperfusion after incomplete forebrain ischemia in the rat: the role of polymorphonuclear leukocytes. *J Cereb Blood Flow Metab.* 1989;9:500-505.

61. Grotta J, Ackerman R, Correia J, et al. Whole blood viscosity parameters and cerebral blood flow. *Stroke.* 1982;13:296-301.

62. Gustafsson L, Appelgren L, Myrvold HE. Effects of increased plasma viscosity and red blood cell aggregation on blood viscosity in vivo. *Am J Physiol.* 1981; 241:H513-H518.

63. Haemodilution in acute stroke: results of the Italian haemodilution trial. *Lancet.* 1988;1:318-320.

64. Ham A, Cormack D. Blood cells: leukocytes. In: *Ham's Histology.* Philadelphia Pa, J B Lippincott; 1979.

65. Harrsion MJG, Pollock S, Kendall BB, et al. Effect of haematocrit on carotid stenosis and cerebral infarction. *Lancet.* 1981;2:114-115.

66. Hellem AJ, Borchgrevink CF, Ames SB. The role of red cells in haemostasis: the relation between haematocrit, bleeding time and platelet adhesiveness. *Br J Haemat.* 1961;7:42-50.

67. The Hemodilutional in Stroke Study Group. Hypervolemic hemodilution treatment of acute stroke: results of a randomized multicenter trial using pentastarch. *Stroke.* 1989;20:317-323.

68. Henriksen L, Paulson OB, Smith RJ. Cerebral blood flow following normovolemic hemodilution in patients with high hematocrit. *Ann Neurol.* 1981;9: 454-457.

69. Hernandez LA, Grisham MB, Twohig BJ, et al. Role of neutrophils in ischemia-reperfusion-induced microvascular injury. *Am J. Physiol.* 1987;253: H699-H703.

70. Heyman A, Patterson JL, Duke TW. Cerebral circulation and metabolism in sickle cell and other chronic anemias, with observations on the effects of oxygen inhalation. *J Clin Invest.* 1952;31:824-828.

71. Hint H. The pharmacology of dextran and the physiological background for the clinical use of rheomacrodex and macrodex. *Acta Anaesthesiol Belg.* 1968; 19:119-138.

72. House SD, Lipowsky HH. Leukocyte-endothelium adhesion: microhemodynamics in mesentery of the cat. *Microvasc Res.* 1987;34:363-379.

73. Huang CR, Pan WD, Chen HQ, et al. Thixotropic properties of whole blood from healthy human subjects. *Biorheology.* 1987;24:795-801.

74. Hudak ML, Koehler RC, Rosenberg AA, et al. Effect of haematocrit on cerebral blood flow. *Am J Physiol.* 1986;251:H63-H70.

75. Humphrey PRD, duBoulay GH, Marshall JW, et al. Cerebral blood-flow and viscosity in relative polycythaemia. *Lancet.* 1979;2:873-876.

76. Humphrey PRD, duBoulay GH, Marshall JW, et al. Viscosity, cerebral blood-flow and haematocrit in patients with paraproteinaemia. *Acta Neurol Scand.* 1980;61: 201-209.

77. Kannel WB, Gordon T, Wolf PA, et al. Hemoglobin and the risk of cerebral infarction: the Framingham study. *Stroke.* 1972;3:409-420.

78. Kee DB, Wood JH. Influence of blood rheology on cerebral circulation. In: Wood JH ed. *Cerebral Blood Flow: Physiologic and Clinical Aspects.* New York, NY: McGraw-Hill;1987:173-185.

79. Kety SS. The physiology of the human cerebral circulation. *Anesthesiology.* 1949;10:610-614.

80. Kiyohara Y, Ueda K, Hasuo Y, et al. Hematocrit as a risk factor of cerebral infarction: long-term prospective population survey in a Japanese rural community. *Stroke.* 1986;17:687-692.

81. Koller M, Haenny P, Hess K, et al. Adjusted hypervolemic hemodilution in acute ischemic stroke. *Stroke.* 1990;21:1429-1434.

82. La Celle P. Alterations by leukocytes of erythrocyte flow in microchannels. *Blood Cells.* 1986;12:179-189.

83. Lacombe C, Bucherer C, Ladjouzi J, et al. Competitive role between fibrinogen and albumin on thixotropy of red cell suspensions. *Biorheology.* 1988;25:349-354.

84. Lammertsma AA, Brooks DJ, Beaney RP, et al. In vivo measurement of regional cerebral haematocrit using positron emission tomography. *J Cereb Blood Flow Metab.* 1984;4:317-322.

85. Lechner H, Ott E, Schmidt R. Present state of hemorheology. *Gerontology.* 1987;33:259-264.

86. Lowe GDD, Jaap AJ, Forbes CD. Relation of atrial fibrillation and high haematocrit to mortality in acute stroke. *Lancet.* 1983;1:784-786.

87. Machi J, Sigel B, Ramos J, et al. Role of red cells in preventing the growth of platelet aggregation. *Thromb Res.* 1984;36:53-66.

88. Mackie IJ, Jones R, Machin SJ. Platelet impedance aggregation in whole blood and its inhibition by antiplatelet drugs. *J Clin Pathol.* 1984;37:874-878.

89. Maeda N, Kon K, Imaizumi K, et al. Alteration of rheological properties of human erythrocytes by crosslinking of membrane proteins. *Biochem Biophys Acta.* 1973;735:104-112.

90. Maeda N, Seike M, Suzuki Y, et al. Effect of pH on the velocity of erythrocyte aggregation. *Biorheology.* 1988;25:25-30.

91. Matthews WB, Oxbury JM, Grainger KMR, et al. A blind controlled trial of dextran 40 in the treatment of ischaemic stroke. *Brain.* 1976;99:193-206.

92. Mayrovitz HN, Rubin R. Leukocyte distribution to arteriolar branches: dependence on microvascular blood flow. *Microvasc Res.* 1985;29:282-294.

93. Meiselman HJ, Merrill EW, Salzman EW, et al. Effect of dextran on rheology of human blood: low shear viscometry. *J Appl Physiol.* 1967;22:480-486.

94. Mercuri M, Ciuffetti G, Robinson M, et al. Blood cell rheology in acute cerebral infarction. *Stroke.* 1989; 20:959-962.

95. Merrill EW. Rheology of blood. *Physiol Rev.* 1969; 49:863-888.

96. Merrill EW, Benis AM, Gilliland ER, et al. Pressure flow relations of human blood in hollow fibers at low flow rates. *J Appl Physiol.* 1965;20:954-967.

97. Merrill EW, Gilliland ER, Cokelet G, et al. Rheology of human blood, near and at zero flow: effects of temperature and hematocrit level. *Biophys J.* 1963; 3:199-213.

98. Messmer K, Görnandt L, Jesch R, et al. Oxygen transport and tissue oxygenation during hemodilution with dextran. In: Braley DF, Bicher HI, eds. *International Symposium on Oxygen Transport to Tissue. Oxygen Transport to Tissue: Pharmacology, Mathematical Studies and Neonatology.* New York, NY: Plenum Press, 1973;37B:669-680.

99. Murata T, Secomb TW. Effects of shear rate on rouleau formation in simple shear flow. *Biorheology.* 1988;25:113-122.

100. Murata T, Secomb TW. Effects of aggregation on the flow properties of red blood cell suspensions in narrow vertical tubes. *Biorheology.* 1989;26:247-259.

101. Nelson D, Fazekas JF. Cerebral blood flow in polycythemia vera. *Arch Intern Med.* 1956;98:328-331.

102. Nobis U, Gaehtgens P. Rheology of white blood cells during blood flow through narrow tubes. *Bibl Anat.* 1981;20:211-214.

103. Ohta K. Increase in red blood cell aggregability following experimental occlusion of the middle cerebral artery in cats. *Keio J Med.* 1989;38:311-318.

104. Ott EO, Lechner H, Aranibar A. High blood viscosity syndrome in cerebral infarction. *Stroke.* 1974;5: 330-333.

105. Palmer AA, Jedrezejczyk HJ. The influence of rouleaux on the resistance of flow through capillary channels at various shear rates. *Biorheology.* 1975; 12:265-270.

106. Paulson OB, Parving HH Olesen J, et al. Influence of carbon monoxide and of hemodilution on cerebral blood flow and blood gases in man. *J Appl Physiol.* 1973;35:111-116.

107. Pearson TC, Wetherley-Mein G. Vascular occlusive episodes and venous haematocrit in primary proliferative polycythaemia. *Lancet.* 1978;2:1219-1222.

108. Pirofsky B. The determination of blood viscosity in man by a method based on Poiseuille's law. *J Clin*

Invest. 1953;32:292-298.

109. Pollock SS, Harrison MJG. Red cell deformability is not an independent risk factor in stroke. *J Neurol Neurosurg Pscychiatry.* 1982;45:369-371.

110. Prentice RL, Szatrowski TP, Kato H, et al. Leukocyte counts and cerebrovascular disease. *J Chron Dis.* 1982;35:703-714.

111. Reinke W, Gaehtgens P, Johnson PC. Blood viscosity in small tubes: effect of shear rate, aggregation, and sedimentation. *Am J Physiol.* 1987;253: H540-H547.

112. Reinke W, Johnson PC, Gaehtgens P. Effect of shear rate variation on apparent viscosity of human blood in tubes of 29 to 94 μm diameter. *Circ Res.* 1986;59: 124-132.

113. Rieger H. The role of hemorheology in the pathophysiology and treatment of arterial occlusive disease. *Int Angiol.* 1986;5:161-167.

114. Sakai F, Igarashi H, Suzuki S, et al. Cerebral blood flow and cerebral hematocrit in patients with cerebral ischemia measured by single-photon emission computed tomography. *Acta Neurol Scand.* 1989; 127(suppl):9-13.

115. Scandinavian Stroke Study Group. Multicenter trial of hemodilution in acute ischemic stroke, I: results in the total patient population. *Stroke.* 1987;18: 691-699.

116. Scandinavian Stroke Study Group. Multicenter trial of hemodilution in acute ischemic stroke, II results of subgroup analyses. *Stroke.* 1988;19:464-471.

117. Schmid-Schönbein G. Leukocyte kinetics in the microcirculation. *Biorheology.* 1987;24:139-151.

118. Schmid-Schönbein GW, Engler RL. Perspectives of leukocyte activation in the microcirculation. *Biorheology.* 1990;27:859-869.

119. Schmid-Schönbein GW, Skalak R, Sung KLP, et al. Human leukocytes in the active state. In: Bagge U, Born GVR, Gaehtgens P, eds. *White Blood Cells: Morphology, and Rheology as Related to Function. Proceedings, with Commentary of the Symposium held at London, England, October 3-4, 1981.* The Hague, Netherlands; Boston, Mass: Martinus Nijhoff Publishers; 1982.

120. Schmid-Schönbein GW, Skalak R, Usami S, et al. Cell distribution in capillary networks. *Microvasc Res.* 1980;19:18-44.

121. Schmid-Schönbein GW, Sung K-LP, Tözeren H, et al. Passive mechanical properties of human leukocytes. *Biophys J.* 1981;36:243-256.

122. Schmid-Schönbein GW, Usami S, Skalak R, et al. The interaction of leukocytes and erythrocytes in capillary and postcapillary vessels. *Microvasc Res.* 1980;19:45-70.

123. Schmid-Schönbein GW, Zweifach BW. RBC velocity profiles in arterioles and venules of the rabbit omentum. *Microvasc Res.* 1975;10:153-164.

124. Schmid-Schönbein H. Macrorheology and microrheology of blood in cerebrovascular insufficiency. *Eur Neurol.* 1983;22(suppl 1):2-22.

125. Schmid-Schönbein H. Fahraeus-effect-reversal (FER) in compaction stasis (CS): microrheological and haemodynamic consequences of intravascular sedimentation of red cell aggregates. *Biorheology.* 1988;25:355-366.

126. Schmid-Schönbein H, Born GVR, Richardson P, et al. Rheology of thrombotic processes in flow: the interaction of erythrocytes and thrombocytes subjected to high flow forces. *Biorheology.* 1981;18:

415-444.

127. Schmid-Schönbeina H, Gaehtgens P, Hirsch H. On the shear rate dependence of red cell aggregation in vitro. *J Clin Invest.* 1968;47:1447-1454.

128. Schneider R, Ringelstein EB, Zeumer H, et al. The role of plasma hyperviscosity in subcortical arteriolsclerotic encephalopathy (Binswanger's disease). *J Neurol.* 1987;234:67-73.

129. Schweinburg FB, Swiddy FG, Fine J. The Granulocytopenic response in hemorrhagic shock. *J Clin Invest.* 1959;38:673-680.

130. Spudis EV, de la Torre E, Pikula L. Management of completed strokes with dextran 40: a community hospital failure. *Stroke.* 1973;4:895-897.

131. Stadler AA, Zilow EP, Linderkamp O. Blood viscosity and optimal hematocrit in narrow tubes. *Biorheology.* 1990;27:779-788.

132. Stoltz JF, Donner M. Erythrocyte aggregation: experimental approaches and clinical implications. *Int Angiol.* 1987;6:193-201.

133. Stoltz JF, Donner M, Larcan A. Introduction to hemorheology: theoretical aspects and hyperviscosity syndromes. *Int Angiol.* 1987;6:119-132.

134. Stone HO, Thompson HK Jr, Schmidt-Nielsen K. Influence of erythrocytes on blood viscosity. *Am J Physiol.* 1968;214:913-918.

135. Strand T, Asplund K, Eriksson S, et al. A randomized controlled trial of hemodilution therapy in acute ischemic stroke. *Stroke.* 1984;15:980-989.

136. Tanahashi N, Gotoh F, Tomita M, et al. Enhanced erythrocyte aggregability in occlusive cerebrovascular disease. *Stroke.* 1989;20:1202-1207.

137. Tanahashi N, Gotoh F, Tomita M, et al. Red blood cell aggregability in occlusive cerebrovascular disease: comparison between deep subcortical infarction and cortical infarction. *Stroke.* 1990;21(suppl 1): 1-126. Abstract.

138. Thomas DJ. The influence of haematocrit on the cerebral circulation. *Acta Neurol Scand.* 1989;127 (suppl):5-8.

139. Thomas DJ, duBoulay GH, Marshall J, et al. Cerebral blood-flow in polycythemia. *Lancet.* 1977;2:161-163.

140. Thomas DJ, Marshall J, Ross Russell RW, et al. Effect of haematocrit on cerebral blood-flow in man. *Lancet.* 1977;2:941-943.

141. Tohgi H, Suzuki H, Tamura K, et al. Platelet volume, aggregation and adenosine triphosphate release in cerebral thrombosis. *Stroke.* 1991;22:17-21.

142. Tohgi H, Yamanouchi H, Murakami M, et al. Importance of the hematocrit as a risk factor in cerebral infarction. *Stroke.* 1978;9:369-374.

143. Tsuda Y, Hartmann A, Weiand J, et al. Comparison of the effects of infusion with hydroxethyl starch and low molecular weight dextran on cerebral blood flow and hemorheology in normal baboons. *J Neuro Sci.* 1987;82:171-180.

144. Tu YK, Heros RC, Karacostas D, et al. Isovolemic hemodilution in experimental focal cerebral ischemia, part 2: effects on regional cerebral blood flow and size of infarction. *J Neurosurg.* 1988;69:82-91.

145. Turitto VT, Baumgartner HR. Platelet interaction with subendothelium in a perfusion system: physical role of red blood cells. *Microvasc Res.* 1975;9:335-344.

146. Vermes I, Strik F. Altered leukocyte rheology in patients with chronic cerebrovascular disease. *Stroke.* 1988;19:631-633.

147. Violi F, Rasura M, Alessandri C, et al. Leukocyte response in patients suffering from acute stroke. *Stroke.* 1988;19:1283-1284.

148. von Kummer R, Back T, Scharf J. Impairment of autoregulatory capacity and the effect of hemodilution on cerebral blood flow and oxygen transport. *Stroke.* 1990;21(suppl 1):I126. Abstract.

149. Wade JPH. Transport of oxygen to the brain in patients with elevated haematocrit values before and after venesection. *Brain.* 1983;106:513-523.

150. Wade JPH, duBoulay GH, Marshall J, et al. Cerebral blood flow, haematocrit and viscosity in subjects with a high oxygen affinity haemoglobin variant. *Acta Neurol Scand.* 1980;61:210-215.

151. Wade JPH, Pearson TC, Ross Russell RW, et al. Cerebral blood flow and blood viscosity in patients with polycythemia secondary to hypoxic lung disease. *Br Med J.* 1981;283:689-692.

152. Wheater P, Burkitt H, Daniels V, Blood. In: Wheater PR, Burkitt HG, Daniels G, eds. *Functional Histology: A Text and Colour Atlas.* New York, NY: Churchill Livingstone Inc., 1979.

153. Wilhelmsen L, Svärdsudd K, Korsan-Bengtsen K, et al. Fibrinogen as a risk factor for stroke and myocardial infarction. *N Engl J Med.* 1984;311:501-505.

154. Wood JH, Fleischer AS. Observations during hypervolemic hemodilution of patients with acute focal cerebral ischemia. *JAMA.* 1982;248:2999-3004.

155. Wood JH, Polyzoidis KS, Epstein CM, et al. Quantitative EEG alterations after isovolemic-hemodilutional augmentation of cerebral perfusion in stroke patients. *Neurology.* 1984;34:764-768.

156. Wood JH, Simeone FA, Fink EA, et al. Correlative aspects of hypervolemic hemodilution: low molecular weight dextran infusions after experimental cerebral arterial occlusion. *Neurology.* 1984;34:24-31.

157. Wood JH, Simeone FA, Snyder LL. Cortical oxygen transport during hypervolemic hemodilutional therapy for focal cerebral ischemia. *Neurosurgery.* 1982;10:781. Abstract.

158. Wood JH, Snyder LL, Simeone FA. Failure of intravascular volume expansion without hemodilution to elevate cortical blood flow in region of experimental focal ischemia. *J Neurosurg.* 1982;56:80-91.

159. Wood JH, Kee DB. Hemorheology of the cerebral circulation in stroke. *Stroke.* 1985;16:765-772.

160. Wood JH, Kee DB Jr. Clinical rheology of stroke and hemodilution. In: Barnett HJM, Stein BM, Mohr JP, Yatsu FM, eds. *Stroke: Pathophysiology, Diagnosis and Management.* New York, NY. Churchill Livingstone Inc.; 1986:97-108.

161. Yamakawa T, Sugiyama I, Niimi H. Behaviors of white blood cells in microcirculatory of the cat brain cortex during hemorrhagic shock: intravital microscopic study. *Int J Microcirc Exp.* 1984;3:554.

CHAPTER 3

Clinical Spectrum and Natural History of Cerebrovascular Occlusive Disease

Marc I. Chimowitz MB, ChB

Cerebrovascular occlusive disease is a heterogeneous disorder. Many vascular pathologies, each with a distinct natural history, may cause ischemic stroke. Furthermore, the clinical features of ischemic stroke differ substantially depending on the underlying vascular pathology. The first section of this chapter introduces a classification system for cerebrovascular occlusive disease; the second section, which is the focus of the chapter, discusses clinical and brain-imaging features that are useful for determining the cause of ischemic stroke; the third section describes selected neurovascular syndromes; and the final section reviews natural history data of the major causes of ischemic stroke.

Classification of Cerebrovascular Occlusive Disease

Various systems have been proposed for classifying cerebrovascular occlusive disease. One system is based on the temporal course of ischemic symptoms and includes categories such as transient ischemic attack (TIA), reversible ischemic neurologic deficit, stroke in evolution, and completed stroke.[26,92] Caplan[15] has argued convincingly that this system fails to provide a useful framework for the clinician since different vascular pathologies may produce similar temporal profiles of symptoms.

A successful classification system for cerebrovascular disease should categorize patients by likely cause of symptoms.[17] This will facilitate clinical studies of patients with homogeneous vascular pathologies and will ultimately lead to development of etiologically specific treatment. The benefits of such an approach are evident when one considers the results of recent multicenter studies of patients with well-defined vascular pathologies. [31,67,77,87]

Classification systems for cerebrovascular occlusive disease have evolved as our understanding of the causes of ischemic stroke has developed. Early studies of the causes of ischemic stroke used a simple classification system — strokes were categorized as either thrombotic or embolic.[3] Further pathologic studies of patients with cerebral infarction showed that thrombosis could occur in large extracranial and intracranial arteries as well as in small arteries that penetrate the brain substance.[37,42] Fisher[37] showed that occlusion of penetrating arteries leads to small subcortical infarctions called lacunes. Using this additional pathologic category in a prospective registry of patients with stroke, Mohr et al[63] classified 40% of ischemic strokes as large-artery thrombotic, 37% as embolic, and 23% as lacunar.

The development of sophisticated technology such as computed tomography (CT), magnetic resonance imaging (MRI), echocardiography, carotid and transcranial Doppler ultrasound, and cerebral angiography has enabled detailed evaluation of patients with ischemic stroke, and it has become apparent that a large percentage of patients with ischemic stroke have normal vascular studies. This has led to the diagnostic category of *stroke of undetermined cause.*[83] Vascular imaging has also enabled in vivo differentiation of atherosclerotic large-artery occlusive disease from nonatherosclerotic large-artery diseases such as dissection, fibromuscular dysplasia, and arteritis.

Based on current knowledge, the following classification system for cerebrovascular occlusive disease is proposed. Six major subgroups, defined largely by the results of vascular and brain-imaging studies, are recognized. *Atherosclerotic large-artery disease* is defined by the presence of moderate or severe stenosis of a major extracranial or intracranial artery. The mechanisms of ischemia in patients with large-artery disease could be artery to artery embolism or low-flow distal to a high-grade stenosis or occlusion. *Nonatherosclerotic large-artery disease* is diagnosed if an arteriopathy other than atherosclerosis is recognized (e.g. dissection, moyamoya disease). *Penetrating artery disease* is diagnosed in the presence of a typical lacunar syndrome, a small subcortical infarction on CT or MRI, and the absence of another potential cause of stroke. *Cardioembolism* is diagnosed if a cardiac source of embolism is recognized (e.g. atrial fibrillation, mitral stenosis). *Stroke of undetermined cause* is diagnosed in the presence of a nonlacunar syndrome and the absence of an identifiable cause of stroke. A *miscellaneous group* is necessary to encompass unusual but identifiable causes of ischemia that cannot be categorized into one of the other diagnostic groups. Examples of these disorders include migraine stroke, a procoagulant state, sickle-cell disease, and antiphospholipid antibody syndrome.

The Stroke Data Bank of the National Institute of Neurological and Communicative Disorders and Stroke used similar definitions to those outlined here in categorizing 1,273 patients with ischemic stroke.[83] Of these 1,273 patients, 508 patients (40%) had stroke of undetermined cause, 337 patients (27%) had penetrating artery disease, 246 patients (19%) had cardioembolism, and 182 patients (14%) had large-artery disease.

Clinical Features Useful for Determing the Etiology of Ischemic Stroke

In patients with cerebral ischemia, an accurate clinical diagnosis facilitates an efficient diagnostic work-up and leads to rapid institution of therapy (e.g. anticoagulation, endarterectomy, thrombolytic therapy) that may prevent further ischemia or ameliorate the effects of ongoing ischemia. Although it is not always possible to make a specific etiologic diagnosis based on clinical and brain-imaging data, it is usually possible to narrow the etiologic differential diagnosis down to a few possible causes.

The following clinical information is useful for determining the etiology of ischemic stroke: vascular risk factor profiles; the characteristics of previous TIAs; the onset and subsequent course of the neurologic deficit; the nature of the neurologic deficit and associated features such as headache and bruits; and the size and location of infarction on CT or MRI.

Vascular Risk Factors

These factors are reviewed in detail in Chapter 5 and will be discussed only briefly in this section. Stroke in patients with advanced age is likely to be caused by atherosclerotic large-artery disease, penetrating artery disease, or cardioembolism. On the other hand, stroke in young patients is frequently of undetermined or miscellaneous causes, or the result of nonatherosclerotic large-artery disease.[1,52] Although males are at higher risk of most types of ischemic stroke, gender is usually not useful for suggesting a particular stroke mechanism in an individual patient.

Blacks have a higher prevalence of hypertension, which increases the likelihood of atherosclerotic large-artery disease and penetrating artery disease. The location of atherosclerotic large-artery disease depends on race; the extracranial internal carotid artery is typically involved in whites, whereas the middle cerebral artery stem is the usual location in blacks and Chinese.[49]

Although hypertension, diabetes, smoking, and hyperlipidemia are established risk factors for large-artery atherosclerotic cerebrovascular disease,[68] they (particularly hypertension and diabetes) are also direct risk factors for penetrating artery disease and indirect risk factors for cardioembolic stroke. For example, patients with one or more of these conditions are at increased risk of myocardial infarction, which in turn is a relatively common cause of cardioembolic stroke.

Patients with mitral stenosis, a prosthetic heart valve, or atrial fibrillation are obviously predisposed to cardioembolic stroke; however, other stroke etiologies also occur more frequently in some of these patients compared to control populations. For example, a recent study showed that the incidence of carotid stenosis greater than 50% was significantly higher in patients with nonvalvular atrial fibrillation than in an age-matched control group.[88]

Transient Ischemic Attacks (TIAs)

From a clinical standpoint, it is vitally important to determine the etiology of TIAs because early recognition of certain vascular lesions (e.g. carotid occlusive disease) offers an opportunity for stroke prevention. It is well recognized that most of the major etiologic subtypes of cerebrovascular occlusive disease may cause TIAs (as they are liberally defined by the 24-hour criterion), and that certain TIAs are commonly associated with a particular etiology, e.g. transient monocular blindness and carotid disease; however, it is still debated whether certain clinical features of TIAs (i.e. the duration of each attack, the

period that the patient has been experiencing attacks, and the frequency of attacks) are useful for predicting their cause.

Fisher,[34] who was the first to recognize the relationship of transient monocular blindness to carotid disease, coined the term TIA. He has studied in detail the clinical features of TIAs in patients with large-artery disease, cardioembolism, and penetrating artery disease. In a study of 135 patients with TIA, Fisher[39] found that transient monocular blindness associated with carotid stenosis resolved in less than 10 minutes in 90% of cases (75% resolved within 1.5-5 minutes), whereas transient monocular blindness in the absence of carotid disease resolved in less than 10 minutes in 62.5% of cases. In the posterior circulation, 70% of TIAs caused by basilar stenosis resolved within 10 minutes. TIAs associated with large-artery stenosis in the anterior or posterior circulation rarely lasted 1 hour. Contrary to this, Fisher suggests that TIAs due to embolism usually last hours, but rarely may last only a few minutes.[39]

The frequency and timing of TIAs, according to Fisher, are also useful for differentiating large-artery occlusive disease from other etiologies. He found that two or more TIAs of the same type predicted tight stenosis of a large cerebral artery as the underlying cause. In 100 patients with TIAs preceding stroke caused by carotid or basilar stenosis, 94% of patients with carotid disease and 88% of patients with basilar disease had two or more TIAs of the same type. The time from first TIA to second TIA in patients with large-artery occlusive disease was within 7 days in 88.5% of cases. Two or more attacks on 1 day signaled that occlusion was imminent. Analysis of 32 other patients with a single TIA revealed that severe arterial stenosis was not present in any of the cases (suggesting a possible cardioembolic mechanism); however, angiography was performed in only 8 patients.[39]

Fisher recognized that penetrating artery disease may on occasion cause TIAs preceding stroke.[41] The attacks almost always occur within 1 week of stroke, as opposed to large-artery disease, which can cause TIAs for weeks or months. The neurologic deficit during a TIA caused by penetrating artery disease is usually one of the classic lacunar patterns, e.g. pure motor hemiparesis, pure hemisensory deficit. A relatively uncommon but specific feature of TIAs associated with penetrating artery disease is a flurry of attacks of pure motor hemiparesis within a 24-hour period.[30]

Studies that have prospectively tested Fisher's criteria for predicting the etiology of TIAs have produced conflicting results. Those supporting Fisher's findings include the following: Pessin et al[72] performed carotid angiography on 95 patients with carotid territory TIAs and found severe carotid stenosis or occlusion in 52%. TIAs lasting more than 1 hour were not associated with notable stenosis of the ipsilateral carotid artery. Harrison et al[50] also found that TIAs lasting more than 1 hour were associated with a widely patent carotid artery. In 81 patients presenting with pure motor, sensorimotor, or pure sensory stroke, Chimowitz et al[24] found that multiple TIAs occurring within only 1 week of stroke were significantly associated with penetrating artery disease compared to other etiologies.

On the other hand, the results of some studies disagree with Fisher's findings. Tsuda[89] found that attacks lasting less than 30 minutes correlated with mild carotid stenosis and longer attacks with carotid occlusion. Bogousslavsky et al[11] studied 205 patients with carotid territory transient ischemic attacks who underwent full angiographic and cardiac investigations and found that short TIAs (less than 15 minutes) and multiple TIAs tended to be more frequent in patients with carotid lesions than in patients with a cardioembolic source, but this difference did not reach statistical significance. In a recent study of patients with "crescendo" TIAs of the anterior circulation, Rothrock et al[81] found that 11 of 23 (48%) patients with a positive carotid angiogram had at least one TIA lasting 15 minutes or longer compared to 6 of 19 (32%) patients with negative carotid angiograms. Five patients with carotid disease (stenosis without thrombus 1, stenosis with intraluminal thrombus 1, deep ulcer without stenosis 3) had attacks lasting 1 hour or longer.

It is difficult to reconcile the conflicting results of these studies. Possible explanations include the variability of the TIA cases chosen for observation, lack of complete vascular evaluations (ultrasound, angiography, echocardiography) in all patients, and failure to use a consistent classification system for defining etiologic subtypes of TIA. For example, some studies considered carotid disease as a potential cause of TIAs only if high-grade stenosis was present, whereas others considered presumed embolism from ulcerative disease without stenosis of the carotid artery as a potential cause of TIA.

The latter point brings up another controversial aspect of TIAs — their pathophysiology. It is widely believed that artery to artery microembolism is the most common cause of TIAs in patients with large-artery occlusive disease; however, Fisher has argued that repetitive, brief, stereotypical TIAs are caused by low-flow distal to high-grade arterial occlusive disease.[39] He bases his argument on the following points: (1) in a pathologic study of carotid endarterectomy plaques, Fisher and Ojemann[44] found that 98% of patients with hemispheric TIAs had a residual luminal diameter of less than 1 mm, whereas only 15% of asymptomatic patients had a residual lumen less than 1 mm. The frequency of ulcers was almost identical in both groups[39,44]; (2) symptoms in patients with hemispheric TIAs produced by embolic mechanisms (e.g. atrial fibrillation, prosthetic heart valves) frequently include hemianopia, paresis of a leg, jargon aphasia, and other cognitive abnormalities, whereas carotid hemispheric TIAs typically involve numbness or weakness of the hand only; (3) carotid stenosis after endarterectomy causes identical TIAs to those preceding endarterectomy despite the fact that the morphology of the stenosis is typically different; (4) according to the embolic theory, stereotypical TIAs are produced by recurrent emboli to the same arterial segment. Fisher believes that it is highly unlikely that consecutive artery to artery emboli would be of similar size and shape and that all these embolic fragments would travel to the same arterial segment.[39] Whisnant[91] has shown that multiple stainless steel bearings approximately 8 mm in diameter injected into one common carotid artery of dogs can embolize to a single MCA branch; however, this embolic model may have little in common with spontaneous emboli from atherosclerotic carotid occlusive disease.

Although there is disagreement on the pathophysiology and clinical features of TIAs, there is a growing consensus that patients with TIAs should be evaluated in the same way as patients presenting with stroke. Indeed the distinction between TIA and stroke, as defined by the 24-hour criterion, is arbitrary. Several recent studies have shown that many patients with TIAs defined by the 24-hour criterion have focal lesions on brain-imaging studies that could account for the neurologic deficits observed during the TIAs.[5,12] Although the pathologies of these lesions are not known, it is likely that some are infarctions.

Temporal Profile of the Neurologic Deficit

In patients with ischemic stroke, the onset and subsequent course of the neurologic deficit are useful for predicting the cause of stroke. Strokes caused by large-artery occlusive disease and penetrating artery disease frequently are present on awaking, whereas cardioembolism typically occurs during daily activities. The hallmark of an embolic mechanism (cardiac or artery to artery) is maximal neurologic deficit at onset. In the Michael Reese and Harvard Stroke Registries,[18,63] 79% to 89% of patients with cardioembolism had a maximal deficit at onset, whereas 38% to 45% of patients with large-artery disease or penetrating artery disease had a maximal deficit at onset (it is probable that artery-to-artery embolism was the underlying mechanism in many of these strokes). Other temporal profiles that are common with large- or small-artery occlusive disease, and rarely associated with embolism, are a stuttering or stepwise course, a smoothly progressive course, or a fluctuant course.

Nature of the Neurologic Deficit

The findings on neurologic examination are important not only for stroke localization but also for making inferences about the cause of stroke. Some neurologic signs enable exclusion of certain causes of stroke from the differential diagnosis (for example, aphasia or hemianopia essentially excludes penetrating artery disease), whereas other signs increase the likelihood of a specific cause of stroke. Examples of neurologic syndromes that favor specific ischemic stroke etiologies are Wernicke's aphasia, alexia without agraphia, and top of the basilar syndromes that favor an embolic mechanism;[14,63] lateral medullary syndrome, which is invariably caused by occlusive disease of the vertebral artery[43]; and pure motor hemiparesis or pure sensory stroke, which are usually caused by penetrating artery disease.[35,41]

Few of these syndromes are 100% specific for individual stroke etiologies. Wernicke's aphasia is sometimes caused by a hemorrhage into the temporal lobe;[63] lateral medullary syndrome is occasionally caused by an embolus; and pure motor hemiparesis has been associated with cardioembolism, carotid artery to lenticulostriate artery embolism, and nonischemic causes.[46,60] In formulating his lacunar hypothesis that pure motor hemiparesis and pure sensory stroke are usually caused by lipohyalinosis (a hypertensive vasculopathy involving penetrating arteries to the brain), Fisher recognized that embolism to a penetrating artery and atherosclerosis at the orifice of a penetrating artery are also potential causes of these clinical syndromes.[35,41] He argued that carotid and vertebrobasilar occlusive disease are rarely, if ever, causes of these syndromes. Fisher's hypothesis has been widely challenged[57,60]; however, few studies have tested the hypothesis by prospectively evaluating the cause of stroke in consecutive patients presenting with pure motor or sensory syndromes.

Recently Chimowitz et al[24] prospectively studied the etiology of stroke in 81 consecutive patients presenting with pure motor, sensorimotor, and pure sensory syndromes. Regardless of the clinical and brain-imaging features, most patients had an extensive diagnostic evaluation, including echocardiography and either cerebral angiography or carotid and transcranial Doppler ultrasound. Penetrating disease was diagnosed if these vascular studies did not reveal another potential cause. Although pure motor hemiparesis (similar involvement of face, arm, and leg) and pure sensory stroke were significantly associated (p < .05) with penetrating artery disease, the positive predictive value of pure motor hemiparesis for penetrating artery disease was only 52% (95% confidence interval: 30% to 74%). Pure motor hemiparesis associated with a subcortical infarction not more than 1.5 cm or negative results on two brain-imaging studies, however, yielded a positive predictive value of 100% (95% confidence interval: 69% to 100%) for penetrating artery disease (i.e. carotid occlusive disease, vertebrobasilar disease, or a cardioembolic source were not found in patients with this combination of features). The positive predictive value of pure sensory stroke involving at least two regions of the body for penetrating artery disease was 95% (95% confidence interval: 66% to 99%).

Associated Features: Bruits and Headaches

The presence of a carotid bruit usually implies that carotid occlusive disease is present; however, it does not necessarily imply that carotid disease is the cause of the patient's symptoms. For example, in a patient with hypertension, pure motor hemiparesis, and a small infarction in the internal capsule, the presence of a carotid bruit ipsilateral to the capsular lesion may signify the coexistence of penetrating artery disease and asymptomatic carotid stenosis. Indeed hypertension is the most important risk factor for both penetrating artery disease and carotid stenosis. Several studies have shown that patients with a lacunar infarction frequently have coexistent carotid stenosis; however, the carotid stenosis occurs as frequently contralateral to the lacunar infarction as it does ipsilateral to the infarction.[54,69]

On the other hand, in a patient who has been experiencing recurrent episodes of right hand weakness and numbness, the presence of a carotid bruit on the left greatly increases the likelihood that the symptoms are caused by carotid occlusive disease. In a study of 205 patients experiencing TIAs, 83 patients had ipsilateral carotid lesions and 50 had cardiac lesions. A carotid bruit ipsilateral to the ischemic region was present in 39.8% of patients with carotid lesions and in only 6% of patients with cardiac lesions (p < .001).[10] The absence of a carotid bruit in a patient experiencing typical carotid territory TIAs should not argue against a diagnosis of carotid occlusive disease since low flow through a tight stenosis may not produce a bruit. Furthermore, the carotid may be occluded. In the latter case, a contralateral orbital bruit may be heard because of increased flow through the contralateral internal carotid artery.[76]

Headache is a relatively common accompaniment of stroke caused by atherosclerotic large-artery occlusive disease, nonatherosclerotic large-artery disease (e.g. dissection), and cardioembolism. In the Michael Reese Stroke Registry, 17% of patients with cardioembolic stroke and 27% of patients with large-artery thrombotic stroke had associated headache.[18,19] On the other hand, headache is associated with stroke caused by penetrating artery disease in only 3% to 16% of patients.[19,63]

It may seem axiomatic, therefore, that the presence of headache in a patient with pure motor hemiparesis or pure sensory stroke favors a cause other than penetrating artery disease; however, in one study of 81 patients presenting with pure motor or sensory syndromes, 9% of patients with penetrating artery disease had an unusual headache less than 24 hours before or within 24 hours after stroke onset, compared to 18% of patients with other causes of stroke — a nonsignificant difference.[24] The relatively low frequency of headache in patients with large-artery disease and cardioembolism in this study is likely due to patient selection. Patients with pure motor or pure sensory syndromes have smaller infarctions than patients with other signs commonly associated with infarction caused by large-artery disease or cardioembolism, e.g. aphasia and hemianopia.

Infarction size is an important factor in the pathophysiology of headache associated with cerebrovascular occlusive disease since edematous ischemic brain causes stretching and compression of pain-sensitive structures such as blood vessels and meninges. Other mechanisms of headache associated with cerebrovascular occlusive disease include the development of collateral circulation and acute distention of an artery by an embolus.[38]

Fisher has described the characteristics of headache associated with occlusive disease of the major cerebral arteries.[38] In some instances the features of a headache may be useful for localizing the vascular pathology to a specific artery. Headache is a necessary condition for the diagnosis of migraine stroke. In this setting it is obligatory for the headache to have the same features as previous migraines.[90]

Features of Infarction on CT or MRI

Several features of an infarction visualized on CT or MRI are useful for making inferences about the etiology of stroke. These include the size, shape, and location of the infarction.[71,79] In addition, the number of infarctions is important.

A subcortical lesion of at least 2 cm rules out penetrating artery disease as a possible cause, whereas a subcortical lesion 1.5 cm or less is highly predictive of penetrating artery

disease.[24] Infarctions caused by penetrating artery disease tend to be round or oval shaped, whereas infarctions caused by large artery disease or cardioembolism tend to have more irregular shapes and margins.[24] In a CT study of 60 consecutive patients with a hemispheral infarction caused by cardioembolism, Ringelstein et al[79] found that 55 patients (92%) had pial artery territory infarctions that usually involved the cerebral cortex and were wedge shaped, and 5 patients (8%) had infarctions resembling lacunes. Four of these lesions could be differentiated from typical lacunar infarctions caused by penetrating artery disease because two were wedge shaped and two others were combined with a pial territory infarction.

Embolism is associated with hemorrhagic infarction on CT in up to 43% of cases,[70] which is substantially higher than the rates of hemorrhagic infarction associated with other causes of ischemic stroke. The probable explanation for the high rate of hemorrhagic infarction associated with embolism is that reperfusion following spontaneous lysis of the embolus leads to bleeding from vessels injured by the preceding ischemia.

Comma-shaped lesions, 2-5 cm in size, involving the internal capsule and caudate, putamen or globus pallidus are called *striato-capsular infarctions*[78] (Figure 1). These lesions have also been termed giant lacunes, an incorrect term since it suggests that the penetrating arteries are directly involved in the pathologic process. In fact striatocapsular infarctions are usually caused by occlusive disease of, or embolism to, the middle cerebral artery proximal to or at the origins of the lateral lenticulostriate arteries.[2,24]

Wedge-shaped cortical infarctions (Figure 2), particularly in the distribution of the middle cerebral artery, are usually caused by an embolic mechanism (either cardioembolism or artery to artery embolism), whereas irregular, patchy infarctions in the border zones between the middle cerebral artery and the anterior cerebral artery or posterior cerebral artery are typically caused by low flow from carotid occlusive disease or global

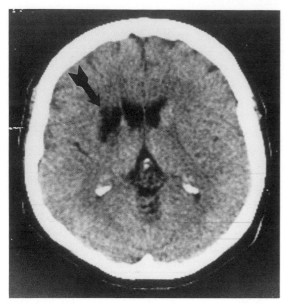

Figure 1. A 57-year-old woman who presented with left hemiparesis. CT shows a 2.5-cm subcortical infarction involving the right caudate nucleus and anterior limb of the internal capsule (striato-capsular infarction). The presumed cause of infarction was atrial fibrillation.

Figure 2. A 68-year-old man with more than 80% stenosis of the right internal carotid artery who presented with sudden onset of agitation and left homonyumous hemianopia. CT shows a wedge-shaped cortical infarction of the right middle cerebral artery. The presumed cause of the infarction was carotid artery to middle cerebral artery embolism.

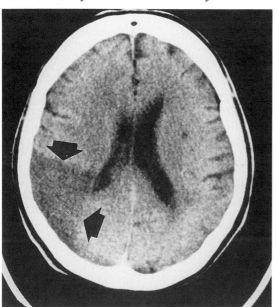

hypoperfusion[93] (Figure 3).

Multiple cortical infarctions in different vascular territories are most suggestive of cardioembolism; however, rarer causes are diffuse atherosclerosis, coagulopathy, or vasculitis.

Selected Neurovascular Syndromes

The typical features of stroke caused by carotid occlusive disease (atherosclerotic and other types), vertebrobasilar disease, penetrating artery disease, and cardioembolism have been described in detail by other investigators.[19,34,35,41,45,61] In this section, less familiar presentations of carotid occlusive disease and penetrating artery disease are discussed briefly, and stroke of undetermined cause is reviewed.

Figure 3. A 62-year-old man with more than 95% stenosis of the left internal carotid artery and total occlusion of the right internal carotid artery who presented with spells of fluctuating left hemiparesis, involving the leg more than the arm. The CT shows two areas of parenchymal infarction, both with indiscreet borders and involving the watershed territory at the border zone of the middle cerebral and the anterior and posterior cerebral arteries. These infarctions are presumed to be due to hemodynamic factors and hypoperfusion.

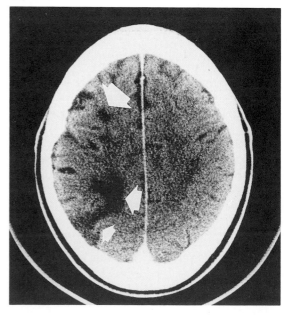

Carotid Occlusive Disease

Fifty to 75% of patients who suffer a stroke from carotid occlusive disease have a history of TIA.[63,74,82] Typical TIAs associated with carotid disease are transient monocular blindness, which is usually described as a blurring, dimming, or darkening of vision, and clumsiness or weakness of the hand. Occasionally patients complain of unilateral visual loss in bright light[48] or arm-shaking spells resembling focal seizures.[94] These TIAs have hemodynamic mechanisms and correlate with high-grade carotid occlusive disease.

The neurologic signs commonly associated with hemispheric stroke caused by carotid occlusive disease are aphasia (or anosognosia and neglect if the nondominant hemisphere is involved), contralateral hemianopia, hemiparesis involving the arm predominantly, and hemisensory loss. These signs correlate with injury to the territory of the brain supplied by the middle cerebral artery, which takes the brunt of the ischemic insult in patients with carotid disease.

Infrequently the contralateral leg may be involved selectively, presumably as a result of an embolus from the internal carotid artery to the anterior cerebral artery.[95] Rarely carotid disease may cause ipsilateral leg weakness if the contralateral anterior cerebral artery is supplied by the ipsilateral carotid artery.[25] Another unusual presentation of carotid disease is ipsilateral occipital infarction. The necessary vascular anatomy for this presentation is a persistent fetal origin of the posterior cerebral artery from the carotid artery instead of the basilar artery.[75]

Penetrating Artery Disease {Lacunes}

Fisher has described four common acute neurologic syndromes that are most frequently caused by penetrating artery disease. These are pure sensory stroke,[35] pure motor hemiparesis,[41] dysarthria (clumsy hand) syndrome,[36] and ataxic hemiparesis.[40] Some authors suggest that the latter three syndromes are variants of each other;[56] however, Fisher maintains that the clinical phenomenology and

usual lesion location associated with each are unique.

Penetrating artery disease may also cause a chronic neurologic syndrome characterized clinically by a history of hypertension, slowly progressive dementia, pseudobulbar palsy, gait difficulties, and urinary incontinence. The pathologic findings, first described by Binswanger, include diffuse areas of periventricular demyelination, numerous white matter and basal ganglia infarctions, dilated ventricles, and marked arteriosclerosis in the penetrating medullary arteries that irrigate the deep white matter.[80]

The development of MRI has rekindled interest in "Binswanger's disease" because periventricular hyperintense lesions are commonly identified on MRI in patients with advanced age, hypertension, and dementia.[6,22] Pathologic studies have shown that these MRI lesions correlate with gliosis, white matter pallor, dilated perivascular spaces, arteriosclerosis, and occasionally infarction.[4] Preliminary blood flow data suggest significantly lower white matter blood flow in patients with these MRI lesions compared to patients without these lesions.[32]

Despite accumulating evidence that ischemia may cause a subgroup of periventricular lesions on MRI, it does not follow that all patients with these lesions have Binswanger's disease, as has been suggested.[80] These lesions are also seen in normal persons and in patients with a variety of other diseases including multiple sclerosis, the leukodystrophies, human immunodeficiency virus infection, progressive multifocal leukoencephalopathy, and toluene exposure.

Stroke of Undetermined Cause

The cause of stroke cannot be established in a high percentage of patients despite every effort to uncover the diagnosis. Clues to the potential causes of infarction in patients currently classified as having stroke of undetermined cause may be found by analyzing the clinical, brain-imaging, and angiographic features of these patients.

A few studies have shown that patients with stroke of undetermined cause commonly have a history of stroke that often involves a different vascular territory; hemispheral syndromes; superficial infarctions on CT or MRI; and distal intracranial occlusions on angiography with normal arteries proximally.[23,83] Based on these observations, Mohr[62] has hypothesized that many strokes of undetermined cause are from cardiac embolism, the source of which evades detection by routine echocardiography. The development of transesophageal echocardiography, which is substantially more sensitive than transthoracic echocardiography for detecting potential embolic sources, may enable Mohr's hypothesis to be tested.

It remains likely, however, that cardioembolism accounts for a minority of these infarctions. The challenge to investigators is to identify new causes of stroke in patients who are currently diagnosed as having stroke of undetermined cause. Some success has already been achieved in this area.[58,85]

Natural History of Cerebrovascular Disease

Atherosclerotic Large-Artery Disease

The risk of stroke from extracranial carotid disease depends largely on the severity of stenosis and whether the lesion is symptomatic. Studies of asymptomatic patients with moderate carotid stenosis (i.e. more than 50%) suggest an ipsilateral stroke risk ranging from less than 1% to 2% per year.[21,27,53] Asymptomatic patients with high-grade carotid stenosis (more than 75%) have an annual stroke risk of 1.7% to 5.5%;[7,21] however, the higher percentage includes strokes that were not ipsilateral to the diseased carotid artery.

Until recently there were limited data on the natural history of symptomatic carotid stenosis because most of these patients undergo carotid endarterectomy. The Joint Study[33] reported that the annual stroke risk was 6% for the first 3 years and 2% thereafter. In a prospective study, Bogousslavsky and colleagues[8] reported 45 patients with symptomatic carotid stenosis of at least 75% who did not undergo endarterectomy because of coexisting systemic illness. The annual stroke rate was 10% the first year and 2.4% thereafter. Recent data from a large randomized multicenter study[67] comparing aspirin therapy to carotid endarterectomy in patients with symptomatic carotid artery stenosis indicate that the stroke rate in patients with greater than 70% stenosis treated with aspirin is substantially higher than the rates suggested by previous natural history studies: Over 24% of patients treated with aspirin had an ipsilateral stroke within 18 months of randomization, whereas 7% of patients undergoing endarterectomy had an ipsilateral stroke in the same period.

Although it has been suggested that carotid occlusion is associated with a benign outcome,[13] a few studies have shown annual stroke rates of 2% to 5% per year.[28,47] Ulcerative disease without stenosis of the extracranial carotid artery appears to be associated with a low risk (less than 1% per year) of ipsilateral stroke.[55] One study by Moore et al[64] suggested that patients with large or compound ulcers have a very high stroke rate of 12.5% per year; however, the retrospective nature of the study and the lack of data regarding the possible progression of ulcerative disease to stenosis before the onset of stroke make these data difficult to interpret.

Patients with atherosclerosis of the intracranial internal carotid artery are at high risk of stroke, particularly if coexistent extracranial artery stenosis is present. Marzewski et al[59] studied 66 patients with angiographically documented intracranial carotid artery occlusive disease. Eight patients (12%) had an ipsilateral stroke during an average of 3.9 years of follow-up. Craig et al[29] found that 11 of 58 patients (19%) had an ipsilateral stroke during an average of 30 months of follow-up.

The natural history of extracranial unilateral vertebral artery disease appears to be benign. Moufarrij et al[65] reviewed the prognosis of 96 patients with asymptomatic unilateral vertebral artery stenosis of at least 50%. Only 2 patients (2%) had brain stem strokes during an average follow-up of 4.6 years, and both patients had coexistent basilar stenosis. Although a benign outcome has also been documented in patients with distal vertebral or basilar stenosis,[9,73] some series suggest that these lesions are associated with a poor prognosis.[16,66] In one study of 44 patients with at least 50% stenosis of a distal vertebral artery or basilar artery, Moufarrij et al[66] found that 5 patients (11%) had a subsequent brain stem stroke during an average follow-up period of 6.1 years.

This discussion has focused on the risk of stroke in patients with atherosclerotic large-artery cerebrovascular disease; however, it is important to note that coronary artery disease is the major cause of death in virtually all studies of patients with cerebrovascular occlusive disease. The extent to which cerebrovascular disease is a marker for coronary artery disease is illustrated by the fact that the incidence of myocardial infarction in the first year following a TIA is similar to the annual incidence of myocardial infarction in patients with stable angina.[86]

Natural History of Cardioembolism, Penetrating Artery Disease, and Stroke of Undetermined Cause

The most common causes of cardioembolism in the United States are nonrheumatic atrial fibrillation (45% of all embolic stroke) and acute myocardial infarction (15%). The presence of nonrheumatic atrial fibrillation increases the risk of stroke five-fold and is associated with an estimated stroke risk of 5% per year. About 3% of patients suffer a stroke within 1 month of acute myocardial infarction.[51] Once a cardioembolic stroke has occurred, the risk of recurrent stroke has been estimated at 1% per day for the first 2

weeks after the initial stroke and is substantially lower thereafter.[20] Up to 20% of atrial fibrillation patients who suffer an initial stroke will have a recurrent stroke within 1 year.[51]

The long-term risk of recurrent stroke in patients with penetrating artery disease and stroke of undetermined cause has not been studied adequately. In the Stroke Data Bank, the risk of recurrent stroke within 30 days of the index stroke was 3.0% for stroke of undetermined cause, and 2.2% for penetrating artery disease.[84]

References

1. Adams HP Jr, Butler MJ, Biller J, et al. Nonhemorrhagic cerebral infarction in young adults. *Arch Neurol.* 1986;43:793-796.
2. Adams HP Jr, Damasio HC, Putman SF, et al. Middle cerebral artery occlusions as a cause of isolated subcortical infarction. *Stroke.* 1983;14:948-952.
3. Aring CD, Merrit HH. Differential diagnosis between cerebral hemorrhage and cerebral thrombosis. *Arch Intern Med.* 1935;56:435-456.
4. Awad IA, Johnson PC, Spetzler RF, et al. Incidental subcortical lesions identified on magnetic resonance imaging in the elderly: II: postmortem pathological correlation. *Stroke.* 1986;17:1090-1097.
5. Awad IA, Modic M, Little JR, et al. Focal parenchymal lesions in transient ischemic attacks: correlation of computed tomography and magnetic resonance imaging. *Stroke.* 1986;17:399-402.
6. Awad IA, Spetzler RF, Hodak JA, et al. Incidental subcortical lesions identified on magnetic resonance imaging in the elderly; 1: correlation with age and cerebrovascular risk factors. *Stroke.* 1986;17:1084-1089.
7. Bogousslavsky J, Despland PA, Regli F. Asymptomatic tight stenosis of the internal carotid artery: long-term prognosis. *Neurology.* 1986;36:861-863.
8. Bogousslavsky J, Despland PA, Regli F. Prognosis of high risk patients with nonoperated symptomatic extracranial carotid tight stenosis. *Stroke.* 1988;19:108-111.
9. Bogousslavsky J, Gates PC, Fox AJ, et al. Bilateral occlusion of vertebral artery: clinical patterns and long-term prognosis. *Neurology.* 1986;36:1309-1315.
10. Bogousslavsky J, Hachinski VC, Boughner DR, et al. Cardiac and arterial lesions in carotid transient ischemic attacks. *Arch Neurol.* 1986;43:223-228.
11. Bogousslavsky J, Hachinski VC, Boughner DR, et al. Clinical predictors of cardiac and arterial lesions in carotid transient ischemic attacks. *Arch Neurol.* 1986;43:229-233.
12. Bogousslavsky J, Regli F. Cerebral infarct in apparent transient ischemic attack. *Neurology.* 1985;35:1501-1503.
13. Bornstein NM, Norris JW. Benign outcome of carotid occlusion. *Neurology.* 1989;39:6-8.

14. Caplan LR. "Top of the basilar" syndrome. *Neurology*. 1980;30:72-79.

15. Caplan LR. Are terms such as completed stroke or RIND of continued usefulness? *Stroke*. 1983; 14:431-433.

16. Caplan LR. Bilateral distal vertebral artery occlusion. *Neurology*. 1983;33:552-558.

17. Caplan LR. TIAs: we need to return to the question, What is wrong with Mr. Jones? *Neurology*. 1988; 38:791-793.

18. Caplan LR, Hier DB, D'Cruz I. Cerebral embolism in the Michael Reese Stroke Registry. *Stroke*. 1983;14:530-536.

19. Caplan LR, Stein RW. *Stroke: A Clinical Approach*. Stoneham, Mass. Butterworths; 1986.

20. Cerebral Embolism Study Group. Immediate anticoagulation of embolic stroke: a randomized trial. *Stroke*. 1983;14:668-676.

21. Chambers BR, Norris JW. Outcome in patients with asymptomatic neck bruits. *N Engl J Med*. 1986; 315:860-865.

22. Chimowitz MI, Awad IA, Furlan AJ. Periventricular lesions on MRI: facts and theories. *Stroke*. 1989; 20:963-967.

23. Chimowitz MI, Furlan AJ, Nayak S, et al. Mechanism of stroke in patients taking aspirin. *Neurology*. 1990;40:1682-1685.

24. Chimowitz MI, Furlan AJ, Sila CA, et al. Etiology of motor or sensory stroke: a prospective study of the predictive value of clinical and radiologic features. *Ann Neurol*. 1991;30:519-525.

25. Chimowitz MI, Lafranchise EF, Furlan AJ, et al. Ipsilateral leg weakness associated with carotid stenosis. *Stroke*. 1990;21:1362-1364.

26. A classification and outline of cerebrovascular disease II. A report of an ad hoc committee established by the Advisory Council for the National Institute of Neurological and Communicative Diseases and Stroke, National Institutes of Health, Besthesda, MD 20014. *Stroke*. 1975;6:564-616.

27. Colgan MP, Kingston W, Shanik DG. Asymptomatic carotid stenosis: is prophylactic carotid endarterectomy justifiable? *Br J Surg*. 1985;72:313-314.

28. Cote R, Barnett HJM, Taylor DW. Internal carotid occlusion: a prospective study. *Stroke*. 1983;14: 898-902.

29. Craig DR, Meguro K, Watridge G, et al. Intracranial internal carotid artery stenosis. *Stroke*. 1982;13: 825-828.

30. Donnan GA, Bladin PF. Capsular warning syndrome: repetitive hemiplegia preceding capsular stroke. *Stroke*. 1987;18:296.

31. The EC-IC Bypass Study Group. Failure of extracranial-intracranial arterial bypass to reduce the risk of ischemic stroke. *N Engl J Med*. 1985;313: 1191-1200.

32. Fazekas F, Niederkorn K, Schmidt R, et al. White matter signal abnormalities in normal individuals: correlation with carotid ultrasonography, cerebral blood flow measurements, and cerebrovascular risk factors. *Stroke*. 1988;19:1285-1288.

33. Fields WS, Lemak NA. Joint study of extracranial arterial occlusion, IX: transient ischemic attacks in the carotid territory. *JAMA*. 1976;235:2608-2610.

34. Fisher CM. Occlusion of the internal carotid artery. *Arch Neurol Psychiatry*. 1951;65:346-377.

35. Fisher CM. Pure sensory stroke involving face, arm, and leg. *Neurology*. 1965;15:76-80.

36. Fisher CM. A lacunar stroke: the dysarthria-clumsy hand syndrome. *Neurology*. 1967;17:614-617.

37. Fisher CM. The arterial lesions underlying lacunes. *Acta Neuropathol*. 1969;12:1-15.

38. Fisher CM. Headache in cerebrovascular disease. In: Vinken PJ, Bruyn GW, eds. *Handbook of Clinical Neurology*. Amsterdam, Netherlands; North Holland Publishing Company; 1972;5:124-156.

39. Fisher CM. Concerning transient ischemic attacks. *Cleve Clin J Med*. 1987;54:3-11.

40. Fisher CM, Cole M. Homolateral ataxia and crural paresis. a vascular syndrome. *J Neurol Neurosurg Psychiatry*. 1965;28:48-55.

41. Fisher CM, Curry HB. Pure motor hemiplegia of vascular origin. *Arch Neurol*. 1965;13:30-44.

42. Fisher CM, Gore I, Okabe N, et al. Atherosclerosis of the carotid and vertebral arteries—extracranial and intracranial. *J Neuropathol Exp Neurol*. 1965; 24:455-476.

43. Fisher CM, Karnes WE, Kubik CS. Lateral medullary infarction—the pattern of vascular occlusion. *J Neuropathol Exp Neurol*. 1961;20:323-379.

44. Fisher CM, Ojemann RG. A clinico-pathologic study of carotid endarterectomy plaques. *Rev Neurol (Paris)*. 1986;142:573-589.

45. Fisher CM, Ojemann RG, Roberson GH. Spontaneous dissection of cervico-cerebral arteries. *Can J Neurol Sci*. 1978;5:9-19.

46. Fisher M, Recht LD. Brain tumor presenting as an acute pure motor hemiparesis. *Stroke*. 1989;20: 288-291.

47. Furlan AJ, Whisnant JP, Baker HL. Long-term prognosis after carotid occlusion. *Neurology*. 1980;30:986-988.

48. Furlan AJ, Whisnant JP, Kearns T. Unilateral visual loss in bright light. *Arch Neurol*. 1979;36:675-676.

49. Gorelick PB, Caplan LR, Hier DB, et al. Racial differences in the distribution of anterior circulation occlusive disease. *Neurology*. 1984;34:54-59.

50. Harrison MJG, Marshall J, Thomas DJ. Relevance of duration of transient ischaemic attacks in carotid territory. *Br Med J*. 1978;1:1578-1579.

51. Hart RG. Prevention and treatment of cardioembolic stroke. In: Furlan AJ, ed. *The Heart and Stroke: Exploring Mutual Cerebrovascular and Cardiovascular Issues*. New York, NY: Springer Verlag; 1987; 7:117-138.

52. Hart RG, Miller VT. Cerebral infarction in young adults: a practical approach. *Stroke*. 1983;14:110-114.

53. Humphries AW, Young JR, Santilli PH, et al. Unoperated, asymptomatic significant internal carotid artery stenosis: a review of 182 instances. *Surgery*. 1976;80:695-698.

54. Kappelle LJ, Koudstaal PJ, van Gijn J, et al. Carotid angiography in patients with lacunar infarction: a prospective study. *Stroke*. 1988;19:1093-1096.

55. Kroener JM, Dorn PL, Shoor PM, et al. Prognosis of asymptomatic ulcerating carotid lesions. *Arch Surg*. 1980;115:1387-1392.

56. Landau WM. Ataxic-hemiparesis: special deluxe stroke or standard brand? *Neurology*. 1988;38: 1799-1801

57. Landau WM. Au clair de lacune: Holy, wholly, holey logic. *Neurology*. 1989;39:725-730.

58. Levine SR, Kim S, Deegan MJ, et al. Ischemic stroke associated with anti-cardiolipin antibodies. *Stroke*. 1987;18:1101-1106.

59. Marzewski DJ, Furlan AJ, St. Louis P, et al. Intracranial internal carotid artery stenosis: longterm prognosis. *Stroke*. 1982;13:821-824.

60. Millikan C, Futrell N. The fallacy of the lacune hypothesis. *Stroke*. 1990;21:1251-1257.

61. Mohr JP. Lacunes. *Stroke*. 1982;13:3-11.

62. Mohr JP. Infarct of unclear cause. In: Furlan AJ, ed. *The Heart and Stroke: Exploring Mutual Cerebrovascular and Cardiovascular Issues*. New York, NY; Springer Verlag; 1987;101-116.

63. Mohr JP, Caplan LR, Melski JW, et al. The Harvard cooperative stroke registry: a prospective registry. *Neurology*. 1978;28:754-762.

64. Moore WS, Boren C, Malone JM, et al. Natural history of nonstenotic, asymptomatic ulcerative lesions of the carotid artery. *Arch Surg*. 1978;113:1352-1359.

65. Moufarrij NA, Little JR, Furlan AJ, et al. Vertebral artery stenosis: long-term follow-up. *Stroke*. 1984; 15:260-263.

66. Moufarrij NA, Little JR, Furlan AJ, et al. Basilar and distal vertebral artery stenosis: long-term follow-up. *Stroke*. 1986;17:938-942.

67. NASCET Investigators. Benefit of carotid endarterectomy for patients with high-grade carotid stenosis of the internal carotid artery. *NINDS Clinical Alert*. February 25, 1991.

68. Norris JW, Hachinski VC. Stroke prevention: past, present, and future. In Norris J.W., Hachinski VC, eds. *Prevention of Stroke*. New York, NY; Springer Verlag; 1991;1:1-15.

69. Norrving B, Cronqvist S. Clinical and radiologic features of lacunar versus nonlacunar minor stroke. *Stroke*. 1989;20:59-64.

70. Okada Y, Yamaguchi T, Minematsu K, et al. Hemorrhagic transformation in cerebral embolism. *Stroke*. 1989;20:598-603.

71. Olsen TS, Skriver EB, Herning M. Cause of cerebral infarction in the carotid territory: its relation to the size and the location of the infarct and to the underlying vascular lesion. *Stroke*. 1985;16:459-466.

72. Pessin MS, Duncan GW, Mohr JP, et al. Clinical and angiographic features of carotid transient ischemic attacks. *N Engl J Med*. 1977;296:358-362.

73. Pessin MS, Gorelick PB, Kwan ES, et al. Basilar artery stenosis: middle and distal segments. *Neurology*. 1987;37:1742-1746.

74. Pessin MS, Hinton RC, Davis KR, et al. Mechanisms of acute carotid stroke. *Ann Neurol*. 1979; 6:245-252.

75. Pessin MS, Kwan ES, Scott RM, et al. Occipital infarction with hemianopsia from carotid occlusive disease. *Stroke*. 1989;20:409-411.

76. Pessin MS, Panis W, Prager RJ, et al. Auscultation of cervical and ocular bruits in extracranial carotid occlusive disease: a clinical and angiographic study. *Stroke*. 1983;14:246-249.

77. Petersen P, Boysen G, Godtfredsen J, et al. Placebo-controlled, randomized trial of warfarin and aspirin for prevention of thromboembolic complications in chronic atrial fibrillation: the Copenhagen AFASAK study. *Lancet*. 1989;1:175-179.

78. Rascol A, Clanet M, Manelfe C, et al. Pure motor hemiplegia: CT study of 30 cases. *Stroke*. 1982; 13:11-17.

79. Ringelstein EB, Koschorke S, Holling A, et al. Computed tomographic patterns of proven embolic brain infarctions. *Ann Neurol*. 1989;26:759-765.

80. Roman GC. Senile dementia of the Binswanger type: a vascular form of dementia in the elderly. *JAMA*. 1987;258:1782-1788.

81. Rothrock JF, Lyden PD, Yee J, et al. 'Crescendo' transient ischemic attacks: clinical and angiographic correlations. *Neurology*. 1988;38:198-201.

82. Russo LS. Carotid system transient ischemic attacks: clinical, racial, and angiographic correlations. *Stroke*. 1981;12:470-473.

83. Sacco RL, Ellenberg JH, Mohr JP, et al. Infarcts of undetermined cause: the NINCDS stroke data bank. *Ann Neurol*. 1989;25:382-390.

84. Sacco RL, Foulkes MA, Mohr JP, et al. Determinants of early recurrence of cerebral infarction: the stroke data bank. *Stroke*. 1989;20:983-989.

85. Sila CA, Chimowitz MI. Elevated plasminogen activator inhibitor (PAI) in cerebral infarction of undetermined cause. *Neurology*. 1990;40(suppl 1):192.

86. Sirna S, Biller J, Skorton DJ, et al. Cardiac evaluation of the patient with stroke. *Stroke*. 1990;21:14-23.

87. Stroke Prevention in Atrial Fibrillation Study Investigators. Preliminary report of the stroke prevention in atrial fibrillation study. *N Engl J Med*. 1990; 322:863-868.

88. Tegeler CH, Stroke Prevention in Atrial Fibrillation Study: Carotid Stenosis Study Group. Carotid stenosis in atrial fibrillation. *Neurology*. 1989;39 (suppl 1):159.

89. Tsuda Y, Kimura K, Yoneda S, et al. Cerebral blood flow and CO_2 reactivity in transient ischemic attacks: comparison between TIAs due to ICA occlusion and ICA mild stenosis. *Neurol Res*. 1983;5(3):17-37.

90. Welch KMA, Levine SR. Migraine-related stroke in the context of the International Headache Society classification of head pain. *Arch Neurol*. 1990; 47:458-462.

91. Whisnant JP. Multiple particles injected may all go to the same cerebral artery branch. *Stroke*. 1982; 13:720.

92. Wiebers DO, Whisnant JP, O'Fallon WM. Reversible ischemic neurologic deficit (RIND) in a community: Rochester, Minnesota, 1955-1974. *Neurology*. 1982;32:459-465.

93. Wodarz R. Watershed infarctions and computed tomography: a topographical study in cases with stenosis or occlusion of the carotid artery. *Neuroradiology*. 1980;19:245-248.

94. Yanagihara T, Klass DW. Rythmic involuntary movement as a manifestation of transient ischemic attacks. *Trans Am Neurol Assoc*. 1981;106:46-48.

95. Yanagihara T, Sundt TM Jr, Piepgras DG. Weakness of the lower extremity in carotid occlusive disease. *Arch Neurol*. 1988;45:297-301.

CHAPTER 4

Diagnostic Evaluation of Ischemic Cerebrovascular Disease

Joseph M. Zabramski, MD, and John A. Anson, MD

The symptoms of occlusive cerebrovascular disease (OCD) are common reasons for neurosurgical referral. OCD may produce a wide range of neurologic syndromes, including amaurosis fugax, transient ischemic attacks (TIAs), reversible ischemic neurologic deficits (RINDs), progressing infarction, and completed stroke. The clinical evaluation of these syndromes has become more complex with an expanding array of radiologic and laboratory tests available. Although computed tomography (CT) revolutionized central nervous system evaluation, it has now been increasingly supplanted by safer and more sensitive magnetic resonance (MR) imaging techniques, and the relative merits and disadvantages of each need to be considered in the work-up of a patient with OCD. Likewise angiography, which has long been considered the "gold standard" for evaluation of the cerebrovascular system, must be weighed against other techniques for visualizing intra- and extracranial blood vessels, including digital subtraction angiography (DSA), MR angiography, and a variety of noninvasive Doppler and ultrasound techniques. Direct tests of cerebral blood flow (CBF) and related parenchymal ischemia also have a bigger role, including xenon CBF, positron emission tomography (PET), and single photon emission CT (SPECT). The goal of this chapter is to outline the appropriate clinical indications for these various tests and to discuss their relative advantages and disadvantages for the imaging and evaluation of ischemic cerebrovascular disease.

General Approaches to Ischemic Cerebrovascular Disease

The initial question to be addressed is who needs evaluation and when? Patients presenting with focal neurologic symptoms of a potentially cerebrovascular origin need to be aggressively, and often urgently, evaluated so that appropriate treatment modalities, including anticoagulants and surgery, can be initiated in a timely fashion. The initial step in evaluating a patient with possible stroke is to rule out a hemorrhagic lesion.

CT scanning is the most reliable and readily available means of distinguishing between acute ischemia and intracerebral hemorrhage in patients who present with the sudden onset of focal neurologic deficits. A basic head CT scan is the logical first step in the evaluation of these patients and should be obtained urgently. The results of the CT scan and the subsequent clinical course of the patient often dictate which additional tests will be needed. Resolution of neurologic deficits, consistent with TIA or RIND, usually warrants complete evaluation of the extracranial and intracranial cerebral vasculature, as well as testing to exclude possible cardiac sources for emboli. Although evaluation of the extracranial carotid circulation with Duplex ultrasound may be helpful as a screening test, we believe that formal angiographic evaluation should be considered in all patients who are potential surgical candidates. Many clinicians also recommend angiography before anticoagulation to rule out intracranial pathology such as an aneurysm or arteriovenous malformation (AVM) that might influence the choice of therapy. Bunt[27] found an 18% incidence of intracranial pathology after the angiographic evaluation of patients with ischemic cerebrovascular disease. Where available, MR imaging can be helpful as a screening test, demonstrating evidence of small-vessel disease not apparent on CT scans and of vascular occlusion on flow-sensitive scans. Recent advances in MR angiography have improved resolution to the point that it may soon replace ultrasound and formal angiography as a screening test in institutions where it is available.

The evaluation of the patient with fixed deficits consistent with completed stroke is more controversial. Repeated CT scans are helpful in managing the potential complications of hemorrhage and progressive edema in these patients, and most authors would agree that noninvasive work-up for cardiac and extracranial vascular disease is warranted. Recommendations regarding the need for angiography and its timing vary considerably. We believe that all patients with symptomatic cerebrovascular disease, including those with completed strokes, benefit from the information obtained by early angiographic evaluation. Angiography may not only confirm the etiology of the ischemic symptoms but can also provide valuable information about the availability of collateral blood flow and the presence of associated vascular pathology that could affect therapeutic decisions. We believe that angiography should be performed early in the patient's hospital course (usually within 24 hours), particularly when deficits are relatively mild. The only exception is when associated disease or the presence of severe deficits limits the potential for useful recovery.

Patients with fluctuating or progressive neurologic deficits who would be potential surgical candidates should be evaluated urgently. Basic head CT scan followed by heparin anticoagulation, when there is no evidence of hemorrhage, will often stabilize neurologic deficits. Complete four-vessel angiography should be performed when the best angiographic team is available (usually within 24 hours of stabilization). Angiography can be considered in patients with continued progression despite anticoagulation; however, angiography in this setting is associated with considerably higher morbidity and mortality (as high as 7.7% in one series).[135]

The evaluation of patients with asymptomatic carotid bruits is more controversial, primarily because the natural history of these lesions is uncertain. Most population-based studies have reported a relatively low risk of stroke in patients with asymptomatic bruits.[64,98,151] In general, this may be true; however, the risk of stroke appears to be increased in the presence of carotid stenosis greater than 75%,[33,48] or with deep, irregular ulcerations.[41,105] Barnett et al[10] have recently demonstrated a direct relationship between the severity of stenosis and risk of stroke in patients with symptomatic carotid artery stenosis. The results of the ongoing Asymptomatic Carotid Artery Stenosis Study should help to clarify this relationship and to identify other factors that affect the natural history of this population. Until then, it would seem prudent to evaluate patients with asymptomatic bruits who would otherwise be good candidates for surgery for the severity of stenosis using noninvasive studies, such as ultrasound and Doppler. When a severe, hemodynamically significant carotid stenosis is identified (greater than 75% reduction or less than 1.5-mm residual lumen diameter), angiography can be pursued. Basic head CT or MR imaging scans in this population may reveal evidence of previously silent infarctions in the distribution of the stenotic artery that would favor surgical intervention. Additionally, patients

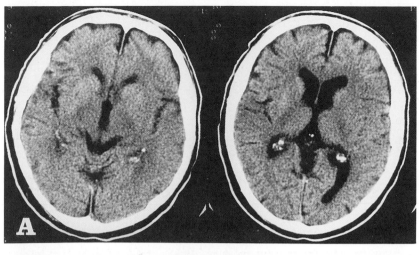

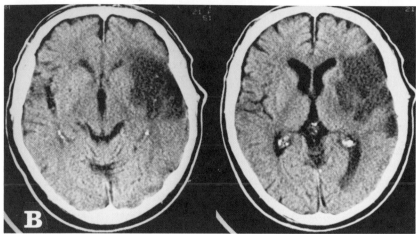

Figure 1. (A) Initial computed tomography (CT) scan performed approximately 6 hours after the onset of marked aphasia and right hemiparesis in a 74-year-old man. There is no evidence of hemorrhage or ischemic changes. (B) Repeat CT scan 48 hours after the onset of deficits reveals a large, well-delineated infarction in the middle cerebral artery distribution.

with asymptomatic carotid bruits should be evaluated for ischemic heart disease as the risk for fatal and nonfatal cardiac events has been shown to be greater than in the general population.[33]

Brain Imaging: CT and MR Imaging

CT Findings in Hemispheric Stroke

Because of its widespread availability, reliability, and safety, CT scanning has become the major diagnostic test for initial evaluation in patients with possible strokes. It is helpful both for localizing and defining lesion topography, for ruling out nonischemic etiologies, and for following infarction development.

Cerebral infarction on CT scan can be divided into three major stages based on their appearance. First is an acute stage, generally 12-24 hours long, during which the CT is usually normal (Figure 1A). Only half of all infarctions are seen on CT in the first 48 hours.[70] The major benefit of CT during this stage is to identify cases with cerebral

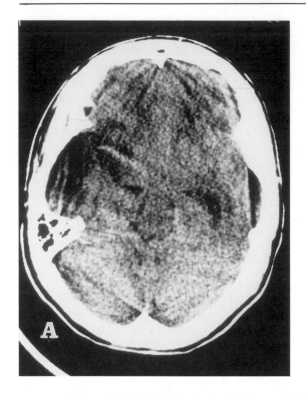
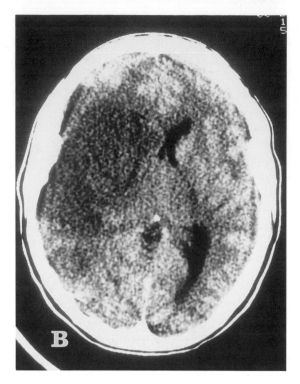

Figure 2. (A & B) Basic head CT scan 24 hours after the onset of left hemiplegia in a 22-year-old woman involved in an all-terrain motor vehicle (ATV) accident. Note the increased CT density (consistent with clotted blood) in the proximal section of the right middle cerebral artery (MCA). *(C)* Lateral view of a selective right internal carotid artery (ICA) angiogram demonstrates findings suggestive of traumatic dissection of the ICA at the base of the skull (curved arrow) and a complete absence of filling of the MCA.

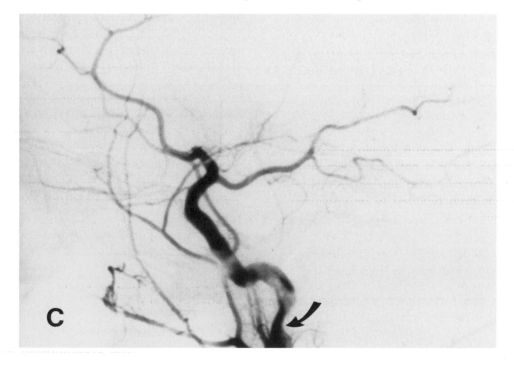

hemorrhage or other lesions (e.g. subdural hematoma, tumor) that may masquerade as stroke or TIA. Occasionally, the underlying vascular pathology responsible for ischemic symptoms may be directly visualized on CT: Giant, partially thrombosed aneurysms may appear as a large hyper- or hypodense mass, whereas thrombosis or embolism of the middle cerebral artery (MCA) trunk may be visualized as a linear area of hyperdensity on a nonenhanced CT (Figure 2).

A subacute stage follows, generally continuing 4-6 weeks, during which the characteristic CT findings of stroke evolve. Hypodensity gradually develops, usually starting about 24 hours after symptoms. Over several days the area of hypodensity becomes more marked and the contours more clearly defined. As the infarction becomes visualized, its topography becomes diagnostically important for its relationship to a particular vascular territory. The MCA territory is most often involved, being affected in 61% to 86% of cerebral infarctions. The entire territory, however, is seldom involved (Figure 1B).[2,20,70,146] The second most common territory involved is the posterior cerebral artery (PCA) (8% to 15%) followed by the anterior cerebral artery (ACA) (3% to 13%), and less commonly, the anterior choroidal (1%) or watershed zones (0.7% to 11%).[2,20,146] The cerebrum is involved in 70% of the cases, the basal ganglia and internal capsule in 20%, the posterior fossa in 10%,[69] and the multiple vascular territories may be involved in about 23% of cases.[146]

Mass effect is often seen during this stage. Pathologically, edema is known to accompany infarctions, but it is not always demonstrable on CT, especially with smaller lesions. Mass effect has been reported to be visualized in only 18% to 47% of cases,[20,31,87] although occasionally it will be seen prior to the appearance of hypodensity.[20] Contrast enhancement may also be noted during this period. It rarely occurs before the third day, peaks in the second to third weeks, and is rare after 2 months. Enhancement may be in a gyral, homogeneous, or ring pattern and can vary considerably depending on volume,

rate, and timing of contrast administration. The mechanism of contrast enhancement is not clear but includes blood-brain barrier breakdown, hyperemic "luxury perfusion," neovascularity, and extravasation. The presence of contrast enhancement has been associated with worse prognosis.[59,115] Additionally, the administration of contrast itself has been suggested to be harmful; it may be associated with worse outcomes, creatine phosphokinase elevations, and hemorrhagic change.[59,79,112,115]

Finally, during the chronic stage, disappearance of the mass effect and contrast enhancement occur, and the hypodense area is further attenuated, approaching the density of cerebrospinal fluid. Although some infarctions may revert to normal density, either temporarily (the so-called fogging effect)[12] or permanently, most necrotic infarctions evolve into cystic cavities, often with focal dilatation of the ipsilateral ventricle.

CT is not as helpful in the evaluation of TIAs and is rarely useful in cases of amaurosis fugax, presumably because these syndromes are not associated with parenchymal destruction. In one recent prospective study,[38] only 27% of CT scans done in patients with TIAs demonstrated a focal hypodense lesion and only 12% were located appropriately to the patient's symptoms.[38] Also no significant difference in outcome between patients with and without CT findings was found. Another series[36] found that the frequency of CT-demonstrable hypodensity with reversible ischemic attacks was related to the duration of deficit. A hypodensity was seen in only 20.5% of those with TIAs, 37.9% of those with RINDs, and 43.6% of those with incompletely resolved RINDs. Nevertheless, as mentioned before, CT is valuable in identifying other intracranial pathology that may present with symptoms masquerading as ischemic cerebrovascular disease.

CT of Lacunar, Vertebrobasilar, and Watershed Infarctions

Lacunar infarctions account for up to 19% of strokes[103] and occur predominantly in deep brain regions. Detection by CT scan is moderately sensitive, visualizing up to 55% within 10 days and 69% within 7 months after onset of symptoms.[42] The absolute limit for detection by current CT scanners is approximately 2 mm,[116,148] and larger ones may be routinely missed because of artifact or scan technique. Comparative studies have shown that MR imaging is more sensitive than CT in the detection of both recent and remote lacunar infarctions.[26]

In the evaluation of vertebrobasilar ischemic syndromes, CT is often limited by bony artifact that interferes with visualization of brain stem structures. The ability of CT to demonstrate posterior fossa infarctions varies from 43% to 75% in several series,[19,69,80] and MR imaging is also proving more useful in this setting. The most clinically valuable use of CT in vertebrobasilar territory infarction is with cerebellar infarctions. In this case, CT may show indirect signs of mass effect such as cisternal effacement, obliteration or displacement of the fourth ventricle, and hydrocephalus. When vertebrobasilar infarctions are visualized on CT, they follow a similar pattern of temporal changes as supratentorial infarctions.

Watershed or border zone infarctions are seen infrequently, accounting for only 2 of 240 cases with infarction on CT in one series.[20] Typically, they appear as a fairly extensive infarction at the border between two vascular territories. Zülch[158] has distinguished three types: (1) superficial watershed infarctions, seen occasionally between the MCA and ACA territories on high CT cuts, and rarely between MCA and PCA areas; (2) deep watershed infarctions, between cortical and deep sylvian branch territories, usually between the putamen and insula, and rarely recognized; and (3) "Dreilandereck" infarctions, located at the angular gyrus where the MCA, ACA, and PCA territories are all adjacent. CT may also be helpful in identifying the etiology of strokes when certain patterns are present. Infarctions in multiple vascular distributions suggest an embolic etiology, typically with a cardiac origin. Likewise, lacunae

suggest small-vessel disease, and the watershed patterns described here argue for a hemodynamic or low-flow mechanism.

Potential Applications: CT of the Carotid Artery

Because of the increasingly high resolution of modern CT scanners, direct examination of the carotid bifurcation and vessels is possible. Both axial and parasagittal reformatted images are available and can demonstrate stenosis, ulceration, calcification, and dissection.[35,60,61,140] A recent report describes the visualization of lucent defects within carotid atheromatous plaques that were found to correlate pathologically with intraplaque necrosis or hemorrhage. Along with severe stenosis, these findings had the most prognostic significance for ipsilateral hemispheric stroke.[35] The incremental dynamic technique for examination of the carotid bifurcation described by Tress[140] added only 5 minutes to a normal contrast-enhanced head CT scan and yielded accurate information about carotid stenosis that was concordant with angiography but was less sensitive for ulceration.[60,61]

Magnetic Resonance Imaging

The clinical use of MR imaging has grown tremendously in the past 10 years, and new applications and examination parameters are being developed, including those utilizing paramagnetic contrast agents such as gadolinium diethylenetriamine penta-acetic acid (Gd-DTPA). MR imaging is clearly more sensitive than CT for imaging most central nervous system pathology. Its ability to provide direct sagittal and coronal views further enhances its versatility. Its disadvantages compared to CT include prolonged scanning time; poor visualization of bone, pathologic calcification, and subarachnoid hemorrhages; and the risk to patients with metallic implants.

MR imaging is extremely sensitive for brain pathology because most lesions in the brain cause a change in the water content of

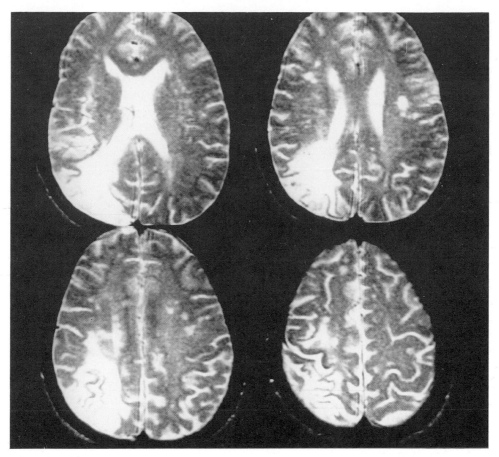

Figure 3. *T2-weighted MRI scan in a 62-year-old man with symptoms of mild left hemiparesis shows a high-signal intensity region characteristic of recent infarction in the watershed distribution between the right MCA and PCA territories. This distribution suggests an ischemic mechanism resulting from hemodynamic insufficiency rather than embolism. Angiographic evaluation in this patient revealed occlusion of the right ICA with poor intracranial collateral blood supply.*

the involved tissue. Cerebral ischemia produces very early changes in local tissue water content, even before infarction. These changes, which progress with time, are easily visualized with MR imaging.

Experimental studies have demonstrated MR imaging changes reliably, appearing within 2-4 hours of ischemia, and potentially as early as 30 minutes.[22,23,117,129,130,143,153] The early stages of ischemia are best seen with T2-weighted images, in which the ischemic area has increased signal intensity because of tissue accumulation of water.[122,129] Later stages of the ischemic process are best appreciated as

low signal intensity on T1-weighted images, and eventually infarctions will appear as areas of low signal intensity on T1-weighted images and as areas of high signal intensity on T2-weighted images (Figure 3). In the subacute to late phase, MR imaging often demonstrates a hyperintense rim surrounding the infarction that may represent persistent ischemia or Wallerian degeneration.[39] MR imaging also has better spatial resolution, allowing better localization of lesions and identifying smaller areas of infarction including lacunar infarctions.[26,81] Absence of bony artifact also allows better resolution of posterior fossa and

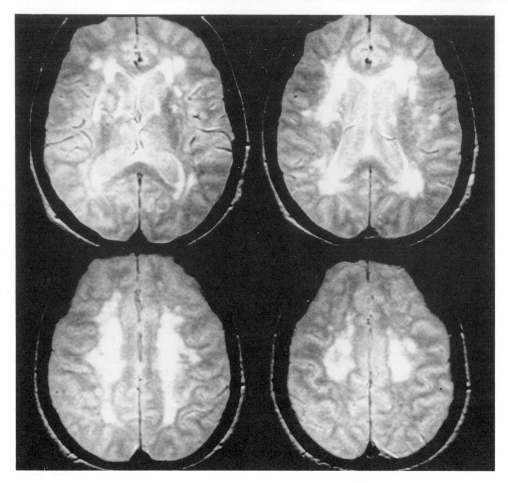

Figure 4. *Proton density (intermediate-weighted) MRIs in a 72-year-old man with progressive dementia and a long history of hypertension. Note the extensive periventricular areas of increased signal intensity consistent with leukemolacia secondary to severe small vessel ischemic disease (Binswanger's Dementia).*

brain stem infarctions than CT. In one series of patients with infarction, MR imaging was positive overall in 80% and in 60% of brain stem infarctions.[70] Administration of the paramagnetic contrast agent, Gd-DTPA, provides additional information. Gd-DTPA shortens T1-relaxation time, causing a brighter signal on T1-weighted images. Areas of cerebral ischemia or infarctions show various degrees of enhancement depending on the amount of collateral circulation, the extent of blood-brain barrier breakdown, and the degree of vasogenic edema. These phenomena also affect contrast-enhanced CT scans, but gado-linium-enhanced MR imaging appears to be a more sensitive measure of vasogenic edema and collateral circulation as well as providing better spatial resolution.[74] Gadolinium enhancement appears as early as 6 days after infarction, compared to 4-18 days for contrast CT.[144] There is also evidence that asymptomatic chronic lacunar or periventricular infarctions do not enhance with Gd-DTPA, whereas symptomatic lacunar infarctions do. This finding provides additional information about the significance of these deep lesions that are often seen in patients with progressive cerebrovascular disease.[144]

Because of early tissue water changes associated with cerebral ischemia, MR imaging is much more sensitive in cases of TIAs (without infarction) than CT. The reported incidence of CT findings with TIAs varies from 0 to 32%,[3,18,30,82,147] whereas MR imaging is positive in 72% to 80% of TIAs.[3,82,124] There is also evidence that MR imaging findings may correlate better with symptoms. In Awad's series[3] comparing CT and MR imaging in patients with TIAs, CT scans were positive in 5 of 15 patients with clinical unilateral carotid TIAs. In 4 of these 5 patients, the abnormality was within the appropriate vascular territory. MR imaging was positive in 12 of the 15, correlated appropriately in 11, and demonstrated additional contralateral lesions in 7.[3]

MR imaging also appears to be a better marker for small-vessel ischemic vascular disease, which often appears as multiple periventricular areas of increased signal intensity or as watershed zone abnormalities (Figure 4). The periventricular changes are believed to be related to subcortical arteriosclerotic encephalopathy (Binswanger's disease), with areas of leukomalacia secondary to hypertensive vascular disease. Several clinical and pathologic studies have confirmed this correlation.[39,81,82] Although these changes are also seen in asymptomatic individuals,[3] they are not common enough to be considered manifestations of normal aging, and they may represent markers of chronic ischemia.

MR imaging also demonstrates ischemic changes in watershed areas better than CT scanning. A study of 27 patients with TIAs identified border zone MR imaging abnormalities in 4 (15%).[81] All patients had increased signal intensity on T2-weighted images between the PCA and MCA distributions that extended from periventricular white matter to the cortex. These findings may represent the residua of low-flow states and should warn of hemodynamic abnormalities potentially traceable to treatable cerebrovascular disease.

The full potential of MR imaging in the clinical evaluation of cerebrovascular disease has yet to be recognized. Recent articles in the literature have demonstrated its usefulness in imaging the extra- and intracranial cerebral vasculature (MR angiography) and in measuring CBF. Two techniques have been described for angiographic imaging, the so-called time-of-flight and phase-contrast techniques, both of which use short radiofrequency-pulse sequences and thus add only 20-30 minutes to a standard examination of the head or neck. Because the signals are sensitive to both velocity and direction of flow, the images can be tuned to demonstrate primarily arterial or venous anatomy (Figures 5 and 6); however, problems still arise with these techniques. The images are degraded by movement and require careful positioning, which makes the patient's cooperation essential. In addition, the signals are extremely sensitive to turbulence, which frequently results in overestimation of the severity of stenosis (Figure 5). Nevertheless, the quality of images has steadily improved, and the technique may soon replace ultrasound and Doppler studies as a screening test for patients with suspected ischemic vascular disease.

In a study of 27 patients with suspected carotid disease, satisfactory MR angiography images were obtained in 50 of 54 carotid bifurcations. MR angiography images corresponded to intra-arterial DSA in all cases with normal carotid arteries, mild to moderate stenosis, or complete occlusion, and in 13 of 15 patients with severe stenosis.[121] In a series of 40 patients with unsuspected cerebrovascular disease, MR angiography with a three-dimensional volume technique provided diagnostic images in 72%.[99] Additionally, aneurysms as small as 4 mm were visualized with this technique.

In a study at our institution, 39 patients with symptoms of ischemic cerebrovascular disease underwent MR angiography as part of their diagnostic evaluation, followed by conventional angiography. The studies were graded for severity of stenosis on a scale of 0-5 by independent examiners. Results between the two techniques correlated for degree of stenosis in 95% of patients (Drayer BP, personal communication, 1991). Subse-

Figure 5. (A) Two views from an MRA of the neck in a 57-year-old man who presented with a history of left hemisphere transient ischemic attacks (TIAs). The MRA study demonstrates severe preocclusive stenosis of the proximal left ICA. Note that the vertebral artery (VA) is superimposed on the images of the ICA and external carotid artery. *(B)* Subsequent angiogram in the same patient reveals less severe stenosis and evidence of ulceration at the same level. Recent experience with MRA suggests that because of its sensitivity to turbulent flow, *it frequently depicts the stenosis in such lesions to be more severe than it actually is*. However, for the same reason, false-negative tests are extremely unlikely, making this an excellent screening tool for the workup of patients with ischemic symptoms. Using present techniques, the MRA study adds only 20 minutes to a routine MRI evaluaton of the brain and requires no contrast or exposure to ionizing radiation.

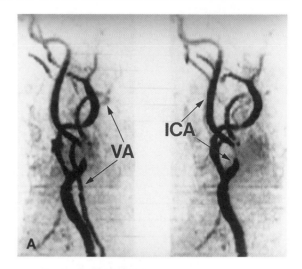

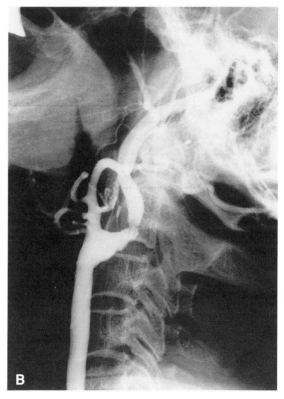

quent carotid endarterectomy in 15 patients confirmed the accuracy of the MR angiography findings. Although MR angiography may occasionally overestimate the severity of stenosis, in our experience false-negative studies of the carotid bifurcations are unlikely.

The combination of MR imaging and MR angiography can be used to study patients presenting with symptoms of cerebral ischemia with a single noninvasive test. MR imaging provides a sensitive study of the brain parenchyma for evidence of ischemic injury, and MR angiography provides a sensitive screening test for large-vessel occlusive disease. We now evaluate most patients with TIAs with this technique.

Recent and Future Applications of MR Imaging

MR imaging techniques have been developed that can provide quantification of blood flow in the carotid arteries. The technique involves sensitizing the phase of the MR signal to blood flow velocity gated to the cardiac cycle. After calibration to a phantom tube system with known constant flows, this technique allows the quantitative determination of blood flow volume and velocity in the carotid artery.[13] This technique may provide additional helpful clinical information in conjunction with MR angiography in the evaluation of patients with ischemic cerebrovascular disease.

Although still primarily investigational, MR spectroscopy has the potential to provide

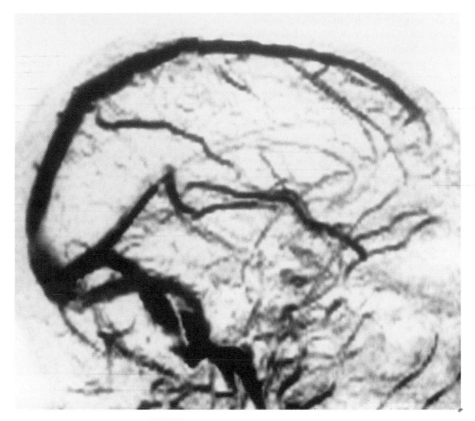

Figure 6. *Normal intracranial venous MRA in a 36-year-old woman who presented with headache and decreased level of consciousness and who was suspected of having possible sagittal sinus thrombosis.*

information about a variety of cerebral metabolic functions. MR imaging can process signals received from nuclei other than hydrogen, in particular phosphate metabolites, carbon, and lactate, and can represent them as separate peaks in a spectrum of the nuclei in a sample. Phosphorus 31 MR spectra demonstrate the relative concentrations of cerebral phosphocreatine (PCr), adenosine triphosphate (ATP), inorganic phosphate (P_i), and intracellular pH that correlate with direct tissue measurements. In addition, experimental animal studies with proton (^{1}H) MR spectroscopy suggest the potential to evaluate lactic acidosis and amino acid alterations.[86] These techniques may allow evaluation of biochemical changes of the brain and structural changes from ischemia by MR spectroscopy.

One recent study[85] of MCA occlusion in cats demonstrated clear evidence of ischemia-induced metabolic changes in ^{31}P MR spectroscopy within 20 minutes. In contrast, T1-weighted MR imaging did not detect changes until 45 minutes after occlusion and T2 images until 60-90 minutes after occlusion.[85] Other studies[4,84] have suggested that the ratio of PCr to P_i (PCr/P_i) on ^{31}P-MR spectroscopy is an indicator of ischemia-induced energy depletion and correlates with outcome and functional recovery. The use of combined MR imaging and MR spectroscopy in clinical settings appears very promising in the evaluation of early ischemic changes. The combination would not only allow earlier and more specific detection, but it may provide information regarding effects of treatment, adequacy of collateral circulation, and prognosis.

*Figure 7. Lateral angiographic views of left common carotid artery injections in a 66 year old woman presenting with cresendo TIAs. Ultrasound evaluation was reported to demonstrate complete occlusion of the internal carotid artery (ICA). **(A)** Preoperative angiogram reveals severe preocclusive stenosis at the ICA origin, with only a thin "string" of contrast visable (arrow). Note also the decrease in distal ICA diameter when compared to the postoperative study; this decrease, which is due to reduced intraluminal pressure past the area of stenosis, is referred to as the "carotid slim sign." **(B)** Postoperative study following an urgent carotid endarterectomy, demonstrates a widely patent carotid bifurcation with increase in ICA diameter well above the level of the dissection.*

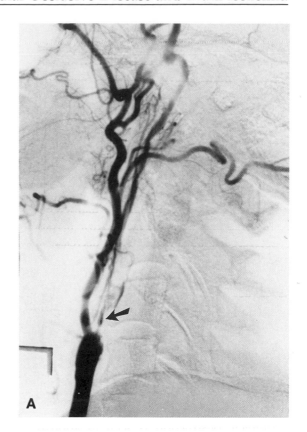

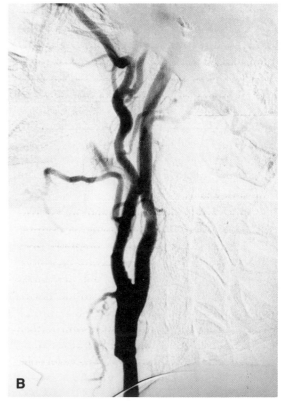

Angiography

Angiography remains the definitive radiologic test for evaluation of the carotid and intracranial vasculature. Although other studies have increasingly supplanted it for screening evaluation, most clinicians consider it necessary before operative intervention, and it remains the gold standard against which other studies must be compared. Angiography for ischemic cerebrovascular disease must include visualization of both carotid bifurcations and the intracranial carotid circulation. The vertebrobasilar circulation should be included as well. It is important to visualize suspicious areas in two planes, as areas of stenosis or ulceration may be underestimated in a single plane. The contrast should be followed on serial films for 10-15 seconds. The circulation time on such studies provides a measure of the adequacy of CBF. In addition, delayed films will often demonstrate filling of the distal territory of intracerebral vessels occluded by embolic disease, or in the case of apparent carotid occlusion, may demonstrate a "string sign" (Figure 7). The latter suggests that occlusion is incomplete and that flow can be readily reestablished by endarterectomy.

Extracranial Carotid Artery

Up to 90% of symptomatic atherosclerotic carotid disease occurs at or near the bifurcation of the carotid artery.[72,152] The remainder involves intracranial vessels in 8% and the inominate or proximal carotid in 2%, thus making it much more important diagnostically to visualize the intracranial vessels on an angiogram than the aortic arch (see Figure 10).[71]

The extent of carotid stenosis should be considered in terms of residual lumen diameter. Although some refer to a percentage narrowing, this value may be difficult to determine as the carotid artery diameter is not uniform and may appear narrow because of decreased blood flow. This decrease in carotid diameter distal to a tight stenosis is referred to as the "carotid slim sign" and is due to decreased intraluminal pressure past the blockage.[96] The slim sign is therefore associated with marginal ipsilateral hemisphere perfusion, and these patients may have a greater risk of hyperperfusion breakthrough complications after endarterectomy.[71] A residual lumen of 2 mm or less typically results in distal hemodynamic change.[34]

Complete obstruction is seen in approximately 12% of patients with chronic or reversible ischemic symptoms.[110,111,113] It may be seen more commonly, however, when patients are studied in the acute phase of a stroke and was noted in 24% of patients within 6 hours of a stroke in one series.[21] Varying degrees of retrograde flow via collaterals may be seen in the distal internal carotid artery. The lowest extent of retrograde carotid flow may predict the success of surgical attempts to reopen the artery. In a recent series at our institution, reopening of the carotid artery was attempted in 26 patients who presented with ischemic symptoms of less than 2 weeks' duration and angiographically documented carotid occlusion. In patients with retrograde flow of contrast to the petrous portion of the carotid, normal flow could be readily re-established in 71% of the vessels. The rate of successful reopening decreased to 50% when the lowest extent of retrograde flow was to the cavernous segment of the carotid and to 25% when contrast filled only the paraclinoid segment

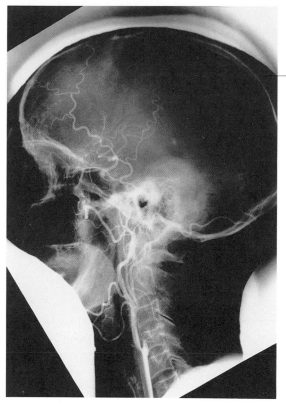

Figure 8. *Left carotid angiogram showing complete occlusion of the proximal internal carotid artery (ICA). Note the presence of external carotid collateral blood supply via the opthalmic artery. Retrograde flow from the opthalmic artery fills only the proximal segment of the cavernous portion of the ICA, suggesting that this is a chronic occlusion (compare with Figure 9).*

(McCormick et al, unpublished data) (Figures 8 and 9). Conversely, flow may be very delayed through an area of severe obstruction (see Figure 7), presenting as a "pseudo-occlusion" on ultrasound evaluation. The configuration of the proximal end of an occluded carotid artery is not an accurate indicator of the age of the occlusion. The three most common configurations are a sharp proximal stump, a virtual absence of the artery, and a rounded blunt stump (see Figures 7, 8, and 9).[110]

Ulceration is another common finding on carotid angiograms and is associated with thromboembolic syndromes such as TIAs and amaurosis fugax. It is usually seen along with

NASCET $\left[\%\ \text{Stenosis} = 1 - \frac{N}{D} \times 100 \right]$

N - site of greatest narrowing
D - diameter of normal artery distil to carotid bulb.

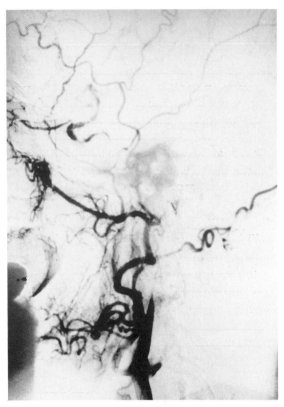

Figure 9. Left common carotid angiogram in a 48-year-old man who presented with sudden onset of right hemiparesis. The patient had a 12-hour history of severe left-sided headache following spinal manipulation for neck pain. The tapered, "flame-like" occlusion of the internal carotid artery (ICA) is characteristic of acute arterial dissections. In addition, note the retrograde flow of contrast filling the distal ICA to the level of its pretrous segment, which is consistent with acute occlusion. (compare with Figure 8.)

some degree of stenosis and is present in most patients with more than 85% stenosis. It is more difficult to visualize when there is more than 90% stenosis.[45] Ulceration can appear as an irregularity of the vessel wall; a niche or outpouching in more severe cases; or a superimposed, well-circumscribed double density when seen *en face* rather than profile. The accuracy of angiographic visualization ulceration has been reported to be about 86%;[16] however, it has been suggested that a significant number of small bifurcation area ulcerations may be missed on angiography,

especially when a subintimal hematoma is present.[45]

Another lesion identified on angiogram is carotid dissection. This is an important consideration, especially in younger individuals with symptoms of headache, amaurosis fugax, focal neurologic deficits, or oculosympathetic palsy. CT scans in these patients are often normal, and angiography should be performed when suspicion of dissections exists. The most typical findings are of very tight stenosis in the mid- to upper cervical internal carotid artery (ICA), the "string sign," or of a tapered, "flame-like" occlusion of the ICA (Figure 9). Less commonly, a pseudoaneurysmal outpouching or a double lumen may be seen.

Intracranial Vessels

A number of angiographic findings involving the ICAs can be seen in patients with ischemic symptoms. These findings have been nicely defined by Sundt and Houser.[71,72,134] Carotid siphon stenosis is usually smooth and nonulcerative. Severe stenosis is found in 3% and mild to moderate stenosis in 20% of patients undergoing carotid endarterectomy.[134] Retrograde ophthalmic flow from the external carotid system is seen in approximately 50% of patients with amaurosis fugax, 50% of those with progressing stroke or generalized ischemia, and 25% of those with TIAs.[72]

Focal alteration of intracranial vessels is found in about 40% of patients with focal infarction and 25% of those with TIAs (Figure 10).[72] They include small-vessel occlusions, focal areas of slow flow, areas of collateral retrograde flow, and reactive hyperemia with early venous drainage. Last, slow internal carotid to middle cerebral artery flow (as compared to the external carotid artery) is associated with decreased CBF.[72]

In Pessin's series[111] of patients undergoing angiography for TIAs, 37% had severe stenosis of the ICA or bifurcation, 12% demonstrated complete ICA occlusion, 3% had severe ICA stenosis, 6% had moderate bifurcation stenosis, 23% had minimal bifurcation stenosis, and 19% had normal carotid arter-

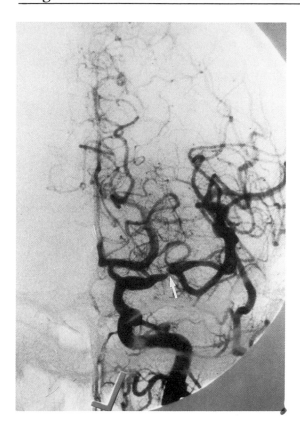

Figure 10. Anterior-posterior view of left common carotid injection in a 62-year-old man who presented with repetitive left hemisphere TIAs. Note the severe focal stenosis of the distal M-1 segment of the MCA (arrow). Cervical views of the carotid revealed no evidence of significant stenosis or ulceration.

ies. Of the patients with normal ICAs and carotid bifurcations, 22% showed evidence of ulceration of the common carotid and 17% had intracranial branch occlusions, whereas patients with minimal ICA stenosis had ulceration present on 27% of the studies and evidence of distal occlusions in 20%.[111]

Normal angiograms are seen in 11% to 19% of patients with TIAs;[111,122] however, as noted before, a number of these will have evidence of embolic disease secondary to ulceration at surgery. Recent studies of patients with TIAs and normal angiograms (and normal cardiac and hematologic studies) have shown that approximately 13% to 18% will progress to a stroke or further TIAs, and 14% to 17% will develop angina pectoris or myocardial infarction.[46,127,128]

Digital Subtraction Angiography

The role of intravenous DSA had been debated over the past few years, and enthusiasm for the technique has waned considerably.[109,141] Problems with intravenous DSA include poor resolution, greater contrast volume, technically inadequate studies, and poor ability to evaluate intracranial collateral circulation.[8] As many as 25% of intravenous DSA studies are technically inadequate.[142] Although intravenous DSA has been proposed as a satisfactory screening test for cerebrovascular disease,[77,155] its technical inadequacies and insufficient intracranial sensitivity make it unsuitable for this role.

IVDSA ✓

Intra-arterial DSA, however, provides several advantages over conventional angiography, including better resolution and less contrast volume.[7,109] Studies can be performed with smaller, softer catheters and can often be done via a transbrachial approach that produces few complications but with technically excellent results.[7,10,65] At our institution, intra-arterial DSA studies are usually performed in addition to regular biplanar angiograms. They are used as a supplementary study to obtain additional oblique views, and specific magnified views of areas of interest. For instance, after biplanar standard images of the carotid arteries are obtained in patients undergoing angiography for a carotid aneurysm, intra-arterial DSA will be used to visualize the posterior circulation or to obtain oblique views to better define the neck of an aneurysm. This decreases the time necessary to obtain the additional images and dramatically reduces costs. The current high-definition system at our institution uses 1024 scanning lines and provides excellent resolution. Systems are now available with twice as many lines and resolution equivalent to standard film images.

IADSA ✓

Risks

Although the development of the transbrachial or transfemoral "Seldinger" technique has made cerebral angiography much safer, it is still an invasive procedure with inherent risks. It is important to consider the risk of angiography both for an individual patient's management and for the evaluation of subsequent procedures such as endarterectomy. The risks of angiography include renal failure, allergic reactions, cardiac complications, stroke, and death. Transient renal failure occurs in up to 10% of patients; as many as 2.5% may require renal dialysis.[54] Idiosyncratic or allergic contrast reactions occur in approximately 2% of patients, but most are minor.[120] Cardiovascular complications include hypotension, myocardial depression or infarction, arterial wall disruption or occlusion, and thrombosis at the catheterization site. The overall incidence of these events has been reported to range from 0.2% to 2%.[63,120]

The neurologic risks of angiography vary considerably with both timing of the study and patient characteristics. Recent studies have estimated the risk of minor or reversible neurologic events as ranging from 1.3% to 4.5% and of permanent deficit or stroke as ranging from 0.6% to 1.3%.[27,44,57,58,135] Mortality has been estimated at 0.1% to 0.3%.[27,58] In his review of five well-defined prospective series between 1977 and 1987, Leow and Murie[93] determined an overall major stroke rate after cerebral angiogram of 2.4%. Morbidity has also been shown to vary with the experience of the angiographer.[100] Patients undergoing angiography for the evaluation of TIAs are at slightly higher risk of neurologic complications,[44,135] and those with stroke in evolution have the highest risk (up to 7.7%).[135] The angiographic contrast agents themselves can also damage endothelial cells in the vessel walls, leading to decreased prostacyclin production and loss of interstitial integrity, which can lead to thrombotic and embolic events.[88,89,107]

Noninvasive Studies

Noninvasive tests of the extracranial carotid circulation can be divided into direct and indirect methods. Direct tests evaluate the carotid artery itself using ultrasound imaging of local blood flow characteristics, whereas indirect tests infer the degree of carotid disease by evaluating the resultant distal hemodynamic changes. Both methods are safe, relatively inexpensive, and easy to perform; the interpretation of both can also be affected by variations in the examiner's technique.

Indirect Tests

Although a number of different types of indirect tests have been developed, including thermography, pulsatility indices, supraorbital photoplethysmography, ophthalmodynamometry, and forehead skin blood pressure, the most important ones in use are periorbital Doppler examination and various types of oculoplethysmography (OPG). The drawbacks of indirect tests are their inability to localize the site of a lesion and that a lesion must be hemodynamically significant to be detected (usually greater than 50% reduction in cross-sectional areas).[47]

Periorbital Doppler examination uses a directional Doppler to determine blood flow patterns in the periorbital arteries.[9,24] A hemodynamically significant carotid stenosis or occlusion reverses flow in the periorbital ophthalmic artery branches from outside to inside the orbit. With temporal artery compression, these changes may diminish or reverse. This test is limited and detects only significant lesions with collateral flow via the external carotid artery, but it is still used as a screening test.[5,47] A negative study, however, does not rule out clinically significant carotid disease.

OPG uses pressure changes in the eye as an indicator of carotid artery flow via the ophthalmic artery. Two different techniques of OPG are commonly used. One is the pulse delay technique in which bilateral corneal suction cups are used to record ocular pulse waves.[76] Hemodynamically significant carotid stenosis is detected by the ocular pulse wave being diminished or arriving later than the contralateral side. Because this technique requires right-left comparisons, detection of bilateral carotid stenosis is a problem. For this reason, pulse delay OPG is usually combined with other techniques. Enthusiasm for this technique has diminished as the accuracy rate has been found to vary widely, and some reports have noted a false-negative rate of as high as 50% in the detection of severe stenosis.[78]

Pressure technique OPG, in contrast, applies a 300- or 500-mm Hg vacuum to the eye via a scleral suction cup that obliterates ocular pulsations. The ophthalmic artery pressure is described by the eye pressure at which ocular pulsations reappear.[50] When performed during ipsilateral common carotid occlusion, this technique may give some measure of collateral circulation as well. The test is considered positive if there is more than a 5-mm Hg difference between the two sides or if the ophthalmic artery/systemic pressure ratio is less than 0.66. It appears that overall accuracy of pressure OPG is better than pulse delay OPG,[1] and it has been reported to have almost 90% sensitivity in detecting stenosis greater than 60%.[6] Like periorbital Doppler, neither OPG technique can distinguish between high-grade stenosis and total occlusion. These techniques are likewise insensitive to lesions that do not significantly reduce pressure and flow. OPG is contraindicated by a variety of eye and retinal problems.

Direct Tests

Quantitative Phonoangiography

This technique uses a transducer and spectrum analyzer to analyze the frequency pattern of a carotid bruit. The frequency at which the amplitude of the bruit sharply drops is closely related to the residual lumen diameter. This technique can determine the residual lumen to within 1.0 mm of angiographic lumen in about 85% of technically possible cases.[43,83] The major limitations are that it is applicable only in patients who have a bruit and that radiating or external carotid bruits can be misinterpreted. Because many patients

can have carotid stenosis without a bruit or a bruit without stenosis, this technique is too limited to be used alone. It is, however, often combined with OPG.

Doppler Ultrasound Arteriography

Doppler ultrasound determines flow information by detecting signals reflected from moving red blood cells. Continuous wave Doppler shows flow characteristics of all vessels within the depth of field, whereas pulsed wave Doppler is range gated to sample flow at any depth. Analysis of flow velocities can identify regions of varying stenosis, and sonolucent areas may correspond to areas of severe stenosis, occlusion, or calcification in an atherosclerotic plaque.

A major limitation of Doppler ultrasound is that the detection of mild stenosis is less than 50%. Other problems include easily induced motion artifact and acoustic shadowing caused by areas of calcification. Despite these limitations, the sensitivity and specificity of these techniques in detecting carotid stenosis have been reported to be as high as 90%.[75,133] A recent report, however, from the Asymptomatic Carotid Atherosclerosis Study showed that 20% of Doppler ultrasound studies at various centers bore no relationship to angiography.[73]

B-Mode Ultrasound

In contrast to the previously described techniques that provide only flow-related information, B-mode ultrasound provides an anatomic image of the carotid arteries with no flow-related information. Scans can be performed in both longitudinal and transverse planes from the distal common carotid artery through the bifurcation to the proximal 1-2 cm of internal and external carotid arteries. The degree of stenosis is identifiable with a resolution of 0.5-1.0 mm and correlates with arteriography in 67% to 86%.[47] Scans are technically unsatisfactory in 5% to

15%, and accuracy is limited in detecting occlusion, ulceration, and thrombus.

Duplex Scanning

Duplex scanning overcomes many of the limitations of Doppler ultrasound and B-mode scans by combining the two techniques into a single unit. The B-mode defines the vessel anatomy and allows accurate placement of the pulse Doppler into the vessel lumen to more accurately measure changes in flow velocity. Duplex scanning has a high degree of sensitivity and specificity. It has been reported to identify 87% to 95% of vessels with more than 50% stenosis and to recognize normal arteries in 84% to 95%.[17,47,53,104] Duplex scanning has become the standard of noninvasive testing in cerebrovascular disease and is at least as accurate as intravenous DSA.[53] Its major limitation is its inability to assess the intracranial circulation; it also requires considerable technical expertise.

Color Flow Imaging

Color flow imaging is a recent development that builds on duplex scanning by using color to demonstrate blood flow direction and velocity to demonstrate Doppler information sampled and displayed from throughout the image. Flow direction is color coded, and flow velocity is indicated by shades of that color.[102] Degree of stenosis is determined quite accurately by this technique,[132] and differentiation of severe obstruction from occlusion may be more successful with color flow imaging.

Clinical Applications

Symptomatic Patients

Considerable controversy regarding the role of noninvasive testing in the evaluation of patients with symptomatic cerebrovascular disease still exists and is further complicated by treatment controversies. Noninvasive testing concentrates primarily on the extracranial carotid artery and will not identify intracranial lesions or embolic sources at the heart or aortic arch. The largest percentage of patients with hemispheric or ocular ischemic symptoms, however, do have carotid lesions, and noninvasive testing can provide a safe and inexpensive means to identify most potential surgical candidates for further study with angiography. Duplex scanning, with color flow imaging if available, is probably the best technique for use in these cases.

Patients with an apparent embolic event who have normal carotid arteries or minimal stenosis rarely have surgical lesions. Although it can be argued that Duplex scanning will not identify ulcerations even in normal cases or cases with minimal stenosis, these patients usually will be candidates for medical therapy once other sources are ruled out. If embolic symptoms recur or persist despite medical therapy, angiography is warranted. In this manner, noninvasive testing can identify patients most likely to benefit from further evaluation with angiography for potential surgery. Given the cost and small but definite risk of angiography, such screening is helpful and appropriate. Intravenous DSA has been proposed as a similar type of screening test; however, the expense and technical disadvantages of intravenous DSA, as well as the apparent superior sensitivity of newer noninvasive techniques, make Duplex scanning a much more appropriate choice. Although it has been suggested that selected patients can undergo endarterectomy on the basis of noninvasive testing alone,[51,137] angiography remains the best preoperative evaluation. Duplex scanning, however, is ideal for continued follow-up of patients after endarterectomy.

Asymptomatic Patients

Although the proper treatment of patients with asymptomatic carotid artery disease remains unclear, noninvasive testing techniques are the most appropriate method of evaluating these patients. Duplex scanning can identify patients with hemodynamically significant lesions that should have further study or follow-up. It is the most accurate and sensitive of the noninvasive tests and provides quantitative values that permit comparison of serial examinations. The greater accuracy of MR angiography makes it a potentially better method of screening asymptomatic patients. As it becomes more widely available, MR angiography may supplant Duplex scanning for the screening and follow-up of asymptomatic patients.

Intra- and Postoperative Assessment

The use of intraoperative ultrasound to assess the technical results of carotid endarterectomy can be quite helpful. Defects such as intimal flaps or stenosis at the arteriotomy site that may contribute to postoperative complications can be readily identified. Both Doppler and B-mode ultrasound can be used intraoperatively and can detect technical defects at the time of endarterectomy.[115,156,158]

Noninvasive testing is also useful in following patients after carotid endarterectomy. Clinically significant recurrent stenosis has been reported to occur in less than 5% of cases.[131] Duplex scanning is useful for following patients with recurrent stenosis to identify those with significant progressive narrowing as opposed to those with mild stenosis due to myointimal hyperplasia that usually follows a benign course.[157]

Intracranial Vessels: Transcranial Doppler

Transcranial Doppler (TCD) uses a directional pulsed range-gated transducer to sample flow velocities at selected sites on the large intracranial vessels. Signals are recorded through the 1)thin "temporal windows" to study the MCA, distal ICA, and proximal ACA and PCA, through a 2)transorbital window to study the carotid siphon and ophthalmic artery, and via a 3) transoccipital approach

for the basilar and vertebral arteries. The uses of TCD in ischemic cerebrovascular disease are continuing to be developed, but it is known that the recorded flow velocities imply proportional changes in lumen size and flow quantity.[15,95]

In patients with ischemic symptoms who have normal extracranial noninvasive studies, TCD may offer a noninvasive means of identifying patients with an intracranial stenotic lesion. Lindegaard[94] demonstrated an inverse relationship between TCD velocity recordings and residual intracranial lumen diameter in 11 patients with intracranial occlusive disease. In severe proximal MCA stenosis, a dampened pulse wave with abnormally low velocities may also be seen. The presence of collateral flow patterns toward the involved artery also confirms an occlusive lesion.[32] MCA occlusions can also be detected by TCD, which shows low velocities proximal to the occlusion and absent signal distal to it.[154] This finding could be important in identifying candidates for emergency thrombolytic therapy.

With regard to extracranial cerebrovascular disease, TCD alone is not particularly useful, but it may be helpful as an adjunct to direct noninvasive study of the carotid arteries. By obtaining velocity recordings from the intracranial vessels, particularly the MCA, TCD may provide an assessment of the final hemodynamic effect of the extracranial disease and often the adequacy of collateral blood supply as well. Extracranial carotid stenosis or occlusion is known to have a variable effect on MCA velocity; some patients maintain normal velocity distal to a carotid occlusion. Schneider et al,[125] however, have demonstrated a statistically significant decrease in ipsilateral MCA velocity and pulsatility in 39 patients with ICA occlusions. They were also able to evaluate sources of collateral flow via the circle of Willis. Another study has used TCD recordings of MCA velocity changes induced by carbon dioxide pressure changes as an index of vasomotor reactivity, which was shown to correlate with symptomatic carotid occlusions.[118]

TCD is also proving to be useful for surgical monitoring of CBF changes. Using a headband and a movable probe, TCD has been used to monitor continuous MCA velocities during both carotid endarterectomy and cardiopulmonary bypass[14,97,108] operations. The extent of decrease in MCA velocities during carotid clamping depends on the collateral flow and may indicate the need for shunting. MCA velocity greater than 20 cm/sec usually indicates adequate collateral circulation. Likewise, reduction of MCA velocity less than 65% from preclamped values is consistent with adequate collateral flow. MCA velocity reductions of more than 65% or below 20 cm/sec, however, are usually associated with changes in the somatosensory evoked potential and suggest a dangerous degree of ischemia. In some cases, however, even complete absence of MCA flow on TCD does not lead to somatosensory evoked potential changes.[14] After restoration of carotid flow at the end of an endarterectomy, MCA velocity typically improves proportional to the degree of stenosis that was relieved.[125,126]

Functional Studies: CBF, SPECT, and PET

Accurate evaluation of cerebral ischemia requires the study of actual cerebral perfusion and resultant functional state, in addition to the structural changes examined in the previously described tests. The most widely available functional test has been xenon CBF studies, but recently SPECT has come into wider use. PET scanners remain expensive and require extensive support, limiting their use primarily to larger research centers. All these studies share the ability to evaluate the result of occlusive cerebrovascular disease, regional brain perfusion on a microcirculatory level, and associated cerebral metabolic parameters.

Xenon Cerebral Blood Flow

The value of measuring rCBF has been apparent since the early work with nitrous oxide and hydrogen clearance techniques in the 1940s and 1950s, respectively. Clinically useful noninvasive measurement of rCBF followed in the 1960s using radiolabeled xenon (^{133}Xe). Radioactive xenon may be administered by either direct intra-arterial or intravenous injection or, more commonly, by inhalation of xenon gas. Scintillation counters positioned over the surface of the head allow monitoring of the gamma radiation in various vascular distributions. Using an indicator dilution technique, rCBF values can be calculated. Fine resolution with this technique is not possible: Mean rCBF values, as well as differential flows in the gray and white matter, can be determined mathematically beneath the various detectors but are subject to numerous possible sources of error. The most common sources of error include variations induced by pulmonary disease when using inhaled ^{133}Xe and errors secondary to the so-called look-through phenomenon, in which normal blood flows in deeper structures mask ischemia in more superficial areas. This second type of error plagues both inhalation and injection methods. One distinct advantage for this technique is that monitoring can be performed at bedside using a portable unit that allows serial determinations of rCBF in seriously ill patients (Simonsen Medical, P.O. Box 666, Chesterland, OH, 44026).

Newly developed CT techniques using cold xenon offer greater precision. The xenon CT technique (Xe-CT) allows the separation of flow values from deep and superficial locations, providing regional blood flow information with a relatively high degree of spatial resolution. This improves one of the major problems with the multiple external probe systems, which is the inability to discriminate between deep and superficial regions and their respective blood flows.

The effect of arterial obstruction or stenosis on rCBF depends, of course, on collateral flow. Xe-CT localizes the diminished rCBF in ischemic areas and may demonstrate surrounding hyperemia of "luxury perfusion," which is a common, but transient, phenomenon that may be seen after acute stroke.[106,139] The relationship of rCBF changes to clinical

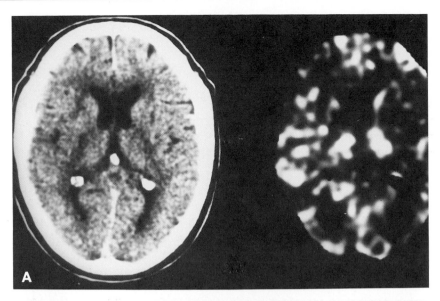

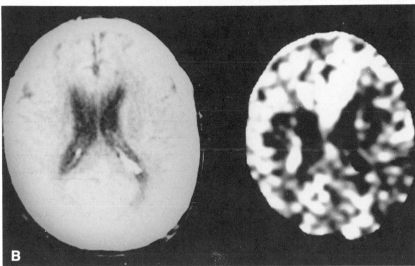

Figure 11. Xenon-enhanced CT cerebral blood flow studies before and after administration of 2 g intravenous Diamox™ in a 64-year-old man with left carotid occlusion and TIAs. The baseline study, before Diamox™, shows diffusely diminished cerebral blood flow (CBF) in the left hemisphere *(A)*. After Diamox™ the CBF in the right hemisphere increases normally, but it remains essentially unchanged in the left MCA distribution, suggesting severe compromise of residual CBF with the presence of little or no functional reserve *(B)*.

findings and prognosis in stroke and TIA has not been completely evaluated. Some studies have shown that lower rCBF after stroke correlates with more severe infarction.[138] Others, however, have found that rCBF is not predictive of outcome in patients with stroke.[28,37] Experimental data also suggest

that some changes in rCBF after infarction may be caused by changes in local neuronal function rather than by cell death.

The utility of CBF evaluation may be increased in the setting of ischemic cerebrovascular disease by combining it with the acetazolamide (Diamox™) challenge test.[29,119] This

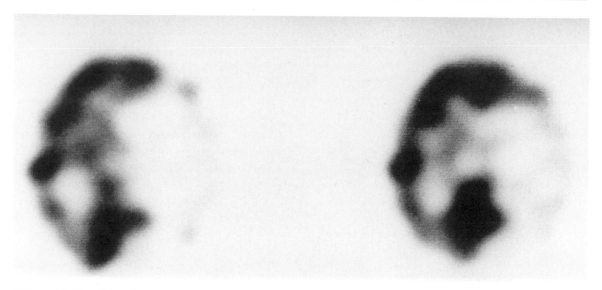

Figure 12. SPECT *study using the IMP tracer demonstrates markedly diminished cerebral blood flow (CBF) in the left MCA distribution of a 57-year-old man 24 hours after the onset of severe hemiparesis and aphasia. SPECT studies often demonstrate earlier and more widespread ischemic changes than shown by CT scans. CBF changes such as those demonstrated in this case carry a poor prognosis for recovery of neurologic function.*

technique identifies patients with diminished or no remaining CBF reserves, so-called misery perfusion, by measuring CBF before and after a flow challenge. Diamox™, given as a 1-gm intravenous injection, will augment CBF 50% to 90% in normal individuals. By demonstrating an absence of augmentation or even decreased rCBF, the Diamox™ test can reveal areas of oligemia with already maximal vasodilatation and no remaining reserves (Figure 11). It has been suggested that this may identify patients who would benefit from surgical revascularization.[55,119,145]

SPECT

SPECT provides metabolic and flow-related information but without the cost and complexity of regular PET scanning. Different radiopharmaceutical tracers allow the study of regional cerebral physiology including blood flow, blood pool, and receptor imaging. The tracer used most often for SPECT is N-isopropyl-[123]P-iodoamphetamine ([123]IMP), which has high first-pass extraction in the

brain and provides quantitative CBF tomograms. Both IMP and another tracer, ^{123}I-labeled propanediamine (HIPDM) cross the blood-brain barrier, then ionize and cannot escape. Their distribution is proportional to blood flow, and they are stable enough to allow the necessary 20 minutes for data acquisition. At our institution we have primarily used IMP SPECT, which provides evidence of perfusion defects in patients with ischemic cerebrovascular disease (Figure 12). A new agent being used increasingly is hexamethylpropyleneamineoxime (HMPAO) labeled with [99m] technetium (^{99m}Tc). [99m]Tc is a better label than ^{123}I because its emission characteristics are more appropriate for scintillation cameras; higher doses can be used; and it is more easily and inexpensively produced than [123]I. The isomers of HMPAO are also distributed in the brain proportional to perfusion and are more stable than the other agents. SPECT shows areas of cerebral infarction after stroke earlier than CT scans and often shows larger areas of abnormality.[25,91] There is some evidence that SPECT studies may provide prognostic information after stroke. Patients with small perfusion defects on early images using the IMP tracer have been shown to have complete or near complete recovery, while almost 50% of patients with large defects have poor outcomes.[68,92] Whether this early prognostic information can be used to improve treatment and outcome, however, has yet to be established.

In the setting of TIAs, in contrast, SPECT studies are often normal or nonspecific.[25,66] This finding provides further evidence that SPECT may primarily reflect neuronal dysfunction rather than blood flow. Another interesting demonstration of functional changes on SPECT is the pattern of decreased flow to the contralateral cerebellar hemisphere as a consequence of a cerebral hemispheric infarction that is distant, but functionally related.[101] This phenomenon, termed *crossed cerebellar diaschisis,* is also demonstrable on PET scans.[11]

SPECT scans utilizing intra-arterial tracer injections have also been used to demonstrate the effects of carotid stenosis and the results of surgery.[67,123] Intra-arterial IMP injection at the time of angiography provides CBF images of the disturbed circulation, whereas contralateral injections may show extensive collaterals. One small series[123] showed improvement in the abnormal region after extracranial-to-intracranial (EC-IC) bypass or carotid endarterectomy.

PET Scanning

Currently, the cost and complexity of PET scanning limit its use in routine clinical evaluation of cerebrovascular disease. There has been considerable study of PET imaging in stroke, however, and it may be useful in select clinical situations. PET scanning allows direct simultaneous measurement of rCBF, oxygen use (rCMRO$_2$), glucose use (rCMRGlu), and the determination of the oxygen extraction ratio (rOER). It has become evident

from PET studies that rCBF alone is a poor indicator of residual tissue function after ischemia. Since oxygen use (rCMRO$_2$) during ischemia is limited by oxygen delivery rather than by cerebral oxygen demand, maximal extraction of available oxygen (rOER) results. Maximal oxygen extraction with continuing ischemia from diminished CBF is another demonstration of misery perfusion, as described earlier, and indicates maximal autoregulatory compensation.

Later, as cellular and mitochondrial functions fail, the rCMRO$_2$ and rOER fall even if rCBF is restored, correlating to the situation of luxury perfusion of an infarcted area.[90,136] Serial studies of acute stroke patients have shown this progression when started early enough, with initial elevation of rOER in scans performed within a few hours of clinical onset. During the subsequent days, rOER drops with associated decreased rCMRO$_2$, even as rCBF stabilizes or improves.[149] Interestingly, rOER tends to drop lower in the white matter and subcortical gray matter in the first few hours or days, then progresses to the overlying cortex, so that deeper structures progress from ischemia to infarction earlier. This progression is probably related to anatomic vascular patterns. Diminished glucose use of ischemic and infarcted areas has been shown to closely parallel and correlate with the drop in rCMRO$_2$.[150] In the late stage, more than 1 month after a cerebral infarction, PET scans demonstrate decreased rCBF and rCMRO$_2$; however, rOER returns to normal, suggesting that the local blood supply, although relatively diminished, is adequate to meet the metabolic requirements of the residual tissue.[114] These findings are seen in cortical or hemispheric strokes only. Studies of lacunar infarctions have failed to show significant cortical metabolic abnormalities.[40] Although SPECT provides some of this information, comparative studies in patients evaluated within 2 hours of TIA or stroke demonstrate that PET has better regional and interhemispheric contrast between high and low metabolic activity and more accurate quantification than SPECT.[62]

PET studies nicely demonstrate the temporal progression of ischemia to infarction. Local rCBF is initially maintained in the setting of large-vessel occlusive disease by autoregulatory dilation of precapillary resistance vessels. Once compensatory vasodilation is maximal (misery perfusion), autoregulation fails and rCBF declines. Local $rCMRO_2$, however, is maintained by increased rOER, which can rise to almost 100%.[49] At that point, a further decrease in rCBF disrupts cellular and mitochondrial function and leads to irreversible infarction. The clinical challenge remains to use the information provided by PET scanning to intervene and reverse this chain of events.

Ideally, the best use of PET would be the identification of patients with misery perfusion who would be best suited for intervention to restore blood flow. Studies have shown that this mismatching of CBF and $CMRO_2$ was present in only a minority of patients considered for EC-IC bypass,[52,56] but that the abnormal pattern of raised rOER can be reversed by surgical intervention.[82,89,107] It has become clear from PET studies that the extent of circulating reserves is more important than absolute CBF in patients with ischemic cerebrovascular disease. Although PET remains primarily a research tool, its ability to measure cerebral circulatory reserves by defining the relationship among CBF, $CMRO_2$, and OER may provide a valuable tool to determine patients most at risk for OCD, patients most likely to benefit from surgical intervention, and the efficacy of therapies.

Conclusion

A wide range of diagnostic tests is available for the evaluation of ischemic cerebrovascular disease, with an equally wide range of efficacy, risk, and cost. Most patients can be adequately evaluated with CT or MR imaging scans, along with initial evaluation of their carotid arteries by Duplex ultrasound or MR angiography where available. We have recently found that MR imaging combined with MR angiography is an ideal initial test for many patients presenting with TIAs or stroke. It provides a sensitive evaluation of cerebral infarctions as well as increasingly accurate information about large-vessel pathology with a single, noninvasive study. At present, we would still recommend intra-arterial angiography before surgical intervention, but further advances in MR angiography may make this test unnecessary in the near future.

A small proportion of patients with less clearly defined ischemic syndromes may benefit from additional testing to detect more subtle changes in cerebral hemodynamics, residual function, or potential collateral. We have found that Xe-CT CBF with a Diamox challenge test is very useful in evaluating many of these patients, although SPECT will also provide the same information. PET scans would obviously offer even greater sensitivity in evaluating these complex patients, but they are not widely available.

The challenge in evaluating ischemic cerebrovascular disease remains to identify patients at risk for stroke before irreversible infarction occurs. Although recent advances in diagnostic studies are providing better means of evaluating and identifying these patients, angiography remains the gold standard test to which all other studies must be compared. It is hoped that improvements in noninvasive studies, particularly MR angiography, will continue to reduce the need for angiography with its attendant risks. The demonstrated potential to reduce the stroke rate by surgical intervention makes it imperative to identify patients at risk before infarction. This goal can only be achieved by an aggressive and thorough approach to the evaluation of patients with ischemic cerebrovascular symptoms.

References

1. AbuRahma AF, Diethrich EB. Comparison of various oculoplethysmography modalities. *J Vasc Surg.* 1985;2:288-291.
2. Aulich A, Wende S, Fenske A, et al. Diagnosis and follow-up studies in cerebral infarcts. In Lanksch W, Kazner E; eds. *Cranial Computerized Tomography.* Berlin, Germany; New York, NY: Springer-Verlag; 1976;273-283.

3. Awad I, Modic M, Little JR, et al. Focal parenchymal lesions in transient ischemic attacks: correlation of computed tomography and magnetic resonance imaging. *Stroke*. 1986;17:399-403.

4. Azzopardi D, Wyatt JS, Cady EB, et al. Prognosis of newborn infants with hypoxic-ischemic brain injury assessed by phosphorus magnetic resonance spectroscopy. *Pediatr Res*. 1989;25:445-451.

5. Baker JD. How vascular surgeons use noninvasive testing. *J Vasc Surg*. 1986;4:272-276.

6. Baker JD, Barker WF, Machleder HI. Ocular pneumoplethysmography in the evaluation of carotid stenosis. *Circulation*. 1980;62(suppl 1):I1-I3.

7. Bakke SJ, Nakstad PH, Aakhus T. Intravenous digital subtraction angiography of the precerebral and cerebral arteries in patients with TIA: a comparison with conventional angiography. *Eur J Radiol*. 1988;8:140-144.

8. Ball JB Jr, Lukin RR, Tomsick TA, et al. Complications of intravenous digital subtraction angiography. *Arch Neurol*. 1985;42:969-972.

9. Barnes RW, Russell HE, Bone GE, et al. Doppler cerebrovascular examination: improved results with refinements in technique. *Stroke*. 1977;8:468-471.

10. Barnett FJ, Lecky DM, Freiman DB, et al. Cerebrovascular disease: outpatient evaluation with selective carotid DSA performed via a transbrachial approach. *Radiology*. 1989;170:535-539.

11. Baron JC, Bousser MG, Comar D, et al. "Crossed cerebellar diaschisis" in human supratentorial brain infarction. *Trans Am Neurol Assoc*. 1980;105:459-461.

12. Becker H, Desch H, Hacker H, et al. CT fogging effect with ischemic cerebral infarcts. *Neuroradiology*. 1979;18:185-192.

13. Bendel P, Buonocore E, Bockisch A, et al. Blood flow in the carotid arteries: quantification by using phase-sensitive MR imaging. *AJR*. 1989;152:1307-1310.

14. Bernstein EF. Role of transcranial Doppler in carotid surgery. *Surg Clin North Am*. 1990;70:225-234.

15. Bishop CCR, Powell S, Rutt D, et al. Transcranial Doppler measurement of middle cerebral artery blood flow velocity: a validation study. *Stroke*. 1986;17:913-915.

16. Blaisdell FW, Glickman M, Trunkey DD. Ulcerated atheroma of the carotid artery. *Arch Surg*. 1974;108:491-496.

17. Blasberg DJ. Duplex sonography for carotid artery disease: an accurate technique. *AJNR*. 1982;3:609-614.

18. Bogousslavsky J, Regli F. Cerebral infarction with transient signs (CITS): do TIAs correspond to small deep infarcts in internal carotid artery occlusion? *Stroke*. 1984;15:536-539.

19. Bonafe A, Manelfe C, Scotto B, et al. Role of computed tomography in vertebrobasilar ischemia. *Neuroradiology*. 1985;27:484-493.

20. Bories J, Derhy S, Chiras J. CT in hemispheric ischaemic attacks. *Neuroradiology*. 1985;27:468-483.

21. Bozzao L, Fantozzi LM, Bastianello S, et al. Occlusion of the extracranial internal carotid artery in the acute stroke: angiographic findings within 6 hours. *Acta Neurochir (Wien)*. 1989;100:39-42.

22. Brant-Zawadzki M, Pereira B, Weinstein P, et al. MR imaging of acute experimental ischemia in cats. *AJNR*. 1986;7:7-11.

23. Brant-Zawadzki M, Weinstein P, Pereira, B, et al. MRI of acute experimental infarction in the cat. *AJNR*. 1985;6:477.

24. Brockenbrough EC. Periorbital Doppler velocity evaluation of carotid obstruction. In Bernstein EF, ed. *Noninvasive Diagnostic Techniques in Vascular Disease*. St. Louis, MO: The C.V. Mosby Company; 1985:335-341.

25. Brott TG, Gelfand MJ, Williams CC, et al. Frequency and patterns of abnormality detected by iodine-123 amine emission CT after cerebral infarction. *Radiology*. 1986;158:729-734.

26. Brown JJ, Hesselink JR, Rothrock JF. MR and CT of lacunar infarcts. *AJR*. 1988;151:367-372.

27. Bunt TJ. Complete cerebral angiography in the evaluation of patients with cerebrovascular insufficiency. *Am Surg*. 1988;54:617-620.

28. Burke AM, Younkin D, Gordon J, et al. Changes in cerebral blood flow and recovery from acute stroke. *Stroke*. 1986;17:173-178.

29. Burt RW, Reddy RV, Mock BM, et al. Acetazolamide enhancement of HIPDM brain flow distribution imaging. *J Nucl Med*. 1986;27:1627-1631.

30. Calandre L, Gomara S, Bermejo F, et al. Clinical-CT correlations in TIA, RIND, and strokes with minimum residuum. *Stroke*. 1984;15:663-666.

31. Campbell JK, Houser OW, Stevens JC, et al. Computed tomography and radionuclide imaging in the evaluation of ischemic stroke. *Radiology*. 1978;126:695-702.

32. Caplan LR, Brass LM, DeWitt LD, et al. Transcranial Doppler ultrasound: present status. *Neurology*. 1990;40:696-700.

33. Chamber BR, Norris JW. Outcome in patients with asymptomatic neck bruits. *N Engl J Med*. 1986;315:860-865.

34. Crowell RM, Ojemann RG. Extracranial cerebrovascular disease. In Hoff JT, ed. *Practice of Surgery*. Philadelphia, Pa: Harper & Row; 1981.

35. Culebras A, Magaña R, Cacayorin ED. Computed tomography of the cervical carotid artery: significance of the lucent defect. *Stroke*. 1988;19:723-727.

36. Dávolos A, Matias-Guiu J, Torrent O, et al. Computed tomography in reversible ischaemic attacks: clinical and prognostic correlations in a prospective study. *J Neurol*. 1988;235:155-158.

37. Demeurisse G, Verhas M, Capon A, et al. Lack of evolution of the cerebral blood flow during clinical recovery of a stroke. *Stroke*. 1983;14:77-81.

38. Dennis M, Bamford J, Sandercock P, et al. Computed tomography in patients with transient ischaemic attacks: when is a transient ischaemic attack not a transient ischemic attack but a stroke? *J Neurol*. 1990;237:257-261.

39. DeWitt LD, Kistler JP, Miller DC, et al. NMR-neuropathologic correlation in stroke. *Stroke*. 1987;18:342-351.

40. DiPiero V, Lenzi GL, Fieschi C. Positron emission tomography: applications in the study of lacunar infarcts. *Eur Neurol*. 1989;29(suppl 2):39-41.

41. Dixon S, Paiz SO, Raviola C, et al. Natural history of nonstenotic, asymptomatic ulcerative lesions of the carotid artery: a further analysis. *Arch Surg*. 1982;117:1493-1498.

42. Donnon GA, Tress BM, Bladin PF. A prospective study of lacunar infarction using computerized tomography. *Neurology*. 1982;32:49-56.

43. Duncan GW, Gruber JO, Dewey CF Jr, et al. Evalua-

tion of carotid stenosis by phonoangiography. *N Engl J Med*. 1975;293:1124-1128.

44. Earnest F IV, Forbes G, Sandok BA, et al. Complications of cerebral angiography: prospective assessment of risk. *AJR*. 1984;142:247-253.

45. Edwards JH, Kricheff II, Riles T, et al. Angiographically undetected ulceration of the carotid bifurcation as a cause of embolic stroke. *Radiology*. 1979; 132:369-373.

46. Evans WE, Hayes JP. Life history of patients with transient ischemic attacks and essentially normal angiograms. *J Vasc Surg*. 1987;6:548-552.

47. Folger WN. Non-invasive studies. In Sundt TM Jr, ed. *Occlusive Cerebrovascular Disease: Diagnosis and Surgical Management*. Philadelphia, Pa: W.B. Saunders Company; 1987:71-81.

48. Ford CS, Frye JL, Toole JF, et al. Asymptomatic carotid bruit and stenosis: a prospective follow-up study. *Arch Neurol*. 1986;43:219-222.

49. Frackowiak RSJ. Clinical application of positron tomographic studies in cerebrovascular disease. *Am J Physiol Imaging*. 1988;3:24-25.

50. Gee W, Oller DW, Wylie EJ. Noninvasive diagnosis of carotid occlusion by ocular pneumoplethysmography. *Stroke*. 1976;7:18-21.

51. Gelabert HA, Moore WS. Carotid endarterectomy without angiography. *Surg Clin North Am*. 1990;70: 213-223.

52. Gibbs JM, Wise RJS, Leenders KL, et al. Evaluation of cerebral perfusion reserve in patients with carotid-artery occlusion. *Lancet*. 1984;1:310-314.

53. Glover JL, Bendick PJ, Jackson VP, et al. Duplex ultrasonography, digital subtraction angiography, and conventional angiography in assessing carotid atherosclerosis. *Arch Surg*. 1984;119:664-669.

54. Gomes AS, Lois JF, Baker JD, et al. Acute renal dysfunction in high-risk patients after angiography: comparison of ionic and nonionic contrast media. *Radiology*. 1989;170:65-68.

55. Grahm TW, Spetzler RF, Hodak JA, et al. The use of computed tomography/cortical blood flow studies to determine patient eligibility for extracranial-intracranial bypass. *BNI Quarterly*. 1990;6:17-21.

56. Grubb RL, Jr, Ratcheson RA, Raichle ME, et al. Regional cerebral blood flow and oxygen utilization in superficial temporal-middle cerebral artery anastomosis patients. *J Neurosurg*. 1979;50:733-741.

57. Hankey GJ, Warlow CP, Molyneux AJ. Complications of cerebral angiography for patients with mild carotid territory ischaemia being considered for carotid endarterectomy. *J Neurol Neurosurg Psychiatry*. 1990;53:542-548.

58. Hankey GJ, Warlow CP, Sellar RJ. Cerebral angiographic risk in mild cerebrovascular disease. *Stroke*. 1990;21:209-222.

59. Hayman LA, Evans RA, Bastion FO, et al. Delayed high dose contrast CT: identifying patients at risk of massive hemorrhagic infarction. *AJNR*. 1981; 2:139-147.

60. Heinz ER, Fuchs J, Osborne D, et al. Examination of the extracranial carotid bifurcation by thin-section dynamic CT: direct visualization of intimal atheroma in man (part 2). *AJNR*. 1984;5:361-366.

61. Heinz ER, Pizer SM, Fuchs H, et al. Examination of the extracranial carotid bifurcation by thin-section dynamic CT: direct visualization of intimal atheroma in man (part 1). *AJNR*. 1984;5:355-359.

62. Heiss W-D, Herholz K, Podreka I, et al. Comparison of [^{99}mTC]HMPAO SPECT with [^{18}F] fluoromethane PET in cerebrovascular disease. *J Cereb Blood Flow Metab*. 1990;10:687-697.

63. Hessel SJ, Adams DF, Abrams HL. Complications of angiography. *Radiology*. 1981;138:273-281.

64. Heyman A, Wilkinson WE, Heyden S, et al. Risk of stroke in asymptomatic persons with cervical arterial bruits: a population study in Evans County, Georgia. *N Engl J Med*. 1980;302:838-841.

65. Hicks ME, Kreipke DL, Becker GJ, et al. Cerebrovascular disease: evaluation with transbrachial intra-arterial digital subtraction angiography using a 4-F catheter. *Radiology*. 1986;161:545-546.

66. Hill TC, Holman BL, Lovett R, et al. Initial experience with SPECT (single-photon computerized tomography) of the brain using N-isopropyl I-123 p-iodoamphetamine: concise communication. *J Nucl Med*. 1982;23:191-195.

67. Hill TC, Holman BL, Magistrette PL. SPECT and N-isopropyl I-123 p-iodoamphetamine (IMP): quantitative assessment of changes in regional brain perfusion related to medical and surgical therapy. In: Raynaud C, ed. *Nuclear Medicine and Biology Advances: Proceedings of the Third World Congress of Nuclear Medicine and Biology, August 29 to September 2 1982, Paris, France*. Oxford, England: Pergamon; 1983:1735-1738.

68. Hill TC, Magistrette PL, Holman BL, et al. Assessment of regional cerebral blood flow (rCBF) in stroke using SPECT and N-isopropyl-(I-123)-p-iodoamphetamine (IMP). *Stroke*. 1984;15:40-45.

69. Houser OW, Campbell JK. Computed tomography in cerebrovascular disease: influences on morphology, topography, clinical factors, and temporal profile. In Moossy J, Reinmuth OM, eds. *Cerebrovascular Diseases, Twelfth Research (Princeton) Conference*. New York, NY: Raven Press; 1981:181-188.

70. Houser OW, Campbell JK, Baker HL Jr. Computed tomography and magnetic resonance imaging, with emphasis on computed tomography. In Sundt TM Jr; ed. *Occlusive Cerebrovascular Disease: Diagnosis and Surgical Management*. Philadelphia, PA: W.B. Saunders Company; 1987:139-162.

71. Houser, OW, Sundt TM Jr. Correlation of angiographic flow patterns with syndromes of ischemic stroke. In Sundt TM Jr, ed. *Occlusive Cerebrovascular Disease: Diagnosis and Surgical Management*. Philadelphia, PA: W.B. Saunders Company; 1987: 101-107.

72. Houser OW, Sundt TM Jr, Holman CB, et al. Atheromatous disease of the carotid artery: correlation of angiographic, clinical, and surgical findings. *J Neurosurg*. 1974;41:321-331.

73. Howard G, Jones AM, Chambless L, et al. A multicenter validation of Doppler ultrasound versus angiogram: the ACAS experience. *Stroke*. 1991;22:147. Abstract.

74. Imakita S, Nishimura T, Naito H, et al. Magnetic resonance imaging of human cerebral infarction: enhancement with Gd-DTPA. *Neuroradiology*. 1987; 29:422-429.

75. Johnston KW, Baker WH, Burnham SJ, et al. Quantitative analysis of continuous-wave Doppler spectral broadening for the diagnosis of carotid disease: results of a multicenter study. *J Vasc Surg*. 1986; 4:493-504.

76. Kartchner, MM, McRae LP, Morrison FD. Noninvasive detection and evaluation of carotid occlusive disease. *Arch Surg.* 1973;106:528-535.

77. Kaye AH, Little JR, Bryerton B, et al. Intravenous digital subtraction angiography in the assessment of patients for carotid endarterectomy. *J Neurosurg.* 1983;59:835-838.

78. Keagy BA, Pharr WF, Thomas DD, et al. Oculoplethysmography/carotid phonoangiography: its value as a screening test in patients with suspected carotid artery stenosis. *Arch Surg.* 1980;115:1199-1202.

79. Kendall BE, Pullicino P. Intravascular contrast injection in ischaemic lesions, II: effect on prognosis. *Neuroradiology.* 1980;19:241-243.

80. Kingsley DPE, Radue EW, Du Boulay EPGH. Evaluation of computed tomography in vascular lesions of the vertebrobasilar territory. *J Neurol Neurosurg Psychiatry.* 1980;43:193-197.

81. Kinkel PR, Kinkel WR, Jacobs L: Nuclear magnetic resonance imaging in patients with stroke. *Semin Neurol.* 1986;6:43-52.

82. Kinkel WR, Jacobs L, Polachini I, et al. Subcortical arteriosclerotic encephalopathy (Binswanger's disease): computed tomographic, nuclear magnetic resonance, and clinical correlations. *Arch Neurol.* 1985;42:951-959.

83. Kistler JP, Lees RS, Miller A, et al. Correlation of spectral phonoangiography and carotid angiography with gross pathology in carotid stenosis. *N Engl J Med.* 1981;305:417-419.

84. Komatsumoto S, Nioka S, Greenberg JH, et al. Cerebral energy metabolism measured in vivo by ^{31}P-NMR in middle cerebral artery occlusion in the cat: relation to severity of stroke. *J Cereb Blood Flow Metab.* 1987;7:557-562.

85. Kucharczyk J, Chew W, Derugin N, et al. Nicardipine reduces ischemic brain injury: magnetic resonance imaging/spectroscopy study in cats. *Stroke.* 1989;20:268-274.

86. Kucharczyk J, Moseley M, Kurhanewicz J, et al. MRS of ischemic/hypoxic brain disease. *Invest Radiol.* 1989;24:951-954.

87. Ladurner G, Sager WD, Iliff LD, et al. A correlation of clinical findings and CT in ischaemic cerebrovascular disease. *Eur Neurol.* 1979;18:281-288.

88. Laerum F. Cytotoxic effects of six angiographic contrast media on human endothelium in culture. *Acta Radiol.* 1987;28:99-105.

89. Laerum F, Dehner LP, Rysavy J, et al. Double blind evaluation of the effects of various contrast media on extremity veins in the dog. *Acta Radiol.* 1987;28:107-113.

90. Lassen NA: The luxury-perfusion syndrome and its possible relation to acute metabolic acidosis localized within the brain. *Lancet.* 1966;2:1113-1115.

91. Lee RGL, Hill TC, Holman BL, et al. N-isopropyl (I-123) *p*-iodoamphetamine brain scans with single-photon emission tomography: discordance with transmission computed tomography. *Radiology.* 1982;145:795-799.

92. Lee RGL, Hill TC, Holman BL, et al. Predictive value of perfusion defect size using N-isopropyl-(I-123)-P-iodoamphetamine emission tomography in acute stroke. *J Neurosurg.* 1984;61:449-452.

93. Leow K, Murie JA. Cerebral angiography for cerebrovascular disease: the risks. *Br J Surg.* 1988; 75:428-430.

94. Lindegaard K-F, Bakke SJ, Sorteberg W, et al. A non-invasive Doppler ultrasound method for the evaluation of patients with subarachnoid hemorrhage. *Acta Radiol.* 1986;369(suppl):96-98.

95. Lindegaard K-F, Lundar T, Wiberg J, et al. Variations in middle cerebral artery blood flow investigated with noninvasive transcranial blood velocity measurements. *Stroke.* 1987;18:1025-1030.

96. Lippman HH, Sundt TM Jr, Holman CB: The poststenotic carotid slim sign: spurious internal carotid hypolasia. *Mayo Clin Proc.* 1970;45:762-767.

97. Lundar T, Lindegaard K-F, Frøysaker T, et al. Cerebral perfusion during nonpulsatile cardiopulmonary bypass. *Ann Thorac Surg.* 1985;40:144-150.

98. Martin NA, Hadley MN, Spetzler RF, et al. Management of asymptomatic carotid atherosclerosis. *Neurosurgery.* 1986;18:505-513.

99. Masaryk TJ, Modic MT, Ross JS, et al. Intracranial circulation: preliminary clinical results with three-dimensional (volume) MR angiography. *Radiology.* 1989;171:793-799.

100. McIvor J, Steiner TJ, Perkin GD, et al. Neurological morbidity of arch and carotid arteriography in cerebrovascular disease. The influence of contrast medium and radiologist. *Br J Radiol.* 1987;60:117-122.

101. Meneghetti G, Vorstrup S, Mickey B, et al. Crossed cerebellar diaschisis in ischemic stroke: a study of regional cerebral blood flow by ^{133}Xe inhalation and single photon emission computerized tomography. *J Cereb Blood Flow Metab.* 1984;4:235-240.

102. Middleton WD, Middleton MA. Color Doppler ultrasonography. *Curr Opin Radiol.* 1990;2:229-236.

103. Mohr JP, Caplan LR, Melski JW, et al. The Harvard cooperative stroke registry: a prospective registry. *Neurology.* 1978;28:754-762.

104. Moneta GL, Taylor DC, Strandness E Jr. Noninvasive assessment of cerebrovascular disease. *Ann Vasc Surg.* 1986;1:489-501.

105. Moore WS, Malone JM, Boren C, et al. Asymptomatic ulcerative lesions of the carotid artery: natural history and effect of surgical therapy compared. *Stroke.* 1979;10:96.

106. Olsen TS, Larsen B, Skriver EB, et al. Focal cerebral hyperemia in acute stroke: incidence, pathophysiology, and clinical significance. *Stroke.* 1981;12:598-607.

107. Osborne RW, Malone JM, Hunter GC, et al. Endothelial fibrinolytic activity: the key to postangiographic thrombosis? *Surg Forum.* 1981;32:328-330.

108. Padayachee TS, Gosling RG, Bishop CC, et al. Monitoring middle cerebral artery blood velocity during carotid endarterectomy. *Br J Surg.* 1986;73:98-100.

109. Pelz DM, Fox AJ, Vinuela F. Digital subtraction angiography: current clinical applications. *Stroke.* 1985;16:528-536.

110. Pessin MS, Duncan GW, Davis KR, et al. Angiographic appearance of carotid occlusion in acute stroke. *Stroke.* 1980;11:485-487.

111. Pessin MS, Duncan GW, Mohr JP, et al. Clinical and angiographic features of carotid transient ischemic attacks. *N Engl J Med.* 1977;296:358-362.

112. Pfeiffer FE, Homburger HA, Houser OW, et al. Elevation of serum creatine kinase B-subunit levels by radiographic contrast agents in patients with neurologic disorders. *Mayo Clin Proc.* 1987; 62:351-357.

113. Pistolesi GF, Maso R, Filosto L, et al. Le rôle de l'angiographie numerique par voie intra-veineuse

dans l'étude de l'ischémie cérébrale régressive. *J Radiol.* 1986;67:87-94. English abstract.

114. Powers WJ, Raichle ME. Positron emission tomography and its application to the study of cerebrovascular disease in man. *Stroke.* 1985;16:361-376.

115. Pullicino P, Kendall BE. Contrast enhancement in ischaemic lesions, I: relationship to prognosis. *Neuroradiology.* 1980;19:235-239.

116. Pullicino P, Nelson RF, Kendall BE, et al. Small deep infarcts diagnosed on computed tomography. *Neurology.* 1980;30:1090-1096.

117. Ramadan NM, Deveshwar R, Levine SR. Magnetic resonance and clinical cerebrovascular disease: an update. *Stroke.* 1989;20:1279-1283.

118. Ringelstein EB, Sievers C, Ecker S, et al. Noninvasive assessment of CO_2-induced cerebral vasomotor response in normal individuals and patients with internal carotid artery occlusions. *Stroke.* 1988; 19:963-969.

119. Rogg J, Rutigliano M, Yonas H, et al. The acetazolamide challenge: imaging techniques designed to evaluate cerebral blood flow reserve. *AJR.* 1989; 153:605-612.

120. Rose JS. Contrast media, complications, and preparation of the patient. In Rutherford RB, ed. *Vascular Surgery.* 2nd ed. Philadelphia, PA: W.B. Saunders Company; 1984:244-252.

121. Ross JS, Masaryk TJ, Modic MT, et al. Magnetic resonance angiography of the extracranial carotid arteries and intracranial vessels: a review. *Neurology.* 1989;39:1369-1376.

122. Rothrock JF, Lyden PD, Yee J, et al. 'Crescendo' transient ischemic attacks: clinical and angiographic correlations. *Neurology.* 1988;38:198-201.

123. Royal HD, Hill TC, Holman BL. Clinical brain imaging with isopropyl-iodoamphetamine and SPECT. *Semin Nucl Med.* 1985;15:357-375.

124. Salgado ED, Weinstein M, Furlan AJ, et al. Proton magnetic resonance imaging in ischemic cerebrovascular disease. *Ann Neurol.* 1986;20:502-507.

125. Schneider PA, Rossman ME, Bernstein EF, et al. Effects of internal carotid artery occlusion on intracranial hemodynamics: transcranial Doppler evaluation and clinical correlation. *Stroke.* 1988;19: 589-593.

126. Schneider PA, Rossman ME, Otis SM, et al. Transcranial Doppler monitoring during carotid arterial surgery. *Surg Forum.* 1987;38:333.

127. Shuaib A, Hachinski VC. Carotid transient ischemic attacks and normal investigations: a follow-up study. *Stroke.* 1990;21:525-527.

128. Shuaib A, Hachinski VC, Oczkowski WJ. Transient ischemic attacks and normal cerebral angiograms: a follow-up study. *Stroke.* 1988;19:1223-1228.

129. Spetzler RF, Zabramski JM, Kaufman B, et al. Preliminary laboratory and clinical evaluation of focal cerebral ischemia. *J Cereb Blood Flow Metab.* 1983;3(suppl 1):S87-S88.

130. Spetzler RF, Zabramski JM, Kaufman B, et al. Acute NMR changes during MCA occlusion: a preliminary study in primates. *Stroke.* 1983;14:185-191.

131. Stoney RJ, String ST. Recurrent carotid stenosis. *Surgery.* 1976;80:705-710.

132. Sumner DS. Use of color-flow imaging technique in carotid artery disease. *Surg Clin North Am.* 1990; 70:201-211.

133. Sumner DS, Moore DJ, Miles RD. Doppler ultrasonic arteriography and flow velocity analysis in carotid artery disease. In Bernstein EF, ed. *Noninvasive Diagnostic Techniques in Vascular Disease.* St. Louis, Mo: The C.V. Mosby Company; 1985:349-366.

134. Sundt TM Jr, Houser OW, Fode NC, et al. Correlation of postoperative and two-year follow-up angiography with neurological function in 99 carotid endarterectomies in 86 consecutive patients. *Ann Surg.* 1986;203:90-100.

135. Theodotou BC, Whaley R, Mahaley MS. Complications following transfemoral cerebral angiography for cerebral ischemia: report of 159 angiograms and correlation with surgical risk. *Surg Neurol.* 1987; 28:90-92.

136. Thomas DGT, Gibbs JM, Wise RJS. Use of positron emission tomography scanning in cerebral ischemia. *Clin Neurosurg.* 1985;32:51-69.

137. Thomas GI, Jones TW, Stavney LS, et al. Carotid endarterectomy after Doppler ultrasonographic examination without angiography. *Am J Surg.* 1986;151: 616-619.

138. Tolonen U, Ahonen A, Sulg A, et al. Serial measurements of quantitative EEG and cerebral blood flow and circulation time after brain infarction. *Acta Neurol Scand.* 1981;63:145-155.

139. Traupe H, Kruse E, Heiss W-D. Reperfusion of focal ischemia of varying duration: postischemic hyper- and hypo-perfusion. *Stroke.* 1982;13:615-622.

140. Tress BM, Davis S, Lavain J, et al. Incremental dynamic computed tomography: practical method of imaging the carotid bifurcation. *AJR.* 1986;146: 465-470.

141. Turner WH, Murie JA. Intravenous digital subtraction angiography for extracranial carotid artery disease. *Br J Surg.* 1989;76:1247-1250.

142. Turnipseed WD, Acher CW. The diagnostic interface between noninvasive cerebral vascular testing and digital arteriography. *J Vasc Surg.* 1986;3: 486-492.

143. Unger EC, Gado MH, Fulling KF, et al. Acute cerebral infarction in monkeys: an experimental study using MR imaging. *Radiology.* 1987;162:789-795.

144. Virapongse C, Mancuso A, Quisling R. Human brain infarcts: Gd-DTPA-enhanced MR imaging. *Radiology.* 1986;161:785-794.

145. Vorstrup S, Paulson OB, Lassen NA. How to identify hemodynamic cases. In Spetzler RF, Carter LP, Selman WR, et al, eds. *Cerebral Revascularization for Stroke.* New York, NY: Thieme-Stratton, Inc; 1985:120-126.

146. Wang A-M, Lin JC-T, Rumbaugh CL. What is expected of CT in the evaluation of stroke? *Neuroradiology.* 1988;30:54-58.

147. Waxman SG, Toole JF. Temporal profile resembling TIA in the setting of cerebral infarction. *Stroke.* 1983;14:433-437.

148. Weisberg LA. Lacunar infarcts: clinical and computed tomographic correlations. *Arch Neurol.* 1982; 39:37-40.

149. Wise RJS, Berndardi S, Frackowiak RSJ, et al. Serial observations on the pathophysiology of acute stroke: the transition from ischaemia to infarction as reflected in regional oxygen extraction. *Brain.* 1983; 106:197-222.

150. Wise RJS, Rhodes CG, Gibbs JM, et al. Disturbance

of oxidative metabolism of glucose in recent human cerebral infarcts. *Ann Neurol.* 1983;14:627-637.

151. Wolf PA, Kannel WB, Gordon T, et al. Asymptomatic carotid bruit and risk of stroke: the Framingham study. *Stroke.* 1979;10:96.

152. Yates PO, Hutchinson EC. *Cerebral infarction: the role of the stenosis of the extracranial cerebral arteries.* London: *Med Res Counc Spec Rep* (London) 1961;300:1-95.

153. Zabramski JM, Spetzler RF, Kaufman B. Magnetic resonance imaging: comparative study of radiofrequency pulse techniques in the evaluation of focal ischemia. *Neurosurgery.* 1985;16:502-510.

154. Zanette EM, Fieschi C, Bozzao L, et al. Comparison of cerebral angiography and transcranial Doppler sonography in acute stroke. *Stroke.* 1989;20:899-903.

155. Zeitler E, Seyfarth W, Richter EJ, et al. The value of angiography in cerebrovascular disease. *Thorac Cardiovasc Surg.* 1989;37:259-263.

156. Zierler RE, Bandyk DF, Thiele BL: Intraoperative assessment of carotid endarterectomy. *J Vasc Surg.* 1984;1:73-83.

157. Zierler RE, Bandyk DF, Thiele BL, et al. Carotid artery stenosis following endarterectomy. *Arch Surg.* 1982;117:1408-1415.

158. Zülch KJ. Cerebrovascular pathology and pathogenesis as a basis of neuroradiological diagnosis. In: Diethelm L, Wende S, eds. *Rontgendiagnostik des Zendralnervensystems. Teil 1A.*Berlin, Germany: Springer-Verlag; 1985:1-192.

CHAPTER 5

Doppler Ultrasonography in Occlusive Cerebrovascular Disease

Pierre B. Fayad, MD, and Lawrence M. Brass, MD

Since the introduction of continuous-wave Doppler ultrasound, noninvasive testing of the cerebral circulation has become an integral part in the management of occlusive cerebrovascular disease. The benign nature of the technique, the ease of its application, and its low cost have made it widely available and applied. Advances in instrumentation and imaging quality, have significantly decreased interexaminer variability and improved reliability. Duplex scans are used routinely in the evaluation of cerebral ischemia, while the recent addition of color Doppler imaging has further enhanced sensitivity.

The recent introduction of Transcranial Doppler (TCD) in 1982 by Aaslid,[2] has expanded the potentials of ultrasound for the evaluation of the intracranial circulation, previously accessible only to contrast angiography. TCD's utility in assessing many forms of cerebrovascular disease is already established.[16,41] New applications are still being explored and reported each year. Established applications are further strengthened by these technologic advancements.

With the increasing reliance on noninvasive techniques for the assessment of the cerebral circulation, knowledge and familiarity with ultrasound techniques become a necessity. This chapter reviews the basic concepts of ultrasound, the different techniques available, and their current clinical applications in the evaluation and management of occlusive cerebrovascular diseases.

Principles of Doppler Ultrasound

Vascular ultrasound imaging is based on characteristics differentials between incident and reflected sound beams as they interact with tissue. Interaction is influenced by the acoustic variables of the tissue, which include pressure, density, temperature, and particle motion.[32] Sound *propagation* velocity increases with higher tissue stiffness (resistance to compression). Intensity and amplitude *attenuation* of the traveling sound by tissues, is due to absorption and scattering of sound energy. Greater sound attenuation occurs with higher frequencies and longer travel paths. Although higher frequencies provide improved resolution, lower frequencies penetrate tissues better and allow the insonation of deep vessels, especially when located behind the skull.

When the insonated object is in motion (e.g. red blood cells, platelets), the reflected signal travels with a different frequency (frequency or Doppler shift) than the incident sound beam (Doppler principle). This Doppler effect can be compared to the change in energy in a baseball after it has been hit by a bat. The frequency shift is directly proportional to the velocity of the traveling reflector. The latter can be calculated when the angle of insonation is known. For technical reasons, the angle of insonation is either measured or estimated by the instruments used.

Two techniques of sound generation are used. The emitted signal can be either uninterrupted (continuous-wave), or intermittent (pulsed-wave). The frequency shift measured by continuous-wave Doppler is caused by all the structures on the path of the sound beam. These measurements are less focused, since the effects of heterogeneous structures not intended as part of the exam are also represented. In pulsed-wave ultrasound, the transmission consists of short bursts of sound, separated by periods of silence. By activating the receiver at a particular time after pulse emission, the reflected sound from structures at certain depths can be selectively measured (range gating). This technique allows the study of relatively small selected volumes of tissue or vessel segments at different depths.

The spectrum of sounds captured by the probe represents the sound reflections from many cells. This spectrum is filtered and divided into frequency ranges through a Fast Fourier Transform Spectral Analyzer. The frequency range can be analyzed acoustically as in conventional Doppler or displayed on a screen. Knowledge of the angle of insonation, allows the calculation of velocities from the measured frequency. Analysis of the amplitude of each frequency is represented as density, or brightness.

Measurements in Ultrasonography

Cerebral blood velocities, like cerebral blood flow (CBF), are determined by the pressure gradient, the cross-sectional area, and the blood viscosity across the vessel. A major determinant of blood viscosity is the hematocrit,[13] which accounts for 60% of its effect; while fibrinogen may be an important factor in older individuals.[5] Other variables that may affect cerebral blood velocities include age, end-tidal CO_2, intracranial pressure (ICP), and brain activation (metabolic demands).

Peak-systolic, end-diastolic, and mean blood velocities can be measured directly from the time-velocity waveform. The direction of blood flow toward or away from the probe can be determined. Under certain conditions, peak-systolic velocities tend to correlate with the severity of arterial narrowing, while end-diastolic velocities correlate better with blood flow.[27]

The resistance (impedance) that blood encounters is inversely related to flow. Several pulsatility indices (PIs) provide crude semiquantitative measurements of flow impedance. The most commonly used is Gosling's Index. It equals the difference between systolic and diastolic velocities, divided by the mean velocity.[24] Pourcelot's Resistivity Index avoids the use of mean velocities and equals the difference between systolic and diastolic velocities divided by the systolic velocity.[39] Distal high impedance to flow correlates with elevated PI, although cardiac and systemic variables can affect the PI as well.

Flow quantitation with ultrasound is affected by many factors—shape of the vessels, variability of diameter, and the estimation of mean velocity. In restricted circumstances, however, blood velocities can correlate well with blood flow measurements when multiple variables are taken into account.[14] Techniques for blood flow measurements have been applied to carotid artery ultrasonography, although absolute blood flow measurements with ultrasound can be difficult in disease states. Cerebral blood flow (CBF) measurement, however, may not be important in most clinical situations since changes in CBF correlate well with changes in intracranial velocities.[37]

Effects of Luminal Narrowing on Blood Flow and Velocity

Blood hemodynamics are described by several formulas as follows:

$$Q = A \times Vm$$

(where Q = flow, A = vessel cross-sectional area, and Vm = mean velocity).

Moreover, blood flow depends on the pressure gradient across the vessel segment and the resistance it encounters.

$$Q = \frac{\Delta P}{R}$$

(where ΔP = pressure gradient across the vessel segment).

Flow resistance is covered by Poiseuille's Law (below), and is significantly increased by a smaller lumen radius:

$$R = \frac{\eta \, 8L}{\pi r^4}$$

(where R = resistance, η = blood viscosity, L = vessel segment length, r = vessel segment radius).

Blood cells travel normally within a narrow range of velocities, in a laminar pattern, with most cells traveling in the central part of the lumen. Luminal narrowing induces on them a wider range of velocities and energies termed "spectral broadening," disturbing the laminar character of the flow and dispersing cells inside the vessel. Within the stenosis there is a rapid increase in blood velocities. Immediately following, the narrowing energy loss produces low velocities. In the distal segments, laminar flow is reconstituted if the severity of stenosis allows enough blood to go through. If significant flow impairment exists, slowing of velocities persists with narrow differences between diastolic and systolic velocities, causing a decrease in the PI.

Instrumentation

Continuous-Wave Doppler

The reflected signal from continuous-wave emission, is primarily examined according to sound patterns, since sound characteristics of normal and pathologic flow patterns can be distinguished. The display of frequencies on a screen improves accuracy of the exam. The common (CCA), external (ECA), and internal (ICA) carotid arteries can be examined as well as the periorbital arteries, and the subclavian, innominate, and the extracranial segments of the vertebral arteries (VA). The initial direction of the signal, the amplitude, and the direction of blood flow in response to different compression maneuvers, can identify the arteries and detect the presence, absence, or sources of collateral flow. A high degree of skill, experience, and technique is necessary for good results.

Advantages of continuous-wave Doppler include: (1) ability to insonate many vessels, (2) small probe size, and (3) the ability to measure very high blood velocities that pulsed-wave Doppler cannot assess. Disadvantages are related to the large volume of tissues examined as well as inability to visualize the insonated vessel or to obtain a precise angle of insonation.

B-Mode and Duplex Ultrasound

Through the use of pulsed waves in B-mode scanning, a two-dimensional anatomic image based on the sonic qualities of the tissues is reconstructed. It is displayed in real time on a monitor according to a grey scale. Since the structural information alone has shortcomings in high-grade stenoses, B-scans are combined with continuous and pulsed Doppler probes that provide blood velocity at selected points. Combined B-mode and Doppler systems (duplex scans), provide more accurate information than either system alone. The transducer frequency used varies between 5 and 10 MHz, with 7.5 MHz being optimal for resolution and depth of penetration.

Duplex is the ultrasonic technique of choice to examine the region of the carotid bifurcation and the proximal portion of the extracranial ICA. Its superficial location allows the use of higher frequencies for improved anatomic resolution. Despite a deeper location, a limited angle of examination, small size of the VA, and the presence of the vertebral processes, the extracranial portion of the VA can be studied.[56] The B-mode anatomic exam is followed by subsequent pulsed Doppler velocity assessment.

Color Doppler

The analysis of phase and frequency shift through a Doppler channel, allows the detection of flow velocity and direction. Coding of this information in color Doppler systems according to a color scale, and superimposing it on the B-scan real-time image, provides an instantaneous velocity map. The color coding is usually red for blood flow directed away from the probe (usually arterial), with lighter hues reserved for higher velocities and darker hues reserved for lower velocities.[46] Blood that travels in the opposite direction is coded in blue (usually venous). A reversal in the direction of arterial flow as in turbulence, steal, or complete distal occlusion, will appear in blue as well. Color Doppler systems provide guidance on the best sampling location for blood velocities on duplex scans. They improve assessment of flow status around hypoechoic lesions, in critical stenoses, and assessment of turbulence patterns.

Transcranial Doppler (TCD)

Two MHz pulsed-wave Doppler is used to provide better sound penetration through the skull. The intracranial vessels forming the circle of Willis, their major branches, and the vertebral arteries can be insonated. The examination takes advantage of "windows" least obstructive to sound.[41] Through the temporal window (above the zygomatic arch), the MCA, ACA, ICA, and PCA can be insonated. The suboccipital window (foramen magnum) is used to study the VA, and BA, while the ophthalmic artery (OA) and ICA siphon are insonated through the orbital window.[51] The distal portion of the extracranial ICA can be also examined through a submandibular approach. The reflected signal is displayed on a screen as a time-velocity graph, with the frequencies simultaneously heard over a speaker. Peak-systolic, end-diastolic, and mean velocities can be measured in addition to the PI.

The vessels are recognized by six main criteria: (1) window used, (2) direction of the probe, (3) depth of examination, (4) rela-

tionship to the ICA-MCA bifurcation, (5) characteristics of the waveform, and (6) the effects of compression maneuvers.[1] Failure to detect a temporal window in 4% to 15% of individuals examined, increases with age, is more common in women, and may be related to hyperostosis. The available windows restrict the Doppler angle to an optimal value of less than 60° at which the vessels can be insonated.

Disadvantages stem mainly from a blind insonation of the vessels, since individual variabilities and anomalies can interfere with accurate measurements. Technologic improvements, however, are overcoming some of these problems. A three-dimensional map of the intracranial vessels can be obtained by using a specially designed headset and computer analysis.[36] A recently introduced color-coded duplex transcranial scan using a 2.25 MHz probe[10] may add anatomic information as well as a velocity map.

Clinical Applications
Atherosclerotic Disease of the Extracranial Arteries

The extracranial segments of the carotid artery are best studied by duplex scans, which can evaluate wall and luminal abnormalities and velocities. Distal segments of the extracranial ICA are best examined by either TCD or continuous-wave Doppler. The extracranial VA and the innominate and subclavian arteries usually are examined with duplex and continuous-wave Doppler.

Carotid Artery

Ultrasound has several applications in the study of occlusive disease of the extracranial carotid artery.

Detection and Characterization of Plaque Morphology

One major advantage of carotid ultrasound

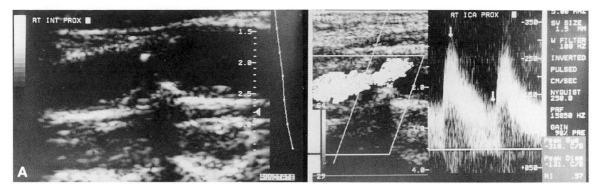

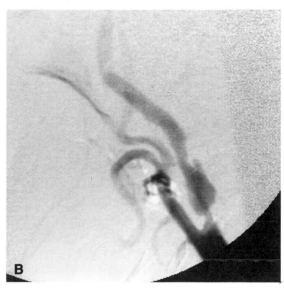

Figure 1. Duplex and color-flow ultrasound of extracranial carotid stenosis of a 65-year-old man with asymptomatic extracranial carotid stenosis. (A) Cross-sectional picture with the B-scan (left) demonstrating narrowing in the proximal portion of the right ICA. A circumferential plaque can be seen with hyperechoic calcification producing a "shadowing" effect on the structures medial to it. The color Doppler scan superimposed on the B-scan (right) is used to identify the best sampling location for velocity measurement. A peak blood velocity of 310 cm is indicative of a critical stenosis. (B) The angiogram reveals a high-grade stenosis at the origin of the ICA. A distal plaque, missed on ultrasound because of the location, is detected with angiography.

over contrast angiography is its detailed evaluation of plaque characterisitics (Figure 1). B-mode imaging can detect most plaques at the bifurcation, as well as mild thickening of the intima and media. Plaques can be characterized as soft, dense, or calcified, according to their echogenic properties. Echolucency with a postenhancement pattern in a plaque is associated with hemorrhage. Cholesterol deposits may appear anechoic as well. Calcifications are hyperechoic and cast a shadow behind them, potentially obscuring adjacent thrombi, and rendering less accurate the assessment of residual lumen. Weakly echogenic material, like fresh thrombi and soft plaques, can be missed with the B-scan alone.

The characteristics of plaque, including its surface regularity, histology, and hemorrhagic component, can have clinical significance.[23] Although plaque ulceration may correlate with clinical symptomatology, its significance re-

mains unclear. Soft, less organized, or heterogeneous plaque correlates highly with ischemic symptoms, particularly when associated with luminal narrowing. Hemorrhage in a carotid plaque is commonly associated with symptomatic cerebral ischemia, more often than endoluminal thrombosis.

Quantification of Luminal Narrowing

Several studies have assessed the correlation between carotid ultrasound and angiographic luminal narrowing.[17] Digital substraction angiography remains superior to duplex in the detection of residual lumen, especially when associated with critical stenosis.[40] A complete occlusion is suggested on duplex or color Doppler by the absence of flow detection. A high impedance signal in the CCA can be an indication of high-grade stenosis or occlusion of the ICA, with either absence or reversal of diastolic blood flow.

Moderate-to-severe luminal narrowing can be graded by ultrasound according to systolic velocities. The limit values of different grades vary among medical centers. Peak-systolic velocity in the ICA ranges between 110-175 cm/sec in stenoses of moderate degree (50% to 75%), and up to 250 cm/sec in stenoses of severe degree. The velocity is higher than 300 cm/sec in critical ICA stenosis.[49]

Diameter narrowing below 50% is not reliably detected by absolute peak blood velocities. The ratio of peak-systolic velocities in the ICA and CCA can be used to estimate the narrowing in low-grade stenoses. Its use may minimize the variability induced by systemic and interindividual factors.[9] A normal ratio is below 1 in normal conditions. Ratios of 2 and 1.5 correspond respectively to 50% and 25% stenosis.

Color Doppler can detect flow disturbances associated with minor and severe lesions thereby enhancing the structural information obtained from duplex scans. Initial validation studies comparing Doppler to angiography are encouraging.[52] The sensitivity of color-flow Doppler in detecting disease can approach 100%, with an accuracy of classifying minor, moderate, and severe stenoses varying from 91% to 97%.

Hemodynamic Effects on the Intracranial Circulation

Assessment of the intracranial circulation in the context of extracranial disease can be important in management decisions (Figure 2). TCD demonstrates slow MCA velocities distal to an ICA with 75% to 100% stenosis,[31] and faster or reversed flow in patent collateral channels. Systolic velocity in the OA ipsilateral to an ICA occlusion, is 17% less than the contralateral one. Pulsatility transmission index (PTI), a ratio of the PI on the side of carotid stenosis over the PI

from the reference vessel, may be more reliable than absolute velocities in unilateral carotid stenoses.[34] Interpretation of the information provided by TCD is more accurate when the status of the extracranial carotid artery is known.

Patency, patterns, and efficiency of the collateral circulation also can be evaluated. An increase in ACA velocities with reversal of flow ipsilateral to a stenosis suggests collateral flow from the opposite ICA through the anterior communicating artery. Similarly, increased velocities in the PCA or BA suggest collateral flow through the posterior circulation. Compared with arteriography, TCD can identify major collateral pathways with a sensitivity of 89% and a specificity of 80%. In all patients without major intracerebral collaterals, 44% demonstrated reversal of blood flow through the OA ipsilateral to ICA occlusion.[48]

Vascular Reserve Assessment

The brain uses several mechanisms to maintain blood flow under physiologic and pathologic conditions. Although collateral flow is one of the most important mechanisms used, it is not always sufficiently adequate to compensate for severe hemodynamic lesions. Although used for short term flow regulation, compensatory arteriolar vasodilatation can act as the last reserve mechanism to maintain adequate blood supply under such circumstances. Cerebral vasodilating stimuli like acetazolamide[38] or CO_2,[43] normally produce a 50% increase in blood flow and velocities under normal conditions. An impairment in vascular reserve capacity due to a continuous vasodilatation, will translate as diminished or unchanged blood velocities. Similar testing allows the selection of patients with hemodynamic compromise, who may benefit most from revascularization.

Vasomotor reactivity is significantly lower than normal on both the occluded and the nonoccluded sides in unilateral ICA disease and on both sides in the bilateral ICA dis-

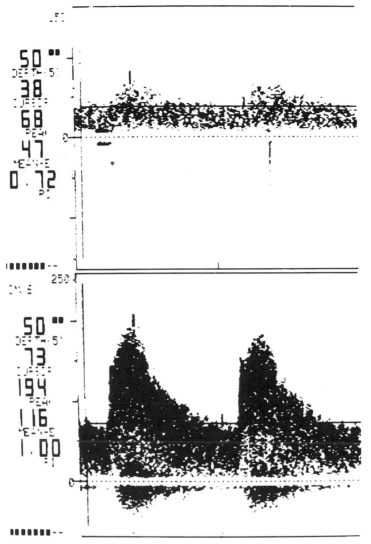

Figure 2. Effects of extracranial carotid stenosis on intracranial blood velocities in a 72-year-old woman with acute occlusion of the left ICA at its origin. Filling of the left MCA, on angiography, was achieved through the contralateral ICA via the anterior circle of Willis. TCD on the abnormal side (top) shows decreased pulsatility, slowed initial upslope, and abnormally low velocities in the MCA distal to the occluded ICA. The contralateral MCA velocities (bottom) are higher than normal, reflecting a compensatory increase in blood flow.

ease.[43] The difference between vasomotor reactivity for symptomatic and asymptomatic unilateral occlusions is also highly significant. There is a striking association between vasomotor reactivities of less than 34% and clinical low-flow status syndromes.

Carotid Disease: a Monitor for Atherosclerotic Activity

Atherosclerosis is a dynamic process accompanied by a continuous modification of content, structure, form, and size of plaque.[44]

Progression of carotid plaque occurs in 17% to 38% of asymptomatic carotid stenosis and correlates strongly with the onset of ischemic symptoms, while regression occurs in 2% to 19%. The sensitivity of B-scans to measure carotid wall thickness, allows the monitoring of an early indicator of occlusive atherosclerotic disease. The noninvasiveness of the technique and the ease of its repetition makes it a valuable research instrument,[55] with potential clinical applications.

The effects of different risk factors in the progression or regression of plaque can be evaluated. Thickness of the CCA intima-media complex is significantly greater in patients with hypercholesterolemia. Progression of carotid narrowing as measured by B-mode, correlates with lipid and hematologic measurements. Cigarette smoking has a strong relationship with carotid wall thickening, and stenosis. Many ongoing epidemiologic studies of risk factors with or without therapeutic interventions are based on carotid medial and intimal thickness, measured by B-mode ultrasound.[11] The potential selection of patients who are at highest risk for progressive occlusive disease and who may benefit most from aggressive medical or surgical therapies, is promising.

Innominate and Vertebral Arteries

Duplex ultrasound has aided investigation of occlusive vascular disease in the innominate, subclavian, and vertebral arteries.[3] Combined duplex, TCD, and continuous-wave Doppler provide information on hemodynamic and steal effects of innominate stenosis.[15] Three grades of innominate artery stenosis of increasing severity can be identified according to blood flow patterns in the vertebral and carotid arteries. A systolic deceleration or alternating flow in the right VA, with minor changes in the carotid arteries, is associated with mild innominate artery stenosis. With moderate stenosis, flow reversal in the ipsilateral VA, and systolic deceleration in the carotid arteries can be seen. The most severe lesions produce alternating flow

or complete steal in the carotid arteries in addition to VA steal.

Ultrasonic examination of the extracranial segments of the VA is more complex and less reliable than in the carotid artery. Although high frequencies and spectral broadening are present in VA stenosis, frequent normal side-to-side asymmetries and tortuosity make them less reliable. Most significant stenoses of the VA occur at its origin, and can be detected in only 60% to 62% of patients because of the depth of insonation required.[18]

Subclavian Artery and Steal Syndrome

Proximal subclavian occlusion is associated with permanent VA flow reversal. With severe stenoses, VA flow direction reverses during systole and returns to normal in diastole. In mild-to-moderate stenoses, a reduction of flow in the VA during systole can be detected with normal flow direction throughout the cardiac cycle. Hyperemic arm tests can increase the sensitivity for detecting mild or moderate lesions.[29]

The effects on intracranial flow can be assessed with TCD. An increase in BA velocities can be demonstrated in subclavian stenosis with reversal of flow in the VA. Also, there is a systolic deceleration of flow velocity, or an alternating flow directed towards the arm in systole and towards the brain in diastole. Basilar flow velocity and direction determined before or after post-ischemic hyperemic test of the upper limb, can improve the assessment of severity of subclavian steal.[19]

Chronic and Subacute Intracranial Occlusive Disease

Atherosclerotic disease and narrowing of the intracranial arteries most commonly affects the ICA and proximal MCA, and to a lesser degree the ACA and PCA. An inverse relationship exists between angiographic residual lumen diameter and flow velocity assessed by TCD, in the carotid siphon, MCA,

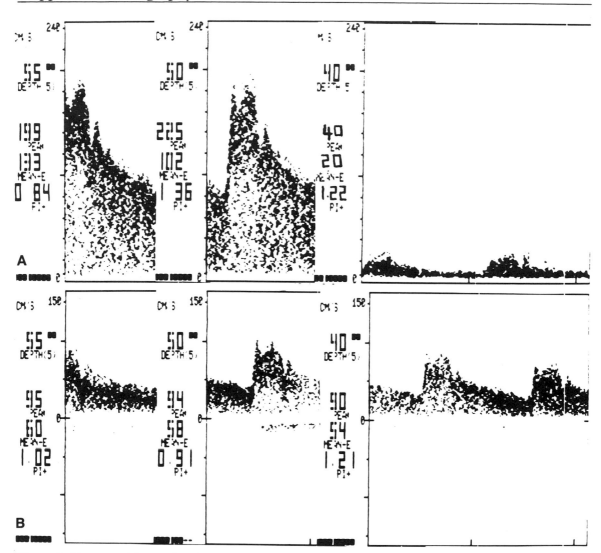

Figure 3. Transcranial Doppler of isolated intracranial MCA stenosis in a 54-year-old Jamaican man with stenosis of the M1 segment of the left MCA. (A) MCA velocities are abnormally high at the level of the narrowing, and drop to abnormally low levels distal to the narrowing. (B) The MCA velocities on the opposite side remain normal in all depths.

ACA, and BA.[33] Concurrent information on the status of the extracranial carotid, allows a 91% sensitivity for TCD in detecting intracranial MCA and ICA stenosis.[25]

MCA narrowing is the most accurately detected intracranial disease.[28] Mild stenosis causes an increase in blood velocities without any other change. Moderate-to-severe stenosis leads to higher peak velocities with spectral broadening (Figure 3). Low velocities are usually present distal to the stenosis. Stenoses

beyond the M1 segment usually are not detected. Doppler findings in MCA disease can be affected by the segment involved (before or after the lenticulostriates), disease of the ipsilateral ICA, and the presence or absence of collateral flow through the ACA.[35]

An ipsilateral ICA occlusion or stenosis can cause marked depression in MCA velocities, and a sharp increase in ACA velocities ipsilaterally or bilaterally. PI and PTI tend to increase in the ICA proximal to central MCA occlusions, and decrease distal to it. The same indices remain stable in peripheral MCA occlusions. Assessment of the hemodynamic effects of MCA disease can enhance TCD sensitivity. ACA velocities, ipsilateral to MCA stem stenosis or occlusion, are higher than the normal side, reflecting collateral blood supply.[12]

Though difficult to quantitate, transorbital diagnosis of intracranial ICA stenosis is detected by TCD with 73% to 94% sensitivity.[51] Occlusive disease in the ACA and PCA is less reliably evaluated. Stenoses of the proximal and middle segments of the BA can be reliably detected.[33] The VA and the posterior inferior cerebellar arteries are normally the subject of anatomic variabilities that produce side-to-side velocity differences and interfere with a reliable interpretation of abnormalities.

Acute Occlusion and Recanalization of Intracranial Vessels

There is a need for noninvasive detection and monitoring of acute arterial occlusion at the onset of ischemic symptoms and its response to acute therapies. The potential role of TCD in such conditions has been partially explored within 6 hours from the onset of ischemic symptoms.[57] In intracranial ICA and MCA stem occlusions, signal from the MCA generally is not detectable. In peripheral MCA occlusions (after the lenticulostriate branches) a 21% reduction in MCA velocity occurs compared to the contralateral side. When three or more distal MCA branches are occluded, a reduction in MCA velocity generally is seen. MCA velocities are not affected if only one or two MCA branches are occluded. No false-positive results were observed in 39 patients studied.[57]

Knowledge of the delay between onset of symptoms and ultrasound assessment is essential. The dynamic nature of the acute occlusive process in the acute and subacute period will be reflected in the examination.

This can be related to partial or total recanalization of the artery, recurrence of occlusion, or development of collateral flow. Followup of acute MCA occlusion and reperfusion is possible with TCD and compares favorably with contrast angiography.[22] Reperfusion in the vessel can occur within the first 24 hours or as late as one week after the onset of symptoms.

Live Detection of Cerebral Microemboli

The reflective characteristics of sound by emboli are different than blood cells and can be detected as they pass through the ultrasound beam. A distinction between different types of emboli (air, fat, and platelet and blood thrombi) based on their ultrasonic characteristics appears possible.[45] Emboli are associated with intraluminal platelet thrombus, ulcerations in the carotid artery, and transient ischemic attacks or stroke. In 26% of patients undergoing carotid endarterectomy, emboli were detected by TCD, before, during, or after surgical dissection.[50] Emboli can be also detected in patients monitored with continuous-wave Doppler of the extracranial carotid artery, during cardiopulmonary bypass surgery.[53] A relationship is suggested between the number of embolic signals detected by TCD and neuropsychologic changes following cardiopulmonary bypass.[28] The ability for subclinical detection of microemboli with TCD in patients with prosthetic aortic valves[8] and atrial fibrillation[54] is unique. Although its clinical significance remains undetermined, it appears promising.

Intraoperative Monitoring of Blood Velocities

The assessment of intracranial collaterals helps predict hemodynamic consequences of cross clamping.[47] Intraoperative monitoring of MCA blood velocities during carotid endarterectomy, allows a continuous surveillance of flow impairment. Patients who demonstrate a significant decrease in cerebral blood velocities with carotid cross-clamp testing may require a temporary shunt to prevent ischemic complications.[37,42] The ratio of systolic over diastolic velocities and the PI can be more sensitive than mean velocity alone in detecting hemodynamic changes.[26] The combination with somatosensory evoked potentials may improve the sensitivity of TCD for detecting patients at high risk for ischemia.

Arterial Dissection

The extracranial ICA and the VA are the most common locations for dissection of the arterial wall, producing a narrowing of the lumen often associated with thrombosis and distal embolization. The ICA portion most commonly subject to dissection is 1-2 cm beyond the bifurcation where it is difficult to image with the duplex scan. With a smaller probe and the ability to penetrate deeper into the tissues, TCD can insonate a long segment of the ICA before penetrating the intracranial cavity, as well as the carotid siphon where intracranial dissections can occur. The hemodynamic effects of the dissection on the intracranial circulation can also be assessed and monitored.[30]

An investigation of extracranial carotid dissections by continuous-wave Doppler and B-scans reveals good correlation with angiography and allows noninvasive frequent followup.[20] The patterns of dissection on duplex scans can be varied. Although a double channel appearance on B-scans is the most typical finding, it is not commonly seen. A tubular appearance is suggestive, particularly when asymmetrical. Dissection can also present as an elongated ectatic carotid without the presence of a plaque. Distinguishing dissection from fibromuscular dysplasia, which is sometimes a cause of dissection, can be difficult. A decrease in CCA and ICA blood velocities when combined with the absence of a plaque in young adults is suggestive of dissection.[21]

Dolichoectasia

A tortuous elongation and dilatation (dolichoectasia) of the cerebral arteries can produce ischemic symptoms by several mechanisms. Turbulent blood flow produced by the irregular lumen promotes thrombus formation with potential distal embolism. An obstruction of the penetrating vessels at their origin is possible and can be associated with atherosclerosis. TCD demonstrates low blood velocities[7] without a decrease in PI, suggesting normal peripheral resistance and arterial compliance.

Sickle-Cell Vasculopathy

With sickle-cell disease, increase in cerebral blood flow is inversely proportional to the hematocrit. This hyperemia appears related to a compensatory vasodilatation and may be associated with symptomatic ischemia in the distal arterial territories. A high prevalence of intracranial vaculopathy involving the ICA, MCA, or ACA, and may act synergistically with hematocrit elevation to produce ischemia. TCD may prove useful in screening patients with sickle-cell disease and in identifying those prone to ischemic complications. Blood velocities in sickle-cell disease correlate well with CBF.[14] Intracranial stenosis can be also detected.[4] TCD may thus help in screening, detecting, and differentiating the pathophysiology of ischemia in sickle-cell disease, and those at risk of developing it.

Overview and Future Directions

Management of occlusive cerebrovascular disease rests primarily on the ability to detect and identify the underlying pathophysiologic mechanism. The need for noninvasive techniques to answer this question in patients with ischemic symptoms is obvious. Ultrasound instruments allow a comprehensive

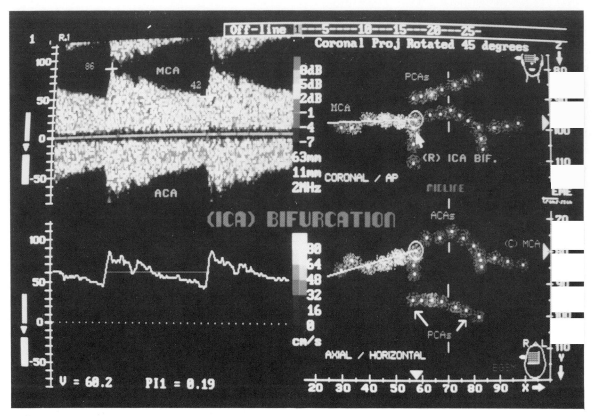

Figure 4. Normal three-dimensional transcranial Doppler mapping of the coronal (top right corner) and axial (bottom right corner) views of the major arteries forming the circle of Willis (Transcan, EME, Uberlingen, Germany). The blood velocity (top left corner) is sampled from the bifurcation of the ICA. Location of the sampled blood velocity is indicated on the vascular map, improving the reliability of the study. (Photo was provided courtesy of C.H. Tegeler, MD)

examination of the extracranial and intracranial vessels with duplex and TCD. Some newer scans incorporate both techniques. Screening, assessment, and followup of occlusive cerebrovascular disease have demonstrated great usefulness. Favorable correlation with contrast angiography has rendered them widely used in varied clinical settings. Their unique capabilities in examining the arterial wall and real-time monitoring of hemodynamics have already proven useful, while further applications are still being explored. Technologic improvements will likely further enhance these capabilities and improve their reliability (Figure 4).

Rapid advances in magnetic resonance angiography (MRA) introduce a challenge to the role of ultrasound in the noninvasive eval-

uation of the cerebral circulation. MRA nonetheless carries some disadvantages compared to ultrasound. It is significantly more expensive, requires large installation space, is not movable, is contraindicated in the presence of certain implanted devices, cannot be used as a monitoring device, and does not appear to assess the arterial wall. Both techniques, however, will probably improve, compensating for some disadvantages, while other limitations will remain. They could complement each other, to answer varied aspects of similar or different clinical situations.

Instruments that will be used in coming years to evaluate occlusive cerebrovascular disease cannot be predicted. Ultrasound has proven practical and useful in screening the vascular segments most frequently subject to occlusive disease. The recent findings of dramatically improved outcomes in symptomatic patients who underwent carotid endarterectomy in the North American and European trials further enhance the role of ultrasound as a noninvasive, low-cost screening technique. Most patients with TIA or minor stroke will need to be screened for carotid stenosis to identify those who would benefit from a proven therapy (carotid endarterectomy) in preventing cerebral infarction.

Despite widescale acceptance in clinical practice, ultrasound techniques may provide false-positive, false-negative, and other occasional erroneous information. They represent excellent modalities for screening and followup of vascular pathology, but should be interpreted in light of the overall clinical situation and other lines of diagnostic information. Results of ultrasound studies are not always sufficiently reliable to exclude a strongly suspected diagnosis or to guide invasive or surgical decisions.

References

1. Aaslid R. Transcranial Doppler examination techniques. In: Aaslid R, ed. *Transcranial Doppler Sonography.* New York, NY: Springer-Verlag; 1986:39-59.
2. Aaslid R, Markwalder T-M, Nornes H. Noninvasive transcranial Doppler ultrasound recording of flow velocity in basal cerebral arteries. *J Neurosurg.* 1982;57:769-774.
3. Ackerstaff RGA, Hoenveld H, Slowikowski JM. Ultrasonic duplex scanning in atherosclerotic disease of the innominate, subclavian, and vertebral arteries. A comparative study with angiography. *Ultrasound Med Biol.* 1984;10:409-418.
4. Adams RJ, Aaslid R, El Gammal T, et al. Detection of cerebral vasculopathy in sickle cell disease using transcranial Doppler ultrasonography and magnetic resonance imaging: case report. *Stroke.* 1988;19:518-520.
5. Ameriso SF, Paganini-Hill A, Meiselman HJ, et al. Correlates of middle cerebral artery blood velocity in the elderly. *Stroke.* 1990;21:1579-1583
6. Assessment: transcranial Doppler. Report of the American Academy of Neurology, therapeutics and technology assessment subcommittee. *Neurology.* 1990;40:680-681.
7. Babikian V, Sloan MA, Burdette D, et al. Transcranial Doppler in dolichoectatic cerebrovascular disease. *J Neuroimag.* 1992;2:19-24.
8. Berger M, Davis D, Lolley D, et al. Detection of subclinical microemboli in patients with prosthetic aortic valves. *J Cardiovasc Technol.* 1990;9:282-283.

9. Blackshear WM Jr, Phillips DJ, Chikas PM, et al. Carotid artery velocity patterns in normal and stenotic vessels. *Stroke.* 1980;1:67-71.
10. Bogdahn U, Becker G, Winkler J, et al. Transcranial color-coded real-time sonography in adults. *Stroke.* 1990;21:1680-1688.
11. Bond MG, Barnes RW, Riley WA, et al. High-resolution B-mode ultrasound scanning methods in the atherosclerosis risk in communities study (ARIC). *J Neuroimag.* 1991;1:68-73.
12. Brass LM, Duterte DL, Mohr JP. Anterior cerebral artery velocity changes in disease of the middle cerebral artery stem. *Stroke.* 1989;20:1737-1740.
13. Brass LM, Pavlakis SG, DeVivo D, et al. Transcranial Doppler measurements of the middle cerebral artery: effect of hematocrit. *Stroke.* 1988;19:1466-1469.
14. Brass LM, Prohovnik I, Pavlakis SG, et al. Middle cerebral artery blood velocity and cerebral blood flow in sickle cell disease. *Stroke.* 1991;22:27-30.
15. Brunhölzl C, von Reutern G-M. Hemodynamic effects of innominate artery occlusive disease. Evaluation by Doppler ultrasound. *Ultrasound Med Biol.* 1989;15:201-204.
16. Caplan LR, Brass LM, DeWitt LD, et al. Transcranial Doppler ultrasound: present status. *Neurology.* 1990;40:696-700.
17. Comerota AJ, Cranley JJ, Katz ML, et al. Real-time B-mode carotid imaging: a three year multicenter experience. *J Vasc Surg.* 1984;1:84-95.
18. Davis PC, Nilsen B, Braun IF, et al. A prospective comparison of duplex sonography vs angiography of the vertebral arteries. *AJNR.* 1986;7:1059-1064.
19. De Bray JM, Blard JM, Tachot C, et al. Transcranial Doppler ultrasonic examination in vertebro-basilar circulatory pathology. *J Mal Vasc.* 1989;14:202-205.
20. De Bray JM, Dubas F, Joseph PA, et al. Ultrasonic study of dissections of the internal carotid artery. 22 cases (in French). *Rev Neurol* (Paris). 1989;145:702-709.
21. Eljamel MSM, Humphrey PRD, Shaw MDM. Dissection of the cervical internal carotid artery. The role of Doppler/Duplex studies and conservative management. *J Neurol Neurosurg Psychiatry.* 1990;53:379-383
22. Fieschi C, Argentino C, Lenzi GL, et al. Clinical and instrumental evaluation of patients with ischemic stroke within the first six hours. *J Neurol Sci.* 1989;91:311-321.
23. Gomez CR. Carotid plaque morphology and risk for stroke. *Stroke.* 1990;21:148-151.
24. Gosling RG, King DH. Arterial assessment by Doppler-shift ultrasound. *Proc R Soc Med.* 1974;67:447-450.
25. Grolimund P, Seiler RW, Aaslid R, et al. Evaluation of cerebrovascular disease by combined extracranial and transcranial Doppler sonography: experience in 1,039 patients. *Stroke.* 1987;18:1018-1024.
26. Halsey JH, McDowell HA, Gelman S. Transcranial Doppler and rCBF compared in carotid endarterectomy. *Stroke.* 1986;17:1206-1208.
27. Halsey JH, McDowell HA, Gelman S, et al. Blood velocity in the middle cerebral artery and regional cerebral blood flow during carotid endarterectomy. *Stroke.* 1989;20:53-58.
28. Harrison MJG, Pugsley W, Newman S, et al. Detection of middle cerebral emboli during coronary

artery bypass surgery using transcranial Doppler sonography. *Stroke.* 1990;21:1512.

29. Hennerici M, Rautenberg W, Schwartz A. Transcranial Doppler ultrasound for the assessment of intracranial arterial flow velocity, II: evaluation of intracranial arterial disease. *Surg Neurol.* 1987; 27:523-532.

30. Kaps M, Dorndorf W, Damian MS, et al. Intracranial haemodynamics in patients with spontaneous carotid dissection: transcranial Doppler ultrasound follow-up studies. *Eur Arch Psychiatry Neurol Sci.* 1990;239:246-256.

31. Kelley RE, Namon RA, Juang SH, et al. Transcranial Doppler ultrasonography of the middle cerebral artery in the hemodynamic assessment of internal carotid artery stenosis. *Arch Neurol.* 1990;47:960-964.

32. Kremkau FW. *Diagnostic Ultrasound: Principles, Instrumentation, and Exercises.* Orlando, Fla: Grune & Stratton, Inc; 1984.

33. Lindegaard K-F, Bakke SJ, Aaslid R, et al. Doppler diagnosis of intracranial artery occlusive disorders. *J Neurol Neurosurg Psychiatry.* 1986;49:510-518.

34. Lindegaard K-F, Bakke SJ Grolimund P, et al. Assessment of intracranial hemodynamics in carotid artery disease by transcranial Doppler ultrasound. *J Neurosurg.* 1985;63:890-898.

35. Mattle H, Grolimund P, Huber P, et al. Transcranial Doppler sonographic findings in middle cerebral artery disease. *Arch Neurol.* 1988;45:289-295.

36. Niederkorn K, Myers LG, Nunn CL, et al. Three-dimensional transcranial Doppler blood flow mapping in patients with cerebrovascular disorders. *Stroke.* 1988;19:1335-1344.

37. Padayachee TS, Gosling RG, Bishop CC, et al. Monitoring middle cerebral artery blood velocity during carotid endarterectomy. *Br J Surg.* 1986;73:98-100.

38. Piepgras A, Schmiedek P, Leinsinger G, et al. A simple test to assess cerebrovascular reserve capacity using transcranial Doppler sonography and acetazolamide. *Stroke.* 1990;21:1306-1311.

39. Pourcelot L. Applications cliniques de l'examen Doppler transcutané. In: Peroneau P, ed. *Velocimetrie ultrasonore Doppler.* Paris, France: Editions INSERM; 1975:213-240.

40. Price R, Bonsor G. A comparison of Doppler duplex scanning with digital substraction angiography. In: Anderson WJ, Sheldon CD, Barbenel JC, et al, eds. *Blood Flow in the Brain.* Oxford, England: Oxford University Press; 1989:109-113.

41. Ringelstein EB. A practical guide to transcranial Doppler sonography. In: Weinberger J, ed. *Noninvasive Imaging of Cerebrovascular Disease.* New York, NY: Alan R Liss; 1989:75-121.

42. Ringelstein EB, Richert F, Bardos S, et al. Transcranial sonographic monitoring of the blood flow of

the middle cerebral artery in recanalizing operations of the extracranial internal carotid artery (in German). *Nervenarzt.* 1985;56:423-430.

43. Ringelstein EB, Sievers C, Ecker S, et al. Noninvasive assessment of CO_2-induced cerebral vasomotor response in normal individuals and patients with internal carotid artery occlusions. *Stroke.* 1988; 19:963-969.

44. Roederer GO, Langlois YE, Jager KA, et al. The natural history of carotid arterial disease in asymptomatic patients with cervical bruits. *Stroke.* 1984;15:605-613.

45. Russell D, Madden KP, Clark WM, et al. Detection of arterial emboli using Doppler ultrasound in rabbits. *Stroke.* 1991;22:253-258.

46. Satiani B, Porter R, Biggers K, et al. Evaluation of the color coded Doppler ultrasound in detecting carotid bifurcation disease. *J Cardiovasc Surg* (Torino). 1988;29:196-200.

47. Schneider PA, Ringelstein EB, Rossman ME, et al. Importance of cerebral collateral pathways during carotid endarterectomy. *Stroke.* 1988;19:1328-1334.

48. Schneider PA, Rossman ME, Bernstein EF, et al. Noninvasive assessment of cerebral collateral blood supply through the ophthalmic artery. *Stroke.* 1991; 22:31-36.

49. Scoutt LM, Zawin ML, Taylor KJW. Doppler US, Part II: clinical applications. *Radiology.* 1990; 174:309-319.

50. Spencer MP, Thomas GI, Nicholls SC, et al. Detection of middle cerebral artery emboli during carotid endarterectomy using transcranial Doppler ultrasonography. *Stroke.* 1990;21:415-423.

51. Spencer MP, Whisler D. Transorbital Doppler diagnosis of intracranial arterial stenosis. *Stroke.* 1986;17:916-921.

52. Steinke W, Kloetzch C, Hennerici M. Carotid artery disease assessed by color Doppler flow imaging: correlation with standard Doppler sonography and angiography. *AJNR.* 1990;11:259-266.

53. Stump DA, Stein CS, Tegeler CH, et al. Validity and reliability of an ultrasound device for detecting carotid emboli. *J Neuroimaging.* 1991;1:18-22.

54. Tegeler CH, Hitchings LP, Eicke M, et al. Microemboli detection in stroke associated with atrial fibrillation. *J Cardiovasc Technol.* 1990;9:283-284.

55. Tell GS. Cigarette smoking, lipids, lipoproteins, and extracranial carotid artery atherosclerosis. *Mayo Clin Proc.* 1991;66;327-331.

56. Trattnig S, Hübsch P, Schuster H, et al. Color-coded Doppler imaging of normal vertebral arteries. *Stroke.* 1990;21:1222-1225.

57. Zanette EM, Fieschi C, Bozzao L, et al. Comparison of cerebral angiography and transcranial Doppler sonography in acute stroke. *Stroke.* 1989;20:899-903.

CHAPTER 6

Risk Factor Modification and Medical Therapy for Stroke Prevention

Robert J. Dempsey, MD, and Robert W. Moore, PhD

The first section of this chapter addresses basic concepts about risk factors for brain ischemia secondary to occlusive artery disease. The second section discusses the individual risk factors. The third section consists of recommendations for reducing the risk of occlusive disease, subsequent brain ischemia, and its complications.

Ways to Think About Risk Factors

Three Phases of Prevention

Prevention of a chronic disabling condition, such as stroke, can focus on the gradual development of the condition. The first phase is the prevention of exposure to risk factors in the healthy population. This is primarily a concern of public and environmental health practitioners. Helping children and adolescents avoid acquiring tobacco use habits is an example.

Second is the limitation of exposure to risk factors among people who are identified to be at high risk due to prior risk factor exposure. Medication or diet modification to control or reduce high blood pressure is an example of second-phase prevention. Preventive medicine is concerned with this stage.

Third is the prevention or amelioration of a risk factor in patients who are symptomatic or who have already experienced the adverse condition for which they were at risk—e.g. had a stroke or transient ischemic attack (TIA). Medicine and surgery here focus on treatments to reduce the risk of deterioration or recurrence of an event such as a stroke. Antiplatelet therapy or carotid endarterectomy are examples of preventive measures at this third phase.

At every stage, prevention of stroke has greater benefit and is more economical than dealing with the consequences of unaddressed risk factors.[43]

Systemic Considerations

Treatment of a patient suffering from central nervous system arterial occlusive disease must address associated proliferation of systemic arterial lesions. This approach is essential in surgical therapy for arterial occlusive disease, both in limiting systemic complications and in decreasing postsurgical restenosis. A consideration of the risk factors for systemic arterial occlusive disease, and the medical treatment of these, is primary to any surgical plan.

Subtypes of Stroke

In consideration of risk factors it is essential to explicitly define specifically the disease being studied.[101] Much of the earlier epidemiology of stroke led to equivocal results in the search for modifiable risk factors, partly due to inability to make distinctions among various types of stroke. An important risk factor for one type of stroke may not prove to be significant for all etiologies of cerebral ischemia. The subtypes must be disaggregated in the search for predisposing factors.[83] For example, in the Multiple Risk Factor Intervention Trial, serum cholesterol was negatively related to the risk of death from hemorrhagic stroke, but positively associated with death from nonhemorrhagic stroke.[55] The true importance of such a risk factor is demonstrated in the study of particular subtypes of stroke.

Technological Advances

Technological advances in the clinical applications of computed tomography (CT), magnetic resonance (MR), and ultrasound imaging greatly improved the diagnosis of stroke subtypes and atherosclerotic plaque. This made possible substantial refinement in the research that examines risk profiles for the various types of stroke.

Such advances are reflected in the conventional categories that are used to classify stroke at a given time. For instance, prior to routine arterial studies stroke due to occlusion of precerebral arteries was not acknowledged as a distinct diagnostic entity in the *International Classification of Diseases Version 7* published in 1957; and in the past decade, clinical and subclinical lacunar infarction has gained wider recognition with routine MR scanning, though the description of the phenomenon and use of the term date from as early as 1838.[29]

Risks for Large Artery Occlusive Disease

For purposes of examining risk factors for large vessel occlusive disease resulting in brain ischemia we define the large vessels as the common and internal carotid arteries, the vertebral and basilar arteries and the major branches of the circle of Willis: the anterior, middle, and posterior cerebral arteries.

The question of risk factors in this context is not singular. We must consider: (1) "What are the factors associated with the onset and progress of cerebral artery stenosis and occlusion?", and (2) "Given occlusion of (or emboli to) a large cerebral artery, what concurrent factors are associated with the clinical onset of ischemia?"

Two tasks are implied by these ways of thinking about risk factors: (1) to prevent the onset and progress of occlusion in the cerebral arteries, and (2) to protect the brain from infarction if an occlusion occurs in such vessels.

Causes Versus Signs of Increased Risk

Not every observable correlation between a phenomenon and an adverse event such as artery occlusion or brain ischemia is causally connected with that event. Many factors are signs of increased risk of cerebral artery occlusion and brain ischemia, but only a subset of these are TRULY causally related.

Risk Factors

Not all risk factors lend themselves to intervention, but our culture strongly values an active approach to controlling future events over accepting whatever fate brings. In this section we emphasize those risk factors most susceptible to intervention.

Occlusion of Vessels as a Risk Factor for Brain Ischemia

Johann Jacob Wepfer (1620-1695) was among the first to understand that occlusion of the lumen of the internal carotid or vertebral arteries by fibrous bodies in the vascular wall was capable of producing apoplexy.[29] At approximately the same time, Francois Bayle

(1622-1709) associated apoplexy with atherosclerotic calcification and plaque in the cerebral arteries. Recognition that atherosclerosis could produce bleeding by weakening vessel walls preceded the discovery in 1823 by Leon Rostan (1790-1866) that infarction (softening) of the brain is related to diseased arteries. R. Virchow in 1847 was first to recognize that softening of the brain may be due to emboli from other arterial sources.

Prior to the 1950s, arteriosclerosis was regarded as a generalized disease of the vascular system for which surgery offered little remedy. When it was appreciated that arteriosclerosis often produces localized occlusion in short arterial segments, surgical intervention became feasible.[33]

C. Miller Fisher called attention to the role of occlusion in the extracranial carotid arteries and insufficiency of cerebral blood flow, suggesting that carotid thrombosis is a major cause of brain ischemia.[31] Studies in the 1950s and 1960s on surgically occluded internal and common carotid arteries for giant internal aneurysms showed an ipsilateral stroke rate from 15% to 50%.[36,81]

Thromboendarterectomy, first performed in Europe in the 1940s for treatment of peripheral vascular occlusion,[97] was attempted on the carotid vessels by Hurwitt in 1953 without complete success.[107] A report of successful surgery on the carotid arteries to achieve recovery from an ischemic neurologic deficit appeared in the *British Medical Journal* in 1956.[25]

Having identified carotid atherosclerosis as a risk factor for cerebral ischemia, the next question was: "How can it be identified?" While stenosis has long been followed by angiography, carotid ultrasound techniques are now able to identify and quantify noninvasively the atherosclerotic plaque itself.[26] Noninvasive, low-risk ultrasound imaging and Doppler examination of carotid arteries creates the potential for screening asymptomatic subjects for the presence of disease. The intent is to refer those with a higher risk of brain ischemia (as indicated by the presence of occlusive plaque) to an effective

intervention. Currently, ultrasound technology is largely used to examine symptomatic patients referred for assessment of their vascular status after signs or symptoms of cerebrovascular disease appear.

When a large vessel becomes occlusive or embolizes, the likelihood of subsequent brain ischemia is heavily conditioned by the patient's potential for developing collateral circulation to the areas of the brain supplied by the occluded artery. Estimation of the efficiency of collateral circulation to regions of the brain has been performed by carotid compression,[77] by carotid compression in conjunction with electroencephalography (EEG),[26,53] by measuring carotid artery backpressure,[80] by carotid angiography,[114] by measuring regional cerebral blood flow during temporary carotid clamping,[56] by Doppler ultrasound measurement of the direction of flow in supraorbital arteries during carotid compression,[108] and by carotid cutaneous photoplethysmography during carotid compression.[34]

Attempts to augment collateral flow include use of general anesthesia, induced hypertension, hypercapnia and hypocapnia, use of shunts, and combinations of these.[113] Both the clinical evaluation and effective treatment of a cerebral collateral vascular bed is difficult. For this reason, most risk factor modification emphasizes prevention of the initial vessel occlusive disease.

In North America, large artery occlusive disease is primarily due to progressive atherosclerotic narrowing, as opposed to other sources of occlusion such as fibro-muscular dysplasia.[35,127] Atherosclerosis presents possibilities for modifying stroke risk factors. For example, noninvasive vascular imaging with ultrasound (Figure 1) enhances our ability to determine the presence of carotid artery plaques. Studies have associated carotid bruit with overall increased stroke risk.[126]

However, carotid bruit is more a general marker of increased atherosclerotic disease than a specific indicator of the vessel at risk. The results of the North American Symptomatic Carotid Artery Stenosis Trial[4] confirm that carotid plaque relates to stroke. In this

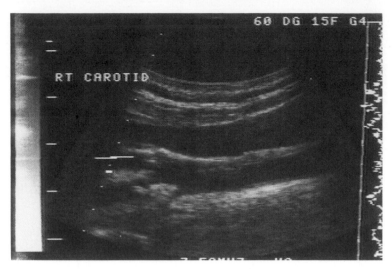

Figure 1. Ultrasound image of the right carotid bifurcation with athero-sclerotic plaque causing flow-sifnificant stenosis of the internal carotid artery (lower-left side).

study, removal of a flow-significant carotid artery plaque in symptomatic patients significantly reduced the incidence of late ipsilateral stroke. The study supports the assumption that increased carotid artery plaque is associated with increased ischemic events, making intervention to reduce carotid plaques a legitimate risk factor modification for stroke prevention.

A substantial proportion of persons with ischemic strokes are found to have no ipsilateral carotid stenosis, indicating that much of the cause of brain ischemia remains to be explained.[128] Further investigations such as the Asymptomatic Carotid Artery Stenosis Study may add to information regarding plaque as a marker of increased risk of ipsilateral stroke.

Heart Disease and Cardiogenic Emboli

Epidemiologic studies consistently find a strong association between stroke and cardiac disease.[104] This association can be interpreted in two ways: (1) heart disease is a factor that increases the risk of stroke; or (2) heart disease and stroke share causes such as hyper-

tension, smoking, and other etiologic agents of occlusive arterial disease.

Emboli from a diseased heart is one mechanism by which heart disease serves as a risk factor for brain ischemia due to occlusive vessel disease. Cardiogenic embolism is suspected to cause approximately 15% of all ischemic strokes,[24] and the majority of these are due to nonvalvular (nonrheumatic) atrial fibrillation,[8,87,106] acute myocardial infarction,[102] left ventricular aneurysm,[12] rheumatic heart disease, or a combination of these.[123]

Risk factors for Cerebral Artery Occlusion

Age

Age is generally regarded as the most important unmodifiable risk factor for cerebral artery atherosclerosis and occlusion.[18,25,32,86,93] Noninvasive studies of 286 subjects in our cerebral vascular laboratories showed a significant (p < .05) independent association between advancing age and progressive thickening of carotid artery plaque.[25] In a study of a representative sample of men from eastern Finland, the proportion of subjects with atherosclerotic carotid plaque increased from 1.1% for 42-year-olds to 4.1% for 48-year-olds, 11.8% for 54-year-olds, and 22.9% for 60-year-olds.[96] Age is also regarded as the most important risk factor for all types of strokes.[23] In the population over age 55, stroke rates double with each increasing decade of life.[91]

It is not certain, however, if atherosclerosis is due to a natural process of aging in the arteries or to the cumulative effect of exposure to other agents or conditions which may initiate or accelerate a pathological process.[112] Since chronological age cannot be modified, subjects should be evaluated in terms of their physiologic ages or of their risk-equivalent ages.[5,44] Much current prevention is based upon effort to modify "age" by improving the apparent physiologic condition or by modifying the risk profile; the implicit rationale is that the subject will have the apparent risk of a younger person. For example, carotid endarterectomy is undertaken to restore a segment of arteries to the appearance and function it had years before the surgery.

While chronological age is not a modifiable risk factor, it highlights the increasing importance of other risk factors in the older population. The deceleration of the atherosclerotic process or its sequela can be studied by noninvasive measures. Thus, the concept of a physiologic age of the vessel in the patient is important in clinical decisionmaking, especially as it pertains to surgical decisions.

Tobacco Use

The relationship of smoking to stroke has become progressively more clear. While smoking was a previously recognized risk factor for cardiac and peripheral atherosclerosis, recent studies have established strong evidence that cigarette smokers suffer from excess risk of stroke.[100] In the Framingham study, cigarette smoking increases risk of stroke independent of age, hypertension, or other cardiovascular disease risk factors.[122] This increased risk itself decreases between 2 and 5 years after cessation of smoking.

Studies from our laboratory suggest that this relationship is mediated through the effect of total smoking exposure on atherosclerotic carotid artery plaque progression. In one study we found that carotid atherosclerosis is accelerated beyond that which was found in nonsmoking patients by the independent influence of smoking and hypertension (Figure 2). In 790 smokers studied by duplex ultrasound, a significant dose-response effect for lifetime smoking exposure to carotid artery atherosclerotic plaque was identified. Smoking, age, and hypertension all contributed independently to progressive thickness of the interluminal plaque. Heavy smokers (more than 60 pack-years of cigarette smoking) had an acceleration of carotid plaque thickening generally beyond that seen in light smokers (less than 30 pack years) who were 10 years their seniors. This effect was, in turn, independent of age, hypertension and diabetes.[19] Such interactions emphasize that no one risk factor should be considered or treated in isolation from other variables of a truly systemic disease.

In another recent study, duration of cigarette smoking was found to be of greater independent significance than age, hypertension, diabetes, sex, or current systolic blood pressure in predicting severe extracranial carotid artery atherosclerosis in patients.[122]

A study of 49 pairs of identical twins who were discordant for cigarette smoking showed that, with a mean life-long smoking dose of only 20 pack-years, carotid artery stenosis was more likely in the smoking co-twins (p = 0.036), the thickness of the inner layer of carotid arteries was greater in the smoking co-twin (p < .001), and the total area of carotid plaques was 3.2 times larger in the smoking co-twins (p < .001).[42] In a representative sample of eastern Finnish men, cigarette-years was the strongest single determinant of carotid atherosclerosis in a multivariate model that included age, body mass index, serum low-density lipoproteins (LDL), high-density

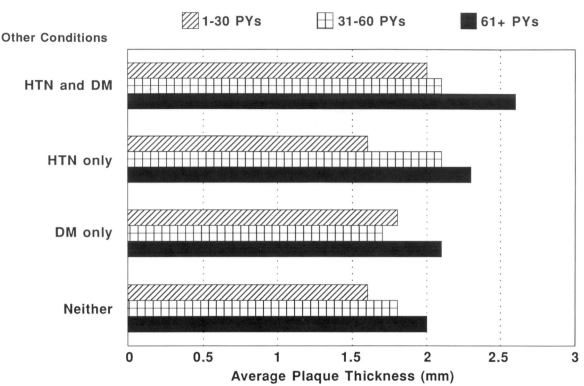

Figure 2. Age-adjusted mean carotid artery plaque thickness by pack-years (PY) of smoking and history of hypertension (HTN) and/or diabetes (DM). From Dempsey RJ and Moore RW. Amount of smoking independently predicts carotid artery atherosclerosis severity. Stroke *1992;23(5):693-696. Reprinted by permission of the American Heart Association.*

liproproteins (HDL$_2$ and HDL$_3$) cholesterol, plasma fibrinogen, and years of hypertension.[96]

In a representative subset of this sample (n = 100), smoking was independently associated with progress of carotid atherosclerosis over a 2-year period.[95] In another study, patients who were former smokers had a carotid plaque distribution that was intermediate to that of nonsmokers and current smokers. This suggests a reduction in the rate of progression of carotid plaque formation among former smokers compared to current smokers.[111]

Hypertension

Due to its strong relationship to both brain infarction and hemorrhage, and to its high prevalence in the population, hypertension is regarded as the most important of all of the modifiable risk factors for stroke.[23]

The role of hypertension in stroke is multifactorial. Systolic pressure has been closely linked to overall stroke rates. In the Framingham study, elevation of blood pressure was positively related to risk of stroke.[63,64]

Control of hypertension appears to contribute to reduction of hemorrhagic and small vessel brain ischemia in the major population.[99] Effective treatment of blood pressure has been correlated with reduction of stroke incidence and mortality in multiple studies.[30,54,115]

Systemic hypertension-related small vessel disease in the brain collateral beds is a key factor in the decrease of the available collaterals needed to tolerate a proximal large arterial occlusion. Hypertension-related aging of the small vessel collaterals appears to be a primary factor in the increasing stroke rate seen with age in carotid occlusion studies and is inferred to be important in the increasing intolerance to transient ischemia in the elderly population.

Recent studies also suggest a positive correlation of increased blood pressure and accelerated carotid atherosclerosis independent of other factors such as age, smoking, or diabetes.[18,25,37,40,120] However, a population-based study did not find that years of hypertension or current blood pressure had an independent effect on the degree of carotid atherosclerosis.[96] The mechanism of this proposed relationship, if it is causal in nature, is obscure. It is theorized that the shear effect of high-pressure flow on existing atherosclerotic plaque may result in progressive damage with resulting proliferative attempts at repair within the arterial plaque. Progressive intimal wall thickening and accelerated stenosis of the involved vessel may result.

Cholesterol

Elevation of blood cholesterol and lipids, particularly that of LDL, are associated with increased risk for both cardiac and cerebral infarction. The overall stroke rate is increased in some types of familial hyperlipidemia.[65] An age-related effect has been noted for increased lipids in the younger patient at risk for stroke.[60] Increasing LDL levels have been associated with increased atherosclerotic plaque as well.

In the Salonen et al population-based study of Finnish men, univariate and age-adjusted analysis revealed that LDL cholesterol was positively associated with severity of carotid atherosclerosis, and HDL was negatively associated with carotid atherosclerosis. However, when LDL and HDL were entered into a regression model with age, cigarette-years of smoking, duration of hypertension, and plasma fibrinogen, only LDL cholesterol remained significantly associated with carotid plaque severity; HDL levels ceased to be significantly associated with carotid plaque.[96]

Tell et al reviewed 24 publications for the relationship between plasma lipid or lipoprotein concentrations protein (total cholesterol, triglycerides, low-density lipoprotein, and/or high-density lipoprotein) and cerebrovascular atherosclerosis. They reported that statistically significant associations were found in all but 4 of these reports.[110] However, only 6 of the 24 studies reviewed performed multivariate analyses. Where multivariate analysis was reported, total cholesterol was associated with atherosclerosis in extracranial carotid arteries in only 1 angiographic correlational study,[86] with atherosclerosis in major intracranial arteries in 1 autopsy study,[51] and with atherosclerosis in large arteries of the circle of Willis in 1 autopsy study.[89] Only 1 autopsy study found that triglyceride levels remained significantly associated with cerebral atherosclerosis (in small vessels of the circle of Willis) after multivariate analysis.[89] Two studies found a statistically significant (negative) association between HDL and severity of carotid atherosclerosis measured by angiography[32] and by ultrasound.[18]

Data relating cholesterol management to stroke reduction are even less clear. Nevertheless, due to the suspected relationship of increased cholesterol and increased stroke risk, treatment suggestions include aggressive lipoprotein management for patients considered to be at risk for cerebral vascular disease. The ongoing Asymptomatic Carotid Artery Plaque Study is investigating this relationship by looking at aggressive lowering of LDL levels in patients known to have established atherosclerotic artery lesions, but who have not yet gone on to manifest symptoms. Serial measurements will determine if aggressive lipoprotein reduction leads to stabilization or regression of atherosclerotic carotid artery lesions. While the relationship of extreme levels of lipoproteins to disease states appears clear, evidence from studies such as this may suggest that even the presently accepted North American levels of cholesterol and lipoproteins may be pathologic.

Alcohol and Other Drugs

A positive association between alcohol consumption and strokes in general, and for brain infarction in men, was found in the Framingham Study.[127] Conversely, it has also been reported that risk of stroke is lessened with low levels of alcohol consumption; only at moderate to high levels of drinking is there an increased risk for stroke.[37]

While some reports have suggested this association is primarily seen in hemorrhagic stroke,[21,69,105] it has also been observed to be correlated with ischemic stroke in some studies.[50,74] In one case-control study, the positive association between alcohol ingestion within the past 72 hours and stroke onset disappeared when statistical controls for smoking and history of hypertension were applied.[39] In a study of similar design, recent alcohol consumption was concluded to have a statistically significant association with stroke after controls for smoking and hypertension; however, duration of smoking was not included in measuring tobacco use, but rather daily consumption was used to assess smoking.[38] These studies demonstrate: (1) the importance of multivariate analysis in assessing risk factors such as alcohol use, and (2) the significance of the nature of measurement of control variables, in this case tobacco use, in determining the outcomes of tests of statistical independence.

In the Whisnant et al study of predictors for extracranial carotid artery atherosclerosis, frequency of alcohol use (never, occasionally, frequently, daily) was significantly related to carotid plaque after controlling for age and sex (p = .04). However, when years of cigarette smoking was introduced as a control variable, alcohol use ceased to be significantly associated with carotid atherosclerotic plaque severity.[120] Additionally, alcohol consumption may effect cardiac arrythmia.[28] The overall effect of alcohol appears to be determined by producing alterations in cerebral blood flow on a cardiac basis and by inhibiting flow at a distal stenotic lesion site.

Other drugs have been associated with hemorrhagic strokes. Cocaine and amphetamine use contribute to elevated blood pressure and vasculitis. Thromboembolic stroke may be related to intravenous drug abuse and an infected route of administration. Such emboli take a similar distribution and anatomic course to those of cardioembolic lesions.

Oral contraceptives have been shown to be associated with an increased risk of cerebral infarction. While the individual risk may be slight, the frequency of use makes the overall population impact profound. In some subgroups stroke risk may be increased considerably and is enhanced by an additional history of hypertension, migraine, diabetes, cigarette smoking, and age greater than 35.[45] The data overall are not completely resolved regarding the risk of estrogen use in postmenopausal women. Separate studies have associated such drugs with a decrease in stroke death[85] and an increase in cerebral vascular disease.[121] Subgroup analysis of particular types of stroke may eventually help to clarify this issue.

Fibrinogen

Elevated fibrinogen levels are considered to increase the risk of stroke.[62,125] Increased fibrinogen also is associated with the progression of carotid stenosis in asymptomatic patients.[41] Exact etiologies are not clear, but intervascular obstruction of flow is postulated. This may damage small vessel flow patterns or may predispose to the increased formation of thrombus at a site of vessel injury or atherosclerotic plaque irregularity. Salonen et al found fibrinogen to be significantly associated with carotid plaque severity when adjusted for age, but not when serum lipids, years of cigarette smoking, and duration of hypertension were added to the regression model.[96].

Diet

The primary elements of diet that are suspected of contributing to an increased risk of stroke are potassium intake, sodium intake (through its influence on hypertension), and fat intake (through its influence on serum lipids). Evidence that reducing levels of salt and fat reduces risk of heart disease has been widely accepted.[3,20,82] However, it has not been demonstrated that dietary fat and sodium intake are independently associated with stroke incidence.[59] A high level of dietary potassium intake appears to be independently associated with a decreased risk of death from stroke.[67]

Modifications of diet are generally undertaken on an individual basis. The purpose is an attempt to intervene with cholesterol, atherosclerotic plaque, or blood pressure as intermediate contributors to decreasing stroke incidence. These individual dietary interventions are more difficult, expensive, and prone to failure than are "structural" interventions, i.e. interventions in which social, cultural, and marketplace conditions are changed to modify opportunities within a population for healthy diet consumption. The impact of diet on atherosclerotic plaque in large cerebral arteries is still under study. The availability of noninvasive assessment of carotid plaque in asymptomatic subjects has created new opportunities for research in this area. The assessment of consumption of various elements in diet remains a technically formidable task.

Sedentary Lifestyle

The observed association between sedentary occupation and increased risk for heart disease has not been seen in relation to stroke.[57,66,76,78,84] Among patients with reversible cerebral ischemic attacks, Passero et al found no association between either work or leisure activity level and the presence or degree of cerebral atherosclerosis in intracranial or extracranial vessels.[86] Similarly, Whisnant et al found that physical activity level was not significantly related to extracranial carotid artery atherosclerosis in patients undergoing carotid arteriography.[120]

Diabetes

Diabetes mellitus is both an independent and an associated risk factor for atherosclerotic stroke.[1] It is commonly associated with hypertension and heart disease in the etiology of stroke. Diabetes also has an independ-

ent impact on atherosclerotic stroke rates.[98] Diabetics appear to be affected both by large vessel atherosclerosis and also by a relative intolerance to ischemia. Hyperglycemia itself is a risk factor for increased infarct size in the setting of cerebral ischemia.[1,15]

Duncan et al found that patients with carotid stenosis were more likely to have a history of diabetes than were age and sex matched controls.[22] However, in similarly designed research, Clagett et al did not find any difference in rates of diabetes among patients with recurrent carotid artery stenosis.[12] Carotid disease progression was more frequent in diabetics than nondiabetics in a prospective study of asymptomatic patients with cervical bruits.[92] Bogousslavsky et al found that diabetes was significantly more common among subjects with internal carotid artery occlusion or stenosis compared to age- and sex-matched controls.[7] The independence of the association of diabetes with carotid atherosclerosis continues to be debated.

History of diabetes was not associated with the presence or degree of extracranial or intracranial atherosclerotic lesions in the Italian Multicenter Study on Reversible Cerebral Ischemic Attacks.[11] Ford et al found that, after controlling for age, diabetes was not significantly associated with the percent of carotid stenosis in patients studied angiographically.[32] Crouse found diabetes to be significantly associated with severity of carotid atherosclerosis in a bivariate analysis, but not in multivariate analysis in which age, hypertension, smoking, HDL cholesterol, uric acid, and Framingham Type A score were included in a regression model.[18] Similarly, Rubens et al found a positive association between diabetes and severity of carotid atherosclerosis in patients with coronary artery disease using bivariate analysis; but, when multivariate analysis was applied, diabetes had no independent relationship to carotid plaque for patients with or without coronary artery disease.[93] On the other hand, Tell et al found that among whites, diabetes was significantly associated with carotid plaque score in a multivariate analysis in which age, sex, hypertension, and smoking history were used as control variables.[111,112] Whisnant et al found diabetes to be associated with extracranial carotid plaque severity in a multivariate analysis in which age, sex, smoking, hypertension history, and current blood pressure were also independently associated with the dependent variable.[120]

Obesity

In a study of men born in 1913 in Gothenburg, Sweden, waist circumference and waist/hip ratio were significantly, independently, and positively associated with the risk of stroke.[119] However, several other reports failed to show a significant age-adjusted association of body mass index or relative weight with stroke risk in prospective population-based studies.[14,59,68,72,73,94,124] Similarly, weight has not been found to be associated with carotid atherosclerosis in multivariate analyses.[18,40,42,86,93,96] It appears that any relationship of obesity to stroke and carotid atherosclerosis is indirect, as through its association with hypertension.

Sex

Although men are more likely to have strokes than women, and to have them at earlier ages, sex is not a well-established risk factor for cerebral artery occlusion. The fact that overall women live longer than men, combined with the fact that age is the major risk factor for stroke, confounds the question. In 1988, when the sex ratio for stroke deaths was 66 (i.e. for every 100 women who died of stroke that year, there were only 66 men who died of stroke), it was nevertheless the case that the age-adjusted death rates for men were higher then for women.[118] In Rochester, Minnesota, during the period 1980-1984, the age-adjusted stroke incidence rate was 168 for men, compared to 110 for women.[9]

Attempts to modify risk that is associated with gender has been based on hormone therapy. It is postulated that the delay in stroke presentation in women may be due to early-life estrogen levels. In two studies, men were treated with female hormones in order to reduce their risk for atherosclerosis to the level of women.[75,90] However, The Veterans Administration Cooperative Study of Atherosclerosis did not show any advantage of estrogen therapy compared to placebo to men with cerebral infarction.[117]

Some of the male-female differential in stroke probably is not due to biologic differences between the sexes, but rather to differences in exposure to environmental risk factors and differential sex-related socialization. Figure 3 shows that the magnitude of the differential between men and women has varied substantially in the population in and around Rochester, Minnesota, in this century.[52] Such variation in the sex difference is consistent with an explanation based on different environmental exposures, such as tobacco use, rather than different biology. This suggests that there is a substantial opportunity in the public and environmental health arena to reduce the differential in stroke rates between men and women.

Race

Physical anthropologists aver that there is no physiologic basis for the racial distinctions that pervade most societies.[6,58] They define racial distinctions as socially constructed realities that vary in the number of racial categories, in the criteria that are used to make distinctions, and even in the permanence of those categories.[70] Further, the practice of hypodescent[47,71] ignores the actual genetic heritage of the individual. From the perspective of a long time frame, it is apparent that all humans have a common origin, and that physiologic variations are transient adaptations to local environmental conditions by relatively isolated populations.

Although genetic factors probably play a role in establishing a person's risk of atherosclerosis, it is doubtful whether these factors

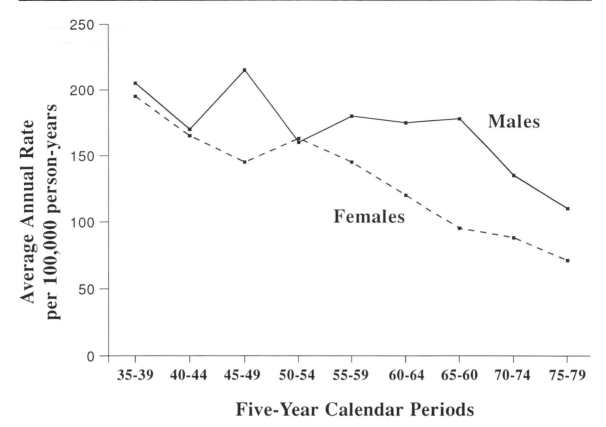

Figure 3. Average annual incidence rates for stroke in men and women from 1935-1979 in Rochester, Minnesota. Reprinted with permission from Annals of Neurology (1987; 22:250).[52]

are linked to social attributions of race. Past and continued social discrimination among races introduces more than enough variation in life chances to account for apparent correlations between race and such conditions as occlusive disease and stroke. The increment of risk for stroke that appears related to race may be due to environmental risk factors. Studies of Japanese subjects reveal that in Japan there is more intracranial than extracranial occlusive artery disease than is experienced by Japanese living in Hawaii or the United States, where they are exposed to different environmental and dietary risk factors.[79,109]

Polycythemia and Hemoglobin

Polycythemia is among associated or concurrent conditions that may predispose to increasing stroke risk. Increased hemoglobin or hematocrit as seen in polycythemia is an indicator of increased risk for stroke. The mechanism is believed to be increased blood viscosity which compresses collateral flow patterns during periods of ischemic stress. This appears also to be associated with hypertension and smoking.[80] Crouse et al did not find hemoglobin to be associated with carotid atherosclerosis.[18]

Sickle-Cell Disease

A similar process may occur in sickle-cell disease. Small-vessel occlusion may occur in widely distributed regions of the brain. The occurrence of stroke in sickle-cell anemia is related to the presentation of the underlying disease with myriad neurologic signs possible in up to 17% of patients homozygous for the disease.[88]

Uric Acid

In the study by Crouse et al, uric acid was negatively associated with carotid plaque severity after adjusting for age, hypertension, coronary stenosis, smoking, HDL cholesterol, Framingham Type A score, and left ventricular hypertrophy.[18]

Bruits

A cervical bruit is known to be a risk factor for stroke in general, but has not been shown to produce stroke in the blood distributional areas of the carotid artery with which it is associated.[23,49] Not all bruits are due to lesions, and there are many substantial lesions without accompanying bruits.

Previous Cerebral Ischemia

An important indicator of markedly increased stroke risk is a history of previous ischemic episodes—either transient ischemia attacks or cerebral infarction. For patients with previous cerebral infarction, the risk of recurrent stroke is markedly increased as compared to an age-matched population.[91] This information may be important in selecting patients who may benefit from more intensive prophylactic therapy. This is especially true if the initial stroke is not devastating and the patient is left with some functional recovery and therefore residual brain at risk.

Recommendations

Of the risk factors and signs of increased risk reviewed above, five present the greatest opportunity for intervention to prevent brain ischemia due to cerebral atherosclerosis: history of tobacco use, hypertension, blood lipids, alcohol, and history of cardiac disease.

Ultrasound Screening for Extracranial Carotid Atherosclerosis

Among men in Eastern Finland, the prevalence of atherosclerotic lesions in carotid arteries increases from 1.1% at age 42 to 4.1% at age 48, 11.8% at age 54, and 22.9% at age 60.[96] Even higher prevalence rates were observed in a representative sample of men and women in Augsburg.[40] The Atherosclerosis Risk in Communities study, now being conducted on four large representative samples in the United States, should provide information which will refine recommendations regarding the age and circumstances under which routine screening for carotid atherosclerosis should be performed.

Early detection offers the advantage of intervention before calamitous events occur and while progress can be arrested or reversed through surgery, medication, or lifestyle modification. Ultrasound investigation of carotid arteries provides an effective screening for carotid atherosclerosis in subjects presenting with cerebrovascular symptoms or major risk factors for large vessel atherosclerosis. Health-hazard appraisals to assess overall risk to health[5,44] as well as relative risk for stroke[2] are available for use in general medical practice.

Reducing Risk by Smoking Cessation

Randomized clinical trials on smoking cessation as an intervention for cerebral vessel stenosis and occlusion have not been implemented and may not be feasible. Correlational studies of patients and representative samples suggest that cigarette smoking has a cumulative, dose-response relationship to carotid artery plaque,[25,96] and that smoking avoidance[42] or cessation[111,112] may retard the progress of extracranial carotid atherosclerosis.

Healthy individuals and patients at every stage of the atherosclerotic process, from those having small, asymptomatic lesions to those trying to avoid a second stroke or restenosis after endarterectomy should be advised to avoid smoking, quit smoking, and expose themselves as little as possible to the tobacco smoke of others. Current smokers or persons who live in a household with a current smoker, should be referred to a specialized smoking cessation program.[16,17] Beyond encouraging patients to stop smoking, neurologists and neurosurgeons will find it more cost-effective and productive to make such referrals rather than undertake to treat their patient's tobacco addiction themselves.

Reducing Risk Through Hypertension Control

One of the best-documented of all stroke prevention strategies in effectiveness is hypertension control. A strong prevention approach aims to keep systolic and diastolic blood pressures below 140 mmHg and 90 mmHg, respectively.

Reducing Risk Through Lipid Control

Evidence relating lipid levels to large cerebral artery occlusion is neither as strong nor as consistent as one might expect, given the well-documented association with coronary artery disease. Difficulties in measuring the combined duration and severity of dyslipidemia produce inconsistent results. The National Heart, Lung, and Blood Institute defines blood cholesterol levels over 200 mg/dL as borderline and over 240 mg/dL as high.[103] Risk of coronary heart disease increases steadily from 200 mg/dL upward.

Low-density lipoproteins appear to elevate risk starting at approximately 130 mg/dL and are regarded as high when they are 160 mg/dL and above. High-density lipoproteins that are less than 35 mg/dL are associated with increased risk. Diet and medication are effective in reducing cholesterol and low-density lipoproteins, and exercise increases the relative proportion of high-density lipoprotein. These interventions should be routine for any patient at risk for atherosclerotic plaque disease.

Reducing Risk Through Medication: Anticoagulants

Anticoagulation medication reduces the risk of stroke and death for patients with cardiac disease. Warfarin and aspirin have been shown in randomized trials of patients with atrial fibrillation to reduce risk compared to placebo[8,87] without substantial increase in bleeding complications. Similarly, the Warfarin Reinfarction Study shows an impressive benefit in stroke risk reduction for patients treated with anticoagulation following myocardial infarction.[102] Patients with left ventricular aneurysm have not been studied in randomized trials for the benefits of anticoagulation therapy, but based on clinical experience physicians generally recommend anticoagulation therapy for such patients who have already had one or more emboli.[24]

Recommendation of anticoagulation therapy for patients with rheumatic heart disease is made on the same basis, except for those patients in whom it occurs in conjunction with atrial fibrillation, producing an 18-fold increase in risk of stroke.[123] For subjects who have experienced cardioembolic stroke, the time of initiation of anticoagulation medication is problematic due to the vulnerability of the recently infarcted brain to hemorrhage. If computed tomography (CT) scanning demonstrates the absence of hemorrhage, some authors recommend starting anticoagulation after a delay of 1-7 days, depending on the size of the infarct, as a compromise between reducing the risk of a second embolus and causing hemorrhage.[24]

Reducing Risk Through Medication: Antiplatelets

The role of aspirin in reducing the risk of stroke is still under study. At least nine prospective, double-blind controlled studies of aspirin and stroke risk reduction have been undertaken. The majority of these studies show some benefit for the use of aspirin, but often this is limited to specific subgroups such as males. A major effect appears to be the reduction of the risk of both stroke and death from all causes, which suggests that the benefit may be systemic or cardiac. The mechanism of action is felt to be antiplatelet activity, but a similar cyclo-oxygenase inhibitor has not been shown to have independent benefit.[10]

Two unresolved issues remain regarding the use of aspirin and stroke prevention. The first is dose. Studies have recommended doses between 50 mg/day and 1.3 g/day. Most reviewers have not been able to conclude which dose is actually preferable. From theoretical and risk considerations, the lowest effective dose should be preferred. The 1988 United Kingdom TIA Trial[116] recommended 300 mg/day as a reasonable dose with minimal complications.

The second issue is whether this agent is effective for women. Several studies have failed to show a significant benefit of aspirin for women. The recent European Stroke Prevention Study,[27] in which women were well represented, did show a benefit for women both in reduction of the risk of stroke and death. Therefore, the use of aspirin for risk reduction of stroke for women is advocated.

Ticlopidine is a second antiplatelet agent under study for potential benefit in cerebral ischemia risk reduction. It appears to function primarily by inhibiting the aggregation of activated platelets. It appears to inhibit the ADP-induced exposure of the fibrinogen-binding site of the glycoprotein IIB-IIIa complex.[46] In the Ticlopidine Aspirin Stroke Study 3,069 patients presenting with cerebral ischemic events were randomized to ticlopidine 500 mg/day or aspirin 1.3 g/day.[48] In both males and females receiving ticlopidine there was a relative reduction of up to 21% for all types of strokes.

While ticlopidine appears to be an effective antiplatelet agent in stroke risk reduction, potential complications need to be considered. Aspirin has a long history of gastrointestinal complications and hemorrhage, which are dose-related. Ticlopidine complica-

tions include diarrhea, rash, urticaria, and elevation serum lipoprotein fractions. The most significant ticlopidine complication is a 0.9% incidence of severe neutropenia, which requires close physician supervision during the early months of ticlopidiine administration.

Reducing Risk Through Surgery

More information now exists regarding the prophylactic surgical removal of carotid atherosclerotic plaque prior to embolization or eventual occlusion. In the results of the North American Symptomatic Carotid Endarterectomy Trial (NASCET),[4] the question of removal of asymptomatic plaques remains open. In the NASCET study, patients with greater than 70% stenosis and ipsilateral symptomatology were substantially benefitted by prophylactic removal of the atherosclerotic carotid lesion. The benefits of surgery exceeded the initial increased morbidity from surgery. The NASCET study continues to assess the benefits of prophylactic surgery for persons with moderate (30% to 69%) carotid stenosis. The Asymptomatic Atherosclerotic Carotid Artery Stenosis Study (AACAS) is endeavoring to answer the question of surgical intervention for patients with flow-significant carotid artery stenosis discovered prior to neurologic presentation.

Conclusions

Brain ischemia due to arterial occlusive disease remains a major cause of death and disability in the North American patient population. A sensible plan of risk factor modification, based on methods to decrease progressive atherosclerotic plaque formation or the adherence of blood products to existing plaques, may substantially decrease the development of potentially devastating neurologic deficit.

References

1. Abbott RD, Donahue RP, MacMahon SW, et al. Diabetes and the risk of stroke: the Honolulu heart program. *JAMA*. 1987;257:949-952.

2. American Heart Association. *Stroke Risk Handbook: Estimating Risk of Stroke in Daily Practice.* New York: American Heart Association, 1974.

3. American Heart Association, Committee on Nutrition. Diet and coronary heart disease. *Circulation.* 1978;58:762A-766A.

4. Barnett HJM. Symptomatic carotid endarterectomy trials. *Stroke.* 1990;21(suppl 3):III-2-III-5.

5. Beery W, Schoenback VJ, Wagner EH, et al. *Description, Analysis and Assessment of Health Hazard/Health Risk Appraisal Programs: Final Report.* Chapel Hill, NC: University of North Carolina, 1981.

6. Bodmer WF, Cavalli-Sforza LL. *Genetics, Evolution, and Man.* San Francisco: W.H. Freeman and Company, 1976.

7. Bogousslavsky J, Regli F, Van Melle G. Risk factors and concomitants of internal carotid artery occlusion or stenosis. *Arch Neurol.* 1985;42:864-867.

8. Boston Area Anticoagulation Trial for Atrial Fibrillation Investigators. The effect of low-dose warfarin on the risk of stroke in patients with nonrheumatic atrial fibrillation. *N Engl J Med.* 1990;323:1505-1511.

9. Broderick JP, Phillips SJ, Whisnant JP, et al. Incidence rates of stroke in the eighties: the end of the decline in stroke? *Stroke.* 1989;20:557-582.

10. Canadian Cooperative Stroke Study Group. A randomized trial of aspirin and sulfinpyrazone in threatened stroke. *N Engl J Med.* 1978;299:53.

11. Candelise L, Bianchi F, Galligoni F, et al. Italian multicenter study on reversible cerebral ischemic attacks: III—Influence of age and risk factors on cerebrovascular atherosclerosis. *Stroke.* 1984; 15:379-382.

12. Cerebral Embolism Task Force. Cardiogenic brain embolism. *Arch Neurol.* 1986;43:71-84.

13. Clagett GP, Rich NM, McDonald PT, et al. Etiologic factors for recurrent carotid artery stenosis. *Surgery.* 1983;93:313-318.

14. Colditz GA, Bonita R, Stampfer MJ, et al. Cigarette smoking and risk of stroke in middle-aged women. *N Engl J Med.* 1988;318:937-941.

15. Combs DJ, Dempsey RJ, Maley M. et al. Relationship between plasma glucose, brain lactate, and intracellular pH during cerebral ischemia in gerbils. *Stroke.* 1990;21:936-942.

16. Cooper TM, Clayton RR. Nicotine reduction therapy and relapse prevention for heavy smokers. Three year follow up of 108 patients. *JADA.* 1990; In press.

17. Cooper TM, Clayton RR. *The Cooper/Clayton Method to Stop Smoking.* Lexington, KY: SBC/SBC Inc., 1988.

18. Crouse JR, Toole JF, McKinney WM, et al. Risk factors for extracranial carotid artery atherosclerosis. *Stroke.* 1987;18:990-996.

19. Dempsey RJ, Moore RW. Amount of smoking predicts carotid artery atherosclerosis independent of age, hypertension, and diabetes. *Stroke.* 1991; 22:150. Abstract.

20. *Dietary Goals for the United States,* 2nd ed. United States Congress. Senate Select Committee on Nutrition and Human Needs; Washington, DC: 1977.

21. Donahue RF, Abbott RD, Reed DM, et al. Alcohol and hemorrhagic stroke: the Honolulu heart program. *JAMA.* 1986;255:2311-2341.

22. Duncan GW, Lees RS, Ojemann RG, et al. Concom-

itants of atherosclerotic carotid artery stenosis. *Stroke.* 1977;8:665-669.

23. Dyken ML. Stroke risk factors. In: Hachinski VC, and Norris JW, eds. *Prevention of Stroke.* New York, NY: Springer-Verlag; 1991;83-101.

24. Easton DJ. *Role of cardiac disease.* International Symposium: Stroke Prevention: Critical Assessment of Today's Strategies. New York, NY: New York University Post-Graduate Medical School, 1991.

25. Edwards C, Rob C. Relief of neurological symptoms and signs by reconstruction of a stenosed internal carotid artery. *Br Med J (Clin Res).* 1956;2: 1265-1267.

26. Eikelboom BC. *Evaluation of Carotid Artery Disease and Potential Circulation by Ocular Pneumoplethysmography.* Utrect: Uitgeversmaatschappij Huisartsenpers BV, 1981.

27. The European Stroke Prevention Study: Principal endpoints. *Lancet.* 1987;2:1351-1354.

28. Ettinger PO, Wu CF, De La Cruz C Jr, et al. Arrhythmias and the "Holiday Heart": Alcohol-associated cardiac rhythm disorders. *Am Heart J.* 1978;95:555-562.

29. Fields WS, Lemak NA. *A History of Stroke: Its Recognition and Treatment.* New York, NY: Oxford University Press; 1989.

30. Fieschi C, Carolei A, Salvetti M, et al. Systemic hypertension as a treatable risk factor for cerebrovascular disease. *Am J Cardiol.* 1989;63:19C-21C.

31. Fisher M. Occlusion of the internal carotid artery. *Arch Neurol Psychiat.* 1951;65:346-377.

32. Ford CS, Crouse JR III, Howard G, et al. The role of plasma lipids in carotid bifurcation atherosclerosis. *Ann Neurol.* 1985;17: 301-303.

33. Foster JH. Arteriography: cornerstone of vascular surgery. *Arch Surg.* 1974;109:605-611.

34. Fuster B. Carotid cutaneous photoplethysmography test: a method to explore the carotid and vertebral basilar systems. *Clin Electroencephalogr.* 1977;8: 6-26.

35. Garraway WM, Whisnant JP, Furlan AJ, et al. The declining incidence of stroke. *N Engl J Med.* 1979; 300:449-452.

36. Giannotta S, McGillicuddy J, Kindt GW. Gradual carotid artery occlusion in the treatment of inaccessible internal carotid artery aneurysms. *Neurosurgery.* 1979;5:417-421.

37. Gill JS, Shipley MJ, Hornby RH, et al. A community case-control study of alcohol consumption in stroke. *Int J Epidemiol.* 1988;17:542-547.

38. Gill JS, Zezulka AV, Shipley MJ, et al. Stroke and alcohol consumption. *N Engl J. Med.* 1986;315: 1041-1046.

39. Gorelick PB, Rodin MB, Langenberg P, et al. Is acute alcohol ingestion a risk factor for ischemic stroke? Results of a controlled study in middle-aged and elderly stroke patients at three urban medical centers. *Stroke.* 1987;18:359-364.

40. Gostomzyk JG, Heller WD, Gerhardt P, et al. B-scan ultrasound examination of the carotid arteries within a representative population (MONICA Project Augsburg). *Klin Wochenschr.* 1988;66(suppl 11):58-65.

41. Grotta JC, Yatsu FM, Pettigrew LC, et al. Prediction of carotid stenosis progression by lipid and hematologic measurements. *Neurology.* 1989; 39:1325-1331.

42. Haapanen A, Koskenvuo M, Kaprio J, et al. Carotid arteriosclerosis in identical twins discordant for

cigarette smoking. *Circulation.* 1989;80:10-16.

43. Hachinski V, Norris JW. *The Acute Stroke.* Philadelphia. Pa: F. A. Davis Company, 1985.

44. Hall JH, Zwemer JD. *Prospective Medicine.* Indianapolis, Ind: Methodist Hospital of Indiana, 1979.

45. Handin RI. Thromboembolic complications of pregnancy and oral contraceptives. *Prog Cardiovas Dis.* 1974;16:395-405.

46. Hardisty RM, Powling MJ, Nokes TJC. The action of ticlopidine on human platelets: studies on aggregation, secretion, calcium mobilization and membrane glycoproteins. *Thromb Haemost.* 1990;64:150-155.

47. Haris M, Kottak CP. The structural significance of Brazilian racial categories. *Sociologia.* 1963;25:203-209.

48. Hass WK, Easton JD, Adams HP Jr, et al. A randomized trial comparing ticlopidine hydrochloride with aspirin for the prevention of stroke in high-risk patients. *N Engl J Med.* 1989;321:501-507.

49. Heyman A, Wilkinson WE, Heyden S, et al. Risk of stroke in asymptomatic persons with cervical arterial bruits: a population study in Evans County, Georgia. *N Engl J Med.* 1980;302:838-841.

50. Hillbom M, Kaste M. Alcohol intoxication: a risk factor for primary subarachnoid hemorrhage. *Neurology.* 1982;32:706-711.

51. Holme I, Enger SC, Helgeland A, et al. Risk factors and raised atherosclerotic lesions in coronary and cerebral arteries: statistical analysis from the Oslo study. *Arteriosclerosis.* 1981;1:250-256.

52. Homer D, Whisnant JP, Schoenberg BS. Trends in the incidence rates of stroke in Rochester, Minnesota since 1935. *Ann Neurol.* 1987;22:250.

53. Horton DA, Fine RD, Lethlean AK, et al. The virtues of continuous EEG monitoring during carotid endarterectomy. *Aust NZ J Med.* 1974;4:32-40.

54. Hypertension Detection and Follow-up Program Cooperative Group. Five-year findings of the hypertension detection and follow-up program: III. reduction in stroke incidence among persons with high blood pressure. *JAMA.* 1982;247:633-638.

55. Iso H, Jacobs DR Jr, Wentworth D, et al. Serum cholesterol levels and six-year mortality from stroke in 350,977 men screened for the Multiple Risk Factor Intervention Trial. *N Engl J Med.* 1989;320:904-910.

56. Jennett WB, Harper AM, Gillespie FC. Measurement of regional cerebral blood-flow during carotid ligation. *Lancet.* 1966;2:1162-1163.

57. Johnson KG, Yano K, Kato H. Cerebral vascular disease in Hiroshima, Japan. *J Chronic Dis.* 1967;20:545-549.

58. Jurman R, Nelson H, Turnbaugh WA. *Understanding Physical Anthropology and Archeology,* 3rd edition. St. Paul, MN: West, 1987.

59. Kagan A, Popper JS, Rhoads GG, et al. Dietary and other risk factors for stroke in Hawaiian Japanese men. *Stroke.* 1985;16:390-396.

60. Kannel WB. Epidemiology of cerebrovascular disease. In: Russell RWR, ed. *Cerebral Arterial Disease.* New York, NY: Churchill Livingstone; 1976:1-23.

61. Kannel WB, Gordon T, Wolf PA, et al. Hemoglobin and the risk of cerebral infarction: the Framingham study. *Stroke.* 1972;3:409-420.

62. Kannel WP, Wolf PA, Castelli WP, et al. Fibrinogen and risk of cardiovascular disease: the Framingham study. *JAMA.* 1987;258:1183-1186.

63. Kannel WB, Wolf PA, McGee DL, et al. Systolic blood pressure, arterial rigidity, and risk of stroke: the Framingham study. *JAMA.* 1981;245:1225-1229.

64. Kannel WB, Wolf PA, Verter J, et al. Epidemiologic assessment of the role of blood pressure in stroke: the Framingham study. *JAMA.* 1970; 214:301-310.

65. Kaste M, Koivisto P. Risk of brain infarction in familial hypercholesterolemia. *Stroke.* 1988;19:1097-1100.

66. Katsuki S, Omae T, Hirota Y. Epidemiological and clinicopathological studies on cerebrovascular disease. *Kyushi J Med Sci.* 1964;15:127-149.

67. Khaw KT, Barrett-Connor E. Dietary potassium and stroke-associated mortality—a 12 year prospective population study. *N Engl J Med.* 1987;316:235-240.

68. Khaw KT, Barrett-Conner E, Suarez L, et al. Predictors of stroke-associated mortality in the elderly. *Stroke.* 1984;15:244-248.

69. Klatsky AL, Armstrong MA, Friedman GD. Alcohol use and subsequent cerebrovascular disease hospitalizations. *Stroke.* 1989;20:741-746.

70. Kottak CP. *Assault on Paradise: Social Change in a Brazilian Village.* New York: Random House, 1983.

71. Kottak CP. *Anthropology: The Exploration of Human Diversity,* 4th edition. New York: Random House, 1987.

72. Lapidus L, Bengtsson C, Larsson B, et al. Distribution of adipose tissue and risk of cardiovascular disease and death: a 12 year follow up of participants in the population study of women in Gothenburg, Sweden. *Bri Med J (Clin Res).* 1984;289:1257-1261.

73. Larsson B, Svärdsudd K, Welin L, et al. Abdominal adipose tissue distribution, obesity, and risk of cardiovascular disease and death: 13 year follow up of participants in the study of men born in 1913. *Bri Med J (Clin Res).* 1984;288:1401-1404.

74. Lee K. Alcoholism and cerebrovascular thrombosis in the young. *Acta Neurol Scand.* 1979;59:270-274.

75. Marmorston J. Effect of estrogen treatment in cerebrovascular disease. In: *Cerebral Vascular Diseases.* New York: Grune & Stratton, 1965.

76. Marquardsen J. The natural history of acute cerebrovascular disease: a retrospective study of 769 patients. *Acta Neurol Scand.* 1969;45(suppl 38):111-192.

77. Matas R. Testing the efficiency of the collateral circulation as a preliminary to the occlusion of the great surgical arteries. *Ann Surg.* 1911;53:1-43.

78. Miller FD, Reed DM, MacLean CJ. A prospective study of mortality and morbidity among carpenters in the Honolulu Heart Program Cohort. *J Occup Med.* 1988;30:879-882.

79. Mitsuyama Y, Thompson LR, Hayashi T, et al. Autopsy study of cerebrovascular disease in Japanese men who lived in Hiroshima, Japan and Honolulu Hawaii. *Stroke.* 1979;10:389-395.

80. Moore WS, Hall AD. Carotid artery back pressure: a test of cerebral tolerance to temporary carotid occlusion. *Arch Surg.* 1969;99:702-710.

81. Nishioka H. Results of the treatment of intracranial aneurysms by occlusion of the carotid artery in the neck. *J Neurosurg.* 1966;25:660-682.

82. *Nutrition and Your Health: Dietary Guidelines for Americans.* U.S. Department of Agriculture and Department of Health, Education and Welfare. USDA-DHEW, Washington, D.C., 1980.

83. Ostfeld AM, Wilk E. Epidemiology of stroke, 1980-1990: progress report. *Epidemiol Rev.* 1990;12:253-256.

84. Paffenbarger RS Jr, Laughlin ME, Gima AS, et al. Work activity of longshoremen as related to death from coronary heart disease and stroke. *N Engl J Med.* 1970;282:1109-1114.

85. Paganini-Hill A, Ross RK, Henderson BE. Postmenopausal estrogen treatment and stroke: a prospective study. *BMJ (Clin Res).* 1988;297:519-522.

86. Passero S, Rossi G, Nardini M, et al. Italian multicenter study of reversible cerebral ischemic attacks, 5: risk factors and cerebral atherosclerosis. *Atherosclerosis.* 1987;63:211-224.

87. Petersen P, Boysen G, Godtfredsen J, et al. Placebo-controlled, randomized trial of warfarin and aspirin for prevention of thromboembolic complications in chronic atrial fibrillation: the Copenhagen AFASAK study. *Lancet.* 1989;1:175-178.

88. Portnoy BA, Herion JC. Neurological manifestations in sickle-cell disease: with a review of the literature and emphasis on the prevalence of hemiplegia. *Ann Intern Med.* 1972;76:643-652.

89. Reed DM, Resch JA, Hayashi T, et al. A prospective study of cerebral artery atherosclerosis. *Stroke.* 1988;19:820-825.

90. Rivin AU, Dimitroff SP. The incidence and severity of atherosclerosis in estrogen-treated males, and in females with hypoestrogenic or a hyperestrogenic state. *Circulation.* 1954;9:533-539.

91. Robins M, Baum HM. The national survey of stroke: incidence. *Stroke.* 1981;12(suppl):I45-I57.

92. Roederer GO, Langlois YE, Jager KA, et al. The natural history of carotid arterial disease in asymptomatic patients with cervical bruits. *Stroke.* 1984;15:605-613.

93. Rubens J, Espeland MA, Ryu J, et al. Individual variation in susceptibility to extracranial carotid atherosclerosis. *Arteriosclerosis.* 1988;8:389-397.

94. Salonen JT, Puska P, Tuomilehto J, et al. Relation of blood pressure, serum lipids, and smoking to the risk of cerebral stroke: a longitudinal study in eastern Finland. *Stroke.* 1982;13:327-333.

95. Salonen R, Salonen JT. Progression of carotid atherosclerosis and its determinants: a population-based ultrasonography study. *Atherosclerosis.* 1990;81:33-40.

96. Salonen R, Seppänen K, Rauramaa R, et al. Prevalence of carotid atherosclerosis and serum cholesterol levels in eastern Finland. *Arteriosclerosis.* 1988;8:788-792.

97. Santos dos JC. Sur la desobstruction des throboses arterilles anciennes. *Mem Acad de Chir.* 1947;73:409-411.

98. Schoenberg BS, Schoenberg DG, Pritchard DA, et al. Differential risk factors for complete stroke and transient ischemic attacks TIA): study of vascular diseases (hypertension, cardiac disease, peripheral vascular disease) and diabetes mellitus. *Am Neurol Assoc.* 1980;105:165-167.

99. Shimizu Y, Kato H, Lin CH et al. Relationship between longitudinal changes in blood pressure and stroke incidence. *Stroke.* 1984;15:839-946.

100. Shinton R, Beevers G. Meta-analysis of relation between cigarette smoking and stroke. *BMJ.* 1989;298:789-794.

101. Schoenberg BS. Epidemiology of cerebrovascular disease. *South Med J.* 1979;72:331-336.

102. Smith P, Arnsen H, Holme I. The effect of warfarin on mortality and reinfarction after myocardial infarction. *N Engl J Med.* 1990;323:147-152.

103. *So You Have High Blood Cholesterol....* Bethesda, Md: National Institutes of Health (Publication No. 87-2922), 1987.

104. Stallones RA. Epidemiology of stroke in relation to the cardiovascular disease complex. *Adv Neurol.* 1979;25:117-126.

105. Stampfer MJ, Colditz GA, Willett WC, et al. A prospective study of moderate alcohol consumption and the risk of coronary disease and stroke in women. *N Engl J Med.* 1988;319:267-273.

106. Stroke Prevention in Atrial Fibrillation Study Group Investigators: preliminary report of the stroke prevention in atrial fibrillation study. *N Engl J Med.* 1990;322:863-868.

107. Strully KJ, Hurwitt ES, Blankenberg HW. Thromboendarterectomy for thrombosis of the internal carotid artery in the neck. *J Neurosurg.* 1953;10:474-482.

108. Tada K, Nukoda T, Yoneda S, et al. Assessment of the capacity of cerebral collateral circulation using ultrasonic Doppler technique. *J Neurol Neurosurg Psychiatry.* 1975;38:1068-1075.

109. Takeya Y, Popper JS, Shimizu Y, et al. Epidemiologic studies of coronary heart disease and stroke in Japanese living in Japan, Hawaii and California. *Stroke.* 1984;15:15-23.

110. Tell GS, Crouse JR, Furberg CD. Relation between blood lipids, liproproteins, and cerebrovascular atherosclerosis: a review. *Stroke.* 19:423-430.

111. Tell GS, Howard G, McKinney WM, et al. Cigarette smoking cessation and extracranial carotid atherosclerosis. *JAMA.* 1989;261:1178-1180.

112. Tell GS, Howard G, McKinney WM. Risk factors for site specific extracranial carotid plaque distribution as measured by B-mode ultrasound. *J Clin Epidemiol.* 1989;42:551-559.

113. Thompson JE, Talkington CM. Carotid endarterectomy. *Ann Surg.* 1976;184:1-15.

114. Torkildsen A, Koppang K. Notes on the collateral cerebral circulation as demonstrated by carotid angiography. *J Neurosurg.* 1951;8:269-278.

115. Tuomilehto J, Piha T, Nissinen A, et al. Trends in stroke mortality and in antihypertensive treatment in Finland from 1972 to 1984 with special reference to North Karelia. *J Hum Hypertens.* 1987;1:201-208.

116. UK-TIA Study Group. United Kingdom Transient Ischemic Attack (UK-TIA) aspirin trial: Interim Results. *Br Med J.* 1988;296:315-320.

117. Veterans Administration Cooperative Study Group. Estrogenic therapy in men with ischemic cerebrovascular disease: effect on recurrent cerebral infarction and survival. Final report of the Veterans Administration Cooperative Study of Atherosclerosis, Neurology Section. *Stroke.* 1972;3:427-433.

118. Vital Statistics of the United States, 1988. Volume II, Part B. Hyattsville, MD: United States Department of Health and Human Services, 1990.

119. Welin L, Svärdsudd K, Wilhelmsen L, et al. Analysis of risk factors for stroke in a cohort of men born in 1913. *N Engl J Med.* 1987;317:521-526.

120. Whisnant JP, Homer D, Ingall TJ, et al. Duration of cigarette smoking is the strongest predictor of severe extracranial carotid artery atherosclerosis. *Stroke.* 1990;21:707-714.

121. Wilson PWF, Garrison RJ, Castelli WP. Postmenopausal estrogen use, cigarette smoking, and cardiovascular morbidity in women over 50. *N Engl J Med.* 1985;313:1038-1043.

122. Wolf PA, D'Agostino RB, Kannel WB, et al.

Cigarette smoking as a risk factor for stroke: the Framingham study. *JAMA*. 1988;259:1025-1029.

123. Wolf PA, Dawber TR, Thomas HE Jr, et al. Epidemiologic assessment of chronic atrial fibrillation and risk of stroke: the Framingham study. *Neurology*. 1978;28: 973-977.

124. Wolf PA, Kannel WB. Reduction of stroke through risk factor modification. Semin Neurol. 1986;6: 243-253.

125. Wolf PA, Kannel WB, Meeks SL, et al. Fibrinogen as a risk factor for stroke: the Framingham study. *Stroke*. 1985;16:139.

126. Wolf PA, Kannel WB, Sorlie P, et al. Asymptomatic carotid bruit and risk of stroke: the Framingham study. *JAMA*. 1981;245:1442-1445.

127. Wolf PA, Kannel WB, Verter J. Current status of risk factors for stroke. *Neurologic Clinics,* Philadelphia, Pa: W.B. Saunders Company; 1983;317-343.

128. Zhu CZ, Norris JW. Role of cardotid stenosis in ischemic stroke. *Stroke*. 1990;21:1131-1134.

CHAPTER 7

Medical Management of Acute Brain Ischemia

Stephen Davis, MD

The reported declining incidence of stroke in most Western societies is chiefly attributable to primary stroke prevention, by means of recognizing and modifying risk factors, particularly hypertension.[28] Major advances in stroke management also include the investigation and treatment of transient ischemic attacks (TIAs) and minor strokes, strategies for prevention of recurrent stroke, and coordinated neurologic rehabilitation of stroke survivors.

Although there is also evidence of a decline in stroke mortality,[28] stroke is still associated with a substantial acute mortality rate, in the order of 20%, and remains the prime cause of major neurologic disability. Specific salvage or "tissue rescue" therapy for ischemic and hemorrhagic stroke remains the current goal for improved stroke outcome.

This chapter discusses the initial assessment of the patient presenting with acute cerebral ischemia, management of transient ischemic attacks and minor strokes, management of established cerebral infarction with emphasis on prevention of recurrent stroke,

strategies for management of patients with a progressive neurologic deficit, and experimental approaches for cerebral tissue rescue in acute ischemic stroke.

Initial Assessment and Investigation of Acute Cerebral Ischemia

The historic term "apoplexy" implied "struck with violence as if by a thunderbolt," and thus led to the use of the term "stroke." It indicated the sudden loss of brain function with disturbance of the senses and paralysis, while also implying associated psychological terror for patient and family.[36]

Evaluation of the patient with acute stroke requires precision in diagnosis and understanding of pathogenesis. The diagnosis of stroke implies a sudden or rapid (seconds to hours) focal, cerebral, or brain stem neurologic deficit due to ischemia or hemorrhage, the deficit lasting longer than 24 hours by accepted convention.[43] A TIA indicates a transient neurologic deficit of vascular origin lasting less than 24 hours, although many patients with TIAs have in fact suffered minor strokes. It is now accepted that TIAs and cerebral infarcts represent a pathoanatomic continuum, but the distinction has some clinical value.[43]

Clinical Assessment

Clinical assessment of the patient with acute stroke includes an evaluation of history, specifically including cerebrovascular risk factors, associated diseases (particularly cardiac disease) and any previous history of transient neurologic episodes or strokes. The temporal profile of the onset of the stroke is particularly important. Sudden onset favors an embolic cause or cerebral hemorrhage, while a stuttering or gradual onset, particularly occurring at night, favors an atherothrombotic basis. These distinctions are by no means absolute, however.

Examination should be directed at establishing the anatomic location and presumed pathogenesis of the neurologic deficit. It should include a thorough neurovascular examination: assessment of the patient's hemodynamic condition (including blood pressure, pulse, volume status), cardiac assessment, auscultation of the cervical vessels, and palpation of the facial pulses.

Following the exclusion of cerebral hemorrhage (see below), a differentiation should be made between ischemia in the carotid or in the vertebrobasilar territory. Carotid territory infarction is associated with neurologic deficits that implicate the middle or anterior cerebral artery territories. The presence of one or more cortical deficits such as dysphasia, apraxia, anosognosia (unawareness or denial of the stroke), sensory, motor or visual agnosia, acalculia, right/left confusion, dysgraphia, or cortical sensory loss indicates that the ischemia involves the cerebral cortex. This implies an embolic or atherothrombotic cause rather than lacunar disease, which most often presents with a pure motor

hemiplegia due to a small deep, capsular infarct.[43] Vertebrobasilar ischemia is suggested by a multiplicity of neurologic signs including crossed cranial nerve and long tract signs, bilateral visual disturbances, and various focal neurologic syndromes indicating ischemia in the vertebrobasilar territory.

While the temporal profile and nature of the presenting neurologic deficit usually indicate the diagnosis of stroke, initial assessment requires (1) the exclusion of nonvascular causes of sudden neurologic deficits ("pseudostrokes"), and (2) the vital differentiation between cerebral ischemia and cerebral hemorrhage.

Exclusion of Pseudostroke

Up to 8% of patients seen in our hospital's emergency department, and then referred to the Stroke Service, constitute individuals with noncerebrovascular pathologies. Careful history and examination may lead to the clinical suspicion of alternative neurologic pathology such as cerebral tumor, subdural hematoma, sepsis (encephalitis or meningitis), electrolyte disturbances (particularly hypoglycemia, which can produce strikingly focal neurologic deficits), labyrinthine disorders, migraine, epilepsy, and psychiatric disorders. All of these conditions can mimic the stroke process.

All patients with suspected stroke should have an urgent computed tomography (CT) scan. This will exclude many noncerebrovascular disorders that frequently require urgent specific therapy such as the surgical drainage of a subdural hematoma or cerebral abscess. Other essential initial investigations should include (1) a blood glucose to rule out hypoglycemia or hyperglycemia, (2) blood urea and electrolytes for electrolyte disturbances such as hyponatremia, (3) full blood examination to detect anemia, elevated hematocrit or other hematologic disturbance, (4) chest x-ray to detect pneumonia, cardiomegaly, cardiac failure or tumor, and (5) and an electrocardiogram (ECG) to detect or confirm arrhythmias or acute myocardial ischemia.

Differentiation Between Cerebral Ischemia and Hemorrhage

The distinction between cerebral hemorrhage and infarction is also vital, as some patients with cerebral hemorrhage are candidates for urgent surgical evacuation, and selected patients with ischemic stroke are treated by anticoagulation. This differentiation between infarction and hemorrhage is based on clinical, CT, and rarely cerebrospinal fluid (CSF) criteria.

Patients with cerebral hemorrhage have an earlier and more severe elevation of intracranial pressure (ICP) with attendant depression of conscious state, which is the single most useful clinical feature in distinguishing the two chief types of stroke. Severe headache, meningismus, and vomiting favor the diagnosis of cerebral hemorrhage. The gradual or stuttering onset of a neurologic deficit, particularly a patient with preceding TIAs in the same vascular territory, strongly favors a cerebral infarct. However, some patients with cerebral hemorrhage have a rather slow evolution of the clinical deficit, and clinical pointers can be unreliable, even when evaluated by an experienced clinician.

Early CT scan will demonstrate all clinically significant supratentorial and posterior fossa hemorrhages, except for small brain stem bleeds. We usually perform an initial noncontrast CT scan; this provides adequate management information and there is some evidence that intravascular iodinated contrast medium might exacerbate tissue damage in the presence of "leaky" cerebral vessels. Intravenous contrast is administered only if the history is atypical or if the unenhanced scan shows suggestive features of alternative pathology such as focal vasogenic edema that might indiate the presence of tumor.

Although cerebral CT scanning provides rapid diagnostic information concerning the presence of hemorrhage and many alternative pathologies, patients with cerebral infarcts often do not demonstrate abnormalities for 24-48 hours after the onset of the ictus. Early changes, including effacement of sulci and loss of gray/white matter differentiation, are seen within hours in patients with large lesions. In addition, CT may show evidence of old, often "silent" cerebral infarcts, which may provide a clue as to pathogenesis. Multiple infarcts in different vascular territories might suggest a cardiac embolic source, for example, whereas evidence of multiple lacunar infarcts or white matter ischemic changes (leucoaraiosis or subcortical arteriosclerotic encephalopathy) might indicate the presence of widespread small-vessel hypertensive disease.

Magnetic Resonance Imaging (MRI)

Magnetic resonance imaging (MRI) allows earlier detection of the tissue changes due to cerebral ischemia, but the scanning time is longer than CT in most cases, and acute hemorrhages may be missed. MRI is particularly useful for the diagnosis of hindbrain ischemia, with sensitive resolution of small brain stem infarcts (Figure 1), whereas CT is relatively insensitive and hampered by bone-induced artifacts.

MR scanning has several other advantages in the evaluation of selected patients with acute cerebral ischemia, including the ability to analyze blood flow within the cerebral arteries and venous sinuses (high signal on T1 images suggesting sluggish or absent flow). Magnetic resonance angiography (MRA) will have a major role in the future assessment of patients with acute stroke, incorporating both brain imaging and visualization of the underlying arterial anatomy and vascular blood flow. Diffusion MR scanning, while still experimental, has already been shown capable of detecting regions of cerebral ischemia less than 60 minutes after onset.

Physiologic Brain Imaging Technique

Physiologic brain imaging techniques include (1) positron emission tomography (PET), which allows in vivo measurement of both cerebral blood flow and tissue metabo-

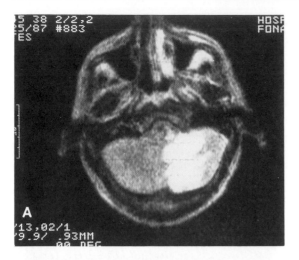

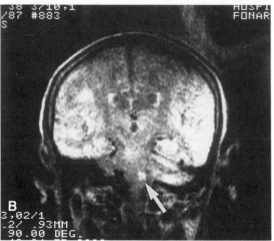

Figure 1. Axial (A) and coronal (B) T2-weighted spin echo MR scans demonstrating high intensity due to infarction in the left cerebellar hemisphere and adjacent left medulla (arrow).

lism, and single photon emission computed tomography (SPECT), which only permits evaluation of cerebral perfusion. Studies using PET,[1,44] provided an insight into relationships between cerebral blood flow and metabolism in acute cerebral ischemia and led to a pathophysiologic "staging" of the stroke process.[1] PET and SPECT are more sensitive than CT in demonstrating acute changes in cerebral ischemia, but have limited practical clinical application at present. In acute stroke, SPECT can provide early prognostic information (Figure 2).

Lumbar Puncture

Lumbar puncture should rarely be used to differentiate between infarct and hemorrhage. The technique is unreliable and can lead to catastrophic deterioration due to transtentorial herniation ("coning"), and to death secondary to the elevation of intracranial pressure associated with the acute stroke process. Lumbar puncture is usually reserved for patients with suspected cerebral sepsis and cerebral vasculitis, and in patients with the clinical suspicion of subarachnoid hemorrhage where an initial CT scan is normal.

Management of the Patient with Transient Ischemic Attack (TIA) or Minor Stroke

Natural History and Pathogenesis

A proportion of patients with acute cerebral ischemia will rapidly recover and fulfil the criteria for TIA, or have only a minor neurologic deficit. Although the majority of TIAs are very brief, usually lasting less than 1 hour,[42] CT and particularly more sensitive brain imaging techniques such as MRI, SPECT, and PET have indicated that many TIAs in fact produce tissue damage and represent small cerebral infarcts.

Many natural history studies have indicated that the risk of stroke after a TIA is approximately 5%-10% per year, compared with about 1% in a control age-matched population.[42] This risk is greatest in the first few weeks after the initial event and is increased in patients with multiple events, particularly "crescendo TIAs," and in those with underlying severe arterial stenosis.

TIAs and minor strokes represent a pathologically heterogeneous group. Clinical evaluation and diagnostic investigation is performed to delineate the precise pathogenesis in each case and to indicate the most appropriate form of prophylactic therapy. TIAs are most often due to artery-to-artery microemboli from atheromatous plaques in large, often extra-

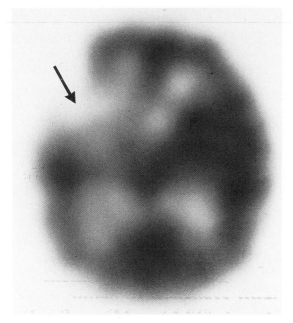

Figure 2. SPECT scan (using technetium-99m HM-PAO) demonstrating severe cortical hypoperfusion (arrow) following ischemia in the right middle cerebral artery territory.

Arterial Territory

The clinical differentiation of TIAs into carotid and vertebrobasilar types has profound implications for investigation and management. Carotid-territory TIAs are subdivided into those affecting the retinal circulation (amaurosis fugax or transient monocular blindness) and those affecting the cerebral hemisphere (transient hemispheric attacks). Vertebrobasilar TIAs are often more complex than carotid territory events and typically include two or more symptoms reflecting transient ischemia of the brainstem, occipital and medial temporal lobes, and the upper spinal cord. The most common symptoms include transient vertigo, binocular visual disturbance, diplopia, and ataxia.

Clinical Evaluation and Investigation

The clinical evaluation of patients with TIAs is based on the identification of the affected arterial territory, the history of the number and frequency of episodes, the assessment of evidence of atherosclerosis and cardiac disease, and the identification and previous treatment of risk factors.

The speed of investigation also depends on such factors as the frequency of events and the timing of the most recent episode. In general, patients with acute cerebral ischemia who recover in the emergency room should be rapidly investigated, as the precise risk in an individual patient remains unknown. Increased short-term risk of completed stroke generally is assumed in patients with multiple episodes over a short period of time ("crescendo TIAs"), and in those with clinical or investigative evidence of an underlying arterial stenosis or a cardiac embolic source such as atrial fibrillation.

In the patient with a carotid-territory TIA, urgent evaluation of the carotid arterial system is usually indicated unless there is an overt cardioembolic source. Duplex Doppler scanning of the carotid artery (the combination of B-mode ultrasound imaging and Dop-

cranial vessels, such as the internal carotid artery in the region of the common carotid bifurcation. They can also be due to distal brain hypoperfusion, particularly in patients with severe hemodynamic arterial stenosis. Multiple, brief TIAs in the same arterial distribution are often due to underlying hemodynamic mechanisms and critical arterial stenosis. TIAs can also be due to cardiac emboli. These episodes are typically more prolonged than those due to extracranial vascular disease,[42] and often occur in different arterial territories. A cluster of TIAs can also precede the development of lacunar infarction, which is most commonly the consequence of localized cerebral perforating artery disease.

Differential Diagnosis

The differential diagnosis of TIAs includes nonvascular pathologies such as partial epilepsy, cerebral tumor, migraine, vestibular disorders, hypoglycemia, drop attacks, and transient global amnesia.

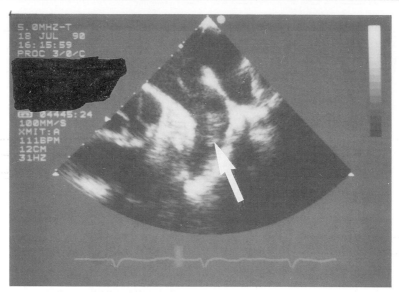

Figure 3. Transesophageal echocardiography demonstrating thrombus (arrow) in the left atrial appendage.

pler frequency analysis) is often performed as a screening, noninvasive technique. This modality provides reasonably accurate information concerning the presence and degree of extracranial carotid stenosis, and some detail related to plaque morphology, such as calcification and intraluminal thrombus. Transcranial Doppler (TCD) noninvasively evaluates erythrocyte flow patterns in the basal intracerebral arteries and provides evidence of the hemodynamic consequences of extracranial stenosis, intracranial arterial lesions, and collateral arterial supply. This newer technique complements duplex Doppler scanning, which only allows evaluation of the extracranial carotid circulation. MRA is increasingly used as an alternative screening technique in this setting.

We often proceed directly to selective intra-arterial digital subtraction angiography (DSA) via the transfemoral route in patients with clearcut carotid-territory TIAs or minor infarcts. DSA is particularly useful if patients have had more than one event in the same territory or a carotid bruit, making them likely candidates for carotid endarterectomy. Arch DSA is an inadequate substitute for

selective arterial catheterization because suboptimal views are obtained of the intracranial vessels in many cases. Cerebral CT scanning should always be peformed to detect recent or old cerebral infarcts, or other pathologies such as cerebral tumors and subdural hematomas that can cause transient neurologic events indistinguishable clinically from TIAs.

Important advances in cardiac evaluation have aided in the diagnosis of a potential cardiac source of cerebral embolism, with implications for stroke prevention. In the absence of clinical signs of heart disease, both M-mode and two-dimensional echocardiography have been relatively insensitive in the diagnosis of cardiac embolic sources in cerebral ischemia. However, color echocardiography and contrast echocardiography (using an intravenous injection of agitated saline) facilitate the detection of small septal defects that potentially permit paradoxical embolism from the venous system. Transesophageal echocardiography (Figure 3) provides high resolution of the cardiac structures, particularly the mitral valve, atrial septum, and left atrium. The latter is an important site of thrombus formation, particularly in patients with atrial fibrillation. Transesophageal echo-cardiography more sensitively diagnoses mitral valve prolapse, a significant cause of ischemic stroke in young adults.[46]

Management Options for Patients with Carotid Territory TIAs

While the precise place of carotid endar-terectomy in patients with TIAs or nondisa-bling stroke and carotid disease remains uncertain, it has been recently proven in North American[34] and European trials that carotid endarterectomy is far more effective in stroke prevention than the best available medical therapy in patients with severe carotid stenosis (greater than 70%).

Several large, multicenter, randomized con-trolled trials indicated that aspirin reduces the incidence of stroke in TIA patients, although the optimal clinical dosage remains controversial. Most of the clinical trials used "large dose" aspirin[7] (1200-1300 mg/day), which effectively inhibits platelet cyclo-oxygenase and hence platelet aggregation, but which is associated with a significant inci-dence of side effects, particularly gastrointes-tinal bleeding.

Smaller doses of aspirin (50-300 mg/day) have a more selective effect on the throm-boxane A_2 (platelet aggregant) pathway than on the prostacyclin (platelet antiaggregant) pathway, and are hence of greater theoretical benefit as well as having a lower incidence of side effects. Ticlopidine hydrochloride is a new antiplatelet agent that inhibits the aden-osine diphosphate platelet aggregant path-way[23] and may be even more effective than aspirin in the prevention of stroke following TIAs. There is a considerably increased inci-dence of side effects, however, particularly diarrhea and reversible neutropenia.[23]

In patients with a suspected cardiac embolic source, anticoagulation with warfarin is generally preferred to the use of antiplatelet therapy.[9]

Management of Vertebrobasilar TIAs

Vertebrobasilar TIAs are also due to a var-iety of underlying pathological lesions, includ-ing localized atherosclerosis in the distal ver-tebral and basilar arteries, basilar branch (small vessel) disease, and embolism from a cardiac source.[8] Stenosis of the proximal ver-tebral artery at its origin is generally consi-dered to be benign, unlike the more sinister distal vertebral and basilar occlusive lesions which carry a poor prognosis. In the past, there was less enthusiasm for investigation of these patients with diagnostic imaging techniques because the underlying arterial lesions are surgically inaccessible.

Many clinicians now use vertebrobasilar DSA in selected patients with vertebrobasilar TIAs and nondisabling vertebrobasilar infarc-tion. Early studies in the 1950s and 1960s[8] indicated that anticoagulation was stroke-protective in patients with vertebrobasilar occlusive lesions, but there has been no ade-quate clinical trial comparing the efficacy of antiplatelet therapy versus formal anticoagu-lation. Nonetheless, many clinicians use war-farin in patients with distal vertebral or basi-lar stenoses in preference to antiplatelet therapy, and use aspirin alone in patients with symptoms due to presumed basilar branch disease.[8]

Carotid endarterectomy has not been shown to be of benefit for patients with vertebro-basilar TIAs. It may have a place in a very small subset of patients with severe bilateral carotid stenosis, and an angiographically normal vertebrobasilar system, where a blood flow "steal" may occur from the hindbrain to the anterior circulation.

Noninvasive evaluation of the vertebrobas-ilar system can also be performed using the transcranial Doppler technique, with insona-tion of the distal vertebral, basilar and poste-rior cerebral arteries via the foramen mag-num "window". MRA is likely to have a major role in the investigation of this group of patients in the future.

Management of the Patient with Established Cerebral Infarction

General Measures

In the patient with established cerebral infarction, general medical and nursing measures are used in initial management and emphasis is placed on precise pathogenetic classification with a view to prevention of further stroke. If the patient has a stable deficit, whether involving part or whole of a cerebral arterial territory, initial management centers upon nursing care rather than any specific medical or surgical intervention.

While there is no proof that the use of stroke intensive care units reduces mortality, there is substantial evidence that the development of stroke units or comprehensive consultative stroke services results in more appropriate coordinated investigation and management of the stroke patient and may well improve functional outcome.

Experienced nursing care should be combined with physiotherapy at an early stage, to prevent complications such as chest infection or muscular contractures and to initiate mobilization and motor relearning. Early speech therapy involvement is particularly useful in the evaluation of bulbar dysfunction and dysphasia. Bulbar palsy is common in patients with acute stroke, particularly vertebrobasilar infarction, and fluid maintenance via an intravenous line or nasogastric tube is often required. Percutaneous gastrostomy is useful in patients with more protracted bulbar palsies.

Adequate hydration is important, as hypovolemia can impair cerebral blood flow. Substantial animal and human evidence indicates that hyperglycemia may be harmful in acute cerebral ischemia.[35] In addition to detection and treatment of hyperglycemia in both known and newly diagnosed diabetic patients, intravenous glucose infusions should be avoided.

Epileptic seizures occur in approximately 4% of acute stroke patients and often require anticonvulsant therapy, but they are not an adverse prognostic factor.[27] No scientific evidence currently supports the use of routine oxygen administration via either mask or intranasal catheters, except in patients where there is known hypoxia.

Treatment of Hypertension

Hypertension is often an acute, yet transient consequence of the stroke process. There has been controversy regarding its management, but it is now generally agreed that aggressive reduction of hypertension in the setting of acute stroke is dangerous. Such therapy may cause further impairment of cerebral perfusion, due to the loss of autoregulation in acute cerebral ischemia. We generally continue the patient's standard antihypertensive therapy and rarely administer parenteral antihypertensive agents, except in patients with either hypertensive encephalopathy or with great caution in those with aneurysmal subarachnoid hemorrhage. Hypotension, due to hypovolemia or cardiac disorders, should be treated with cautious fluid replacement and volume expansion, with careful monitoring to avoid acute pulmonary edema.

Anticoagulation

Following exclusion of cerebral hemorrhage by CT, formal anticoagulation is often used in patients with partial, stable cerebral ischemic deficits, with a view to prevention of stroke progression. While heparin has a more defined and accepted place in stroke prevention in patients who have cardiogenic cerebral embolism (see below), the role of anticoagulation in management of the acute stroke patient remains highly controversial.[13,21]

There is little scientific evidence by way of randomized controlled clinical trials to suggest that heparin prevents the neurological deterioration experienced by approximately one-third of patients with acute cerebral infarction following hospital admission. However, we often use heparin in stable patients with a partial vertebrobasilar infarct, as the consequences of deterioration with basilar thrombosis may be lethal. We do not routinely use heparin in stable atherothrombotic carotid territory infarction unless there is evidence of progression or a possible cardioembolic source, or in selected patients with demonstrated underlying severe stenosis where progressive or propagating thrombosis might be detrimental.

Pathogenetic Classification and Prevention of Recurrent Infarction

Stroke classification has been chiefly based on anatomical location, with the delineation of discrete stroke syndromes associated with ischemia in specific arterial territories. Greater emphasis is now placed on the pathogenesis of cerebral infarction, because of the therapeutic implications, particularly with regard to prevention of recurrent stroke. The three principal pathogeneses include (1) extracranial atherosclerosis and thromboembolism, (2) cardiogenic embolism, and (3) lacunar infarction.

Extracranial Atherosclerosis and Thromboembolism

Although various investigators, including Chiari, Ramsay-Hunt, and Moniz pointed to the importance of extracranial occlusive disease in the pathogenesis of stroke in the early 1900s,[36] in situ middle cerebral thrombosis was considered to be the most important cause of stroke until two landmark papers by C. Miller Fisher in the early 1950s.[15] Fisher re-emphasised the role of extracranial carotid stenosis and thrombosis as the chief cause of ischemic stroke.

The formation of extracranial atherosclerotic plaque most commonly occurs at the common carotid bifurcation, the distal vertebral and basilar arteries, with progressive stenosis of these vessels and turbulence of blood flow. Atherosclerotic plaques later become complicated by the development of ulceration, intraplaque and subintimal hemorrhages, and superimposed formation of platelet-fibrin thrombi. Cerebral infarction due to extracranial atherosclerosis occurs via several mechanisms, including extracranial thrombus formation with distal propagation into the intracranial arteries (atherothrombosis), distal embolization of components of the atherosclerotic plaque or superimposed fibrin-platelet thrombus (artery-to-artery embolism), and hemodynamic failure due to distal cerebral hypoperfusion consequent upon critical stenosis. This hemodynamic mechanism affects internal or external "watershed" territories between the major intracerebral arteries, is related to underlying severe stenosis in most cases, and is potentiated by systemic hypotension or an inadequate collateral circulation.

Clinical features that favor the diagnosis of extracranial atherosclerosis as the cause of cerebral ischemia include a stuttering or nocturnal onset of the stroke, previous TIAs in the same arterial territory, the presence of carotid bruit on cervical auscultation, the presence of cortical neurologic deficits, and the absence of an overt cardiac source.

Duplex Doppler scanning allows more precise, noninvasive diagnosis in these patients. We perform acute angiography only if patients show rapid resolution or substantial improvement of neurological deficits. In general, we use intravenous heparin acutely in selected patients with extracranial atherosclerosis and cerebral infarction if they progress under neurologic observation, or have a proven underlying critical stenosis. We use heparin more routinely in patients with stable but partial vertebrobasilar ischemia.

Urgent carotid thromboendarterectomy in patients with acute cerebral ischemia due to extracranial vascular disease is generally associated with an unacceptably high morbidity and mortality, with deterioration attributed to rapid reperfusion injury which may be associated with cerebral hemorrhage. However, in patients with a fluctuating yet minor interval deficit or in those with frequent ("crescendo")

TIAs, urgent angiography and endarterectomy should be considered (Figure 4).

In patients with acute atherosclerotic infarction and a significant neurologic deficit, we screen the extracranial vessels with duplex Doppler during the acute stroke stage and consider elective carotid endarterectomy following later DSA examination at 4-6 weeks, depending on the degree of stroke recovery. However, this time delay is only used as a guide. Patients with small deficits are often treated earlier and managed along the lines of TIA patients. Some clinicians would anticoagulate patients with heparin and then warfarin for this interval period prior to elective carotid endarterectomy, if there was evidence of an underlying severe arterial stenosis.

Prophylaxis in this group otherwise involves the use of long-term antiplatelet therapy, which is commenced following the exclusion of cerebral hemorrhage by CT.

Cardiogenic Cerebral Embolism

Cardiogenic cerebral embolism also leads to infarction of the cerebral cortex, due to a variety of cardiac diseases affecting the cardiac walls, valves, or chambers. It has been estimated from aggregate clinical studies that about one stroke in six is cardioembolic. The most important causes include nonvalvular atrial fibrillation, rheumatic and other types of valvular heart disease with or without arrhythmias, recent or past myocardial infarction with intraventricular thrombus formation, postcardiac surgery, prosthetic cardiac valves, infective endocarditis, nonbacterial thrombotic (marantic) endocarditis, atrial myxoma, cardiomyopathy and septal defects with paradoxical embolism.

Nonvalvular atrial fibrillation is one of the most important treatable causes of stroke.[9] Several studies have indicated that warfarin reduces the stroke rate in previously asymptomatic patients with nonvalvular atrial fibrillation, while one study also indicated benefit from aspirin at 300 mg per day.[40] These trials demonstrated a reasonably low risk of anticoagulant-precipitated major hemorrhage. This

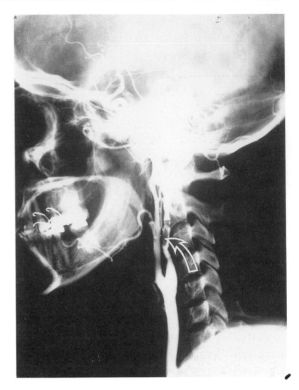

Figure 4. Selective carotid arteriogram demonstrating a stenotic, irregular internal carotid artery and a filling defect (arrow) due to luminal thrombus.

has been attributed to the use of lower intensity anticoagulation, with International Normalized Ratio (INR) values in the range of 2-3. The presence of rheumatic heart disease, previous cerebral infarction and peripheral embolism all convey a much higher risk of recurrent stroke, while the diagnosis of "lone" atrial fibrillation (atrial fibrillation in the absence of any identifiable cardiac disease) is considered to carry a lower risk.[9]

Clinical pointers to the diagnosis of cardiogenic embolism include the suddenness of the ictus, the presence of overt cardiac pathology such as atrial fibrillation or recent myocardial infarction, previous clinical or CT evidence of embolization in different cerebral arterial territories, and evidence of current or previous peripheral embolization. On CT scan, a cardiac source is also suggested by evidence of infarcts in different arterial territories and an increased incidence of hemorrhagic cerebral infarction. The exclusion of infective endocarditis (cardiac murmur, peripheral embolization, fever, elevated erythrocyte sedimentation rate, splinter hemorrhages, eye signs, splenomegaly) is of great importance, as anticoagulants are not used in these cases due to the increased risk of precipitated cerebral hemorrhage and substantial reduction of recurrent embolism by appropriate antibiotic therapy.[9]

Advances in echocardiography and other techniques, including ambulatory cardiac monitoring and electrophysiological stimulation, have increased the yield of potential cardiac sources, even in patients without clinical signs of cardiac disease. Small septal defects, intracardiac thrombi, and prolapsing mitral valve are all examples of cardiac lesions that may not be detected by routine clinical examination. Other new cardiac evaluation techniques include cardiac CT, magnetic resonance imaging, and radio isotope-labeled platelet scintigraphy, but the precise place of these modalities in the detection of a cardiac embolic source is uncertain at present. It is also recognized that many cerebral cardiogenic emboli are subclinical. Notwithstanding these advances in cardiac investigation, reliable clinical diagnostic criteria for cardioembolic stroke remains a clinical problem, and the clinical significance of some cardiological abnormalities is uncertain.

In general, patients with cardiogenic cerebral embolism are managed with acute anticoagulation using intravenous heparin; this is because the risk of early recurrent embolism after cardiogenic brain infarction is estimated to be up to 20% over 3 weeks.[9] However, a confounding factor in management is the knowledge that cardioembolic infarcts are often associated with microscopic areas of hemorrhage, and there is a substantial risk of transformation (conversion of ischemic to hemorrhagic infarction) in patients with large infarcts on clinical or CT criteria. In such patients, or in those with uncontrolled hypertension, it is desirable to delay the use of anticoagulation for 7 to 10 days after the acute ictus. Some authorities[9] recommend the performance of a subacute CT scan (at least 48 hours after the ictus) to pick up the group of patients who might have an early spontaneous hemorrhagic transformation and hence obviate the use of early anticoagulation in that subgroup.

Although the numbers of patients in clinical trials have been relatively small, there is good evidence that anticoagulation in patients with cardiogenic embolic infarction (after the exclusion of hemorrhagic infarction on initial CT scan) reduces the risk of recurrent stroke.[9] We generally do not recommend warfarin as an alternative to heparin in these cases in the first instance, as oral anticoagulation is usually only therapeutically effective after a few days of treatment. Once patients are adequately anticoagulated with heparin, warfarin is usually commenced and given on a long-term basis, the duration dependent on the precise cardiac pathology.

Lacunar Infarction

Lacunar infarcts are small, deep infarcts in the territory of single deep perforating arteries supplying the internal capsule, basal ganglia or brain stem. These are most commonly due to small-vessel hypertensive disease, particularly lipohyalinosis, although other mechanisms including localized microatheroma are sometimes relevant.[14] Some controversy remains concerning the relevance or frequency of embolic causes of such lesions. Millikan and Futrell have criticized what they regard as the therapeutic nihilism induced by the diagnosis of lacunar infarction, and proposed six basic causes for a lacunar syndrome: embolism, hypertension, small-vessel occlusive disease, hematologic abnormalities, small intracerebral hemorrhages and vasospasm.[30]

Five "classical" lacunar syndromes have been described and documented by clinicopathological correlations. These include: (1) pure motor hemiplegia (due to a lacunar infarct in the posterior limb of the internal capsule or pons), (2) pure sensory stroke (often due to a thalamic lacune), (3) sensory-motor stroke (typically thalamus and adjacent capsule), (4) the dysarthria-clumsy hand syndrome and (5) the syndrome of ataxic-hemiparesis. The latter two syndromes can be due to lacunar infarcts in the pons or internal capsule.

We often perform screening duplex Doppler examination in patients with carotid territory lacunar infarcts, but only proceed to further investigation if severe ipsilateral stenosis is identified. This finding, however, is unusual. Norrving and Cronqvist[33] found that severe carotid disease was far more commonly associated with nonlacunar than with lacunar infarcts. Lacunar infarcts are most strongly associated with hypertension, and prophylactic treatment depends on effective modification of this risk factor. The role of antiplatelet therapy is uncertain, but we generally place these patients on long-term aspirin.

On CT scan, lacunar infarcts are less than 1.5 cm in diameter and should be distinguished from larger subcortical infarcts in the capsular region termed striatocapsular infarcts. These "comma-shaped" larger infarcts are often due to embolism to the proximal middle cerebral artery, obliterating the mouths of multiple lenticulostriate vessels, yet with sufficient collateral supply to prevent cortical infarction. In fact, cortical signs are often present, perhaps due to a functional depression of neuronal activity. The diagnosis indicates the need for investigation to exclude a proximal embolic source.

Young Adult and Rare Types of Cerebral Infarction

Approximately 3% of cerebral infarctions occur in adults under the age of 40 years.[2,10,22] Atherosclerosis is a rare cause of brain ischemia in these patients, and various other mechanisms should be considered, including (1) migraine, (2) cardiac sources, (3) cerebral vasculitis, (4) dissection of extracranial arteries, (5) fibromuscular dysplasia, (6) Moyamoya disease, (7) hematologic disorders, and (8) cerebral venous thrombosis.

These patients require more intensive investigation than do many older patients with cerebral infarction, as the underlying pathology often requires specific therapy. Prognosis is generally favorable compared with older stroke patients.[10] Cerebral angiography and detailed cardiac investigation including echocardiography is virtually manditory in all cases. Many patients also require a lumbar puncture to look for evidence of an underlying inflammatory condition, and detailed hematologic investigations to elucidate a possible underlying coagulopathy. Some of the rarer types of cerebral ischemia, with implications for management, are considered below.

Migraine

Migraine is a relatively common cause of stroke in young adults, particularly involving the posterior cerebral artery territory. The precise mechanism of infarction is unclear, although severe vasospasm with ischemia and tissue necrosis is usually postulated. This has only been rarely demonstrated on angiography. Even in the known migraineur with a persisting neurological deficit in the wake of a classical attack, other causes should be excluded by appropriate investigations, including angiography and echocardiography. The use of prophylactic measures in these patients is uncertain, but our practice is to advise long-term antiplatelet therapy, often combined with antimigraine prophylaxis such as propranolol or pizotifen.

Cardiac Causes

While mitral valve prolapse (MVP) is a common echocardiographic finding in young women, it is disproportionately more prevalent in young adult patients with stroke. Whereas the individual risk of cerebral infarction is remote and prophylactic anticoagulation is not usually advocated in patients with asymptomatic mitral valve prolapse, there is a small but increased risk of stroke due to cardiogenic embolism, particularly in those with a primary myxomatous abnormality of the valve leaflets, chordae, and annulus.[9] Increased risk has been shown in males, with advancing age and with specific echocardiographic abnormalities. Antiplatelet therapy has been advocated as an appropriate prophylactic measure in patients with mitral valve prolapse who have sustained a stroke, although many workers would use anticoagulants initially for at least 6-12 months, before long-term aspirin.

The increased use of transesophageal echocardiography has enabled the diagnosis of small septal defects, including the presence of patent foramen ovale, with the attendant risk of paradoxical embolism from the venous circulation. This abnormality is found at a higher rate in young adult stroke patients compared with a control population, but the precise significance and therapeutic implication of the abnormality remains uncertain in many cases.

Cerebral Vasculitis

Cerebral vasculitis can occur secondary to septic, inflammatory conditions, such as tuberculosis or syphilis which are associated with a basal meningitis. Aseptic cerebral vasculitis is more common and can be due to systemic inflammatory conditions such as polyarteritis nodosa or systemic lupus erythematosis, or due to illicit drug use, particularly with cocaine, heroin, or amphetamines. Herpes zoster ophthalmicus is occasionally followed by infarction in the middle cerebral territory due to middle cerebral vasculitis. Giant cell arteritis (temporal arteritis) is rarely associated with extracranial arteritis of the carotid or vertebral arteries, leading to cerebral infarction. Isolated central nervous system angiitis (granulomatous angiitis) is an idiopathic, aseptic arteritis with a high mortality rate due to multiple cerebral infarcts.

Investigations useful in the diagnosis of cerebral vasculitis include angiography showing the characteristic "beading" of small intracerebral arteries, the presence of multifocal infarcts on CT or MR scanning, a CSF lymphocytosis, and an elevated erythrocyte sedimentation rate. Confirmatory brain biopsy is useful in some cases. Management includes the treatment of sepsis, the withdrawal of any toxic agent, and the management of any systemic disorder. The latter often requires the use of corticosteroids or other immunosuppressive agents. Specific antiviral chemotherapy with acyclovir may have a particular role in the middle cerebral angiitis associated with herpes zoster ophthalmicus.

Dissection of the Extracranial Arteries

Dissection of the carotid or vertebral arteries should always be considered a possible cause of cerebral infarction in a young adult, even if there is no history of previous trauma. Some patients have an underlying arteriopathy, such as the Ehlers-Danlos syndrome, or fibromuscular dysplasia. In other cases, preceding (often mild) trauma to the neck is an etiology. Examples of such trauma are motor vehicle accidents and cervical manipulation. Neurologic deficits occur due to thromboembolism superimposed on the intimal tear. Carotid artery dissection is associated with pain in the region of the orbit, with or without Horner syndrome or other neurologic deficits. Vertebral artery dissections can present with various brainstem syndromes, including the lateral medullary syndrome. Diagnosis is made by angiography which shows a range of abnormalities, including a narrowed or tapered artery (the "string sign"), and sometimes arterial aneurysm formation. Anticoagulation may be used to prevent subsequent thromboembolic events, while surgery is rarely indicated.

Fibromuscular Dysplasia

This condition is often associated with renal artery fibromuscular dysplasia and is usually asymptomatic. It can affect the distal portions of the internal carotid artery, with a "saw-tooth" angiographic appearance. There is an increased risk of both TIAs and cerebral

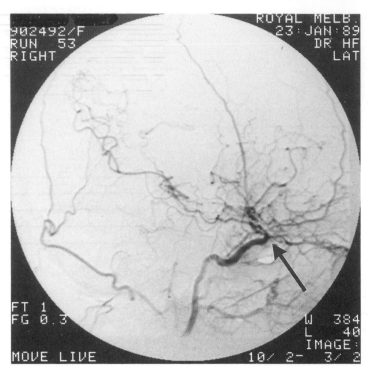

Figure 5. *Selective carotid arteriogram in a patient with moyamoya disease, demonstrating terminal internal carotid occlusion (arrow) and a fine, telangiectatic collateral arterial network.*

infarcts, as well as subarachnoid hemorrhage due to aneurysmal formation. Treatment is generally conservative, including the use of aspirin.

Moyamoya Disease

This rare obliterative arteriopathy, originally described in Japan, is now recognized to have a worldwide distribution. The terminal internal carotid arteries are typically occluded, with an intracranial, fine, telangiectatic "puff of smoke" appearance on angiography, usually sparing the posterior circulation (Figure 5). Patients may present with either cerebral ischemia or hemorrhage. There is no proven medical therapy for this condition, but various surgical procedures, including transcranial bypass anastomosis, may have a role in selected patients.

Hematologic Disorders

In up to 4% of young adults with stroke,

there is an underlying hematologic disorder or coagulopathy.[22] Transient hematologic derangement after stroke frequently occurs, and is a confounding problem in the diagnosis of an underlying hypercoagulability state. Examples of prothrombotic states include: (1) congenital deficiencies of the inhibitors of blood coagulation (antithrombin III, protein C, protein S and heparin cofactor II); (2) hereditary abnormalities of fibrinolysis (such as hereditary plasminogen deficiency and plasminogen activator deficiency); (3) erythrocyte disorders such as polycythemia vera and sickle-cell anemia; (4) thrombocytosis and other platelet abnormalities; (5) underlying cancer with or without an associated nonbacterial thrombotic (marantic) endocarditis; and, (6) a range of autoantibody syndromes, including lupus anticoagulants.

Lupus anticoagulants (LAs) are acquired immunoglobulins that are prothrombotic[22] and are antiphospholipid antibodies. A prolonged activated partial thromboplastin time (APTT) suggests the presence of LA. The abnormality fails to correct when affected plasma is mixed with normal plasma. However, other antiphospholipid antibodies that do not prolong the APTT have also been linked with stroke.[22] Many of the reported cases of stroke in the setting of antiphospholipid antibodies have had an additional possible contributing factor, such as nonbacterial thrombotic endocarditis. The precise risk of the oral contraceptive pill as a prothrombotic agent remains uncertain, but there is considered to be a stronger link between stroke and pills with higher estrogen content.

In practical terms, all young adult patients should be screened for an underlying hemostatic or coagulation disorder unless there is another unequivocal cause of the cerebral infarction, although the yield is usually small.[10] The place for hypercoagulability screening in older patients is less certain and is probably only warranted if there is a prior personal or family history of a thrombotic state. Specific prophylactic therapy depends on the type of abnormality found.[10]

Cerebral Venous Thrombosis

Cerebral venous thrombosis is a rare cause of stroke, with both ischemic and hemorrhagic manifestations. Whereas sepsis was the most common cause in the past, particularly related to underlying sinus disease, ear infection, and meningitis, hypercoagulability states including pregnancy are now far more commonly implicated.

Clinical syndromes are protean and depend on the particular sinus or sinuses thrombosed as well as the distribution of deep venous thrombosis. Focal neurologic signs, fever, elevated ICP, and meningeal irritation can all be present. Specific diagnosis is most important, as the use of urgent heparin anticoagulation has been demonstrated to reduce a high associated mortality rate. Antibiotics are reserved for septic cases. Measures often used to reduce ICP include steroids, mannitol, and lumboperitoneal shunting, but all are of unproven value. Thrombosis in sinuses is sometimes evident on CT scanning with the

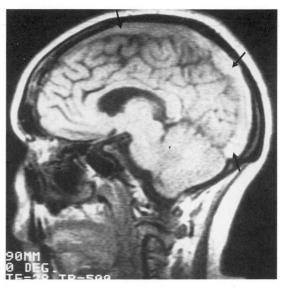

Figure 6. Sagittal T1-weighted spin echo MR scan demonstrating high signal in the superior sagittal sinus (arrows) due to sinus thrombosis.

T1 - ↑ signal intensity.

"delta" sign, due to blood clot filling of the central portion of the sagittal sinus. MRI is particularly useful in demonstrating high signal intensity due to fresh thrombus in nonflowing venous sinuses (Figure 6). Phase contrast MRA also appears to be extremely reliable in this setting.

Management of Stroke in Evolution/Progressing Stroke

Deterioration in patients with cerebral infarction occurs in up to 30% of patients after hospitalization and is due to a variety of causes, including (1) elevation of ICP, (2) progressive cerebral thrombosis and recurrent embolism, (3) secondary biochemical changes in the brain, and (4) systemic complications of stroke such as pneumonia, electrolyte disorders, pulmonary embolism, and acute myocardial infarction.

The cause of early deterioration, and the most important cause of mortality in supratentorial cerebral infarcts, is elevated intracranial pressure and transtentorial herniation. Although corticosteroid therapy is very effective for brain edema associated with cerebral tumors, the edema associated with cerebral infarction is largely unresponsive to steroids. Clinical trials have shown that even high-dose steroid therapy does not improve the prognosis of acute cerebral ischemia and may be harmful.[32] Other antiedema agents such as mannitol may decrease focal tissue pressure and improve cerebral blood flow, although their effectiveness has not been demonstrated in controlled studies.

The controversial role of anticoagulation has been considered. A large cooperative study in the early 1960s[4] found a lower incidence of progression of infarction in patients with thrombosis-in-evolution treated with anticoagulants compared with a control group, but this study was performed before CT was available. More recent studies have not demonstrated any benefit in patients with progressive infarction treated by heparin, where continued neurological deterioration has been observed in approximately 50% of patients despite anticoagulation.[21] Opponents of the use of heparin point to the lack of proven efficacy and emphasize the risks of hemorrhage, as well as the procoagulant effects of heparin in some patients.[39]

The many trials evaluating the role of heparin in stable and progressing atherothrombotic stroke have been flawed by multiple design factors, most particularly the failure to differentiate the various pathogenetic subtypes of cerebral infarction.[13] Many investigators consider that the role of heparin in partial atherothrombotic and progressive stroke remains unsettled. They also consider that heparin is reasonably safe in selected and monitored cases, and believe that adequately designed trials should be organized to address these issues.[13]

Other therapies sometimes used for patients with evolving or deteriorating stroke include volume expansion and thrombolytic therapy. These approaches are considered below.

Stroke units have a particular role in the early detection, prevention, and treatment of secondary systemic complications of stroke such as electrolyte disorders, hyponatremia, cardiac problems, deep venous thrombosis and pulmonary embolism, and pneumonia.

These conditions can contribute to secondary clinical deterioration following an ischemic insult.

Therapeutic Strategies for Tissue Rescue in Acute Ischemia

In acute cerebral ischemia, various levels of brain function derangement can occur, including abnormal perfusion, metabolism, and biochemical alterations.[18]

Studies using positron emission tomography (PET) [1,44] demonstrated a mismatch or uncoupling between cerebral metabolism and perfusion that is characteristic of acute ischemic stroke. Maintenance of cerebral oxygen metabolism was shown to be the hallmark of neuronal viability. In the early stages of the ischemic process, perfusion is typically more severely compromized than oxygen metabolism, indicating that the tissue is underperfused relative to its metabolic requirements ("misery perfusion"). This is reflected by an increase in the oxygen extraction fraction.

In animal models of cerebral ischemia and infarction, an "ischemic penumbra" of viable tissue was shown to surround the infarct core.[29] Reduction of cerebral blood flow (CBF) below a certain threshold leads to electrical and synaptic failure. Further flow reduction as a function of time leads to depletion of energy stores, membrane failure, and irreversible infarction. This penumbra may be present for up to 3 hours after the onset of ischemia. These findings led to therapeutic attempts to increase cerebral tissue perfusion in the "therapeutic window" of time available, in the hope of maintaining sufficient cerebral metabolism to avoid neuronal necrosis and to "rescue" ischemic but potentially viable brain tissue.

Complex metabolic, biochemical, and ultrastructural derangements follow acute ischemia.[19] These effects include an intracellular increase in calcium concentration following its release from intracellular organelles, ion flux into neurons, loss of cellular potassium, and the release of toxic byproducts of the ischemic process, including "free radicals" such as superoxide and leukotrienes. Paradoxically, cerebral damage is more severe following incomplete ischemia than complete ischemia. Hyperglycemia and possibly even blood glucose level in the upper euglycemic range, also have adverse effects.[35]

Experimental strategies for tissue rescue include attempts to increase brain perfusion via thrombolysis with reperfusion, and hemodilutional, hypervolemic therapy. Attempts were made to modify the consequences of the ischemic process by the administration of calcium antagonists and other experimental agents.[18] These therapeutic strategies were or are being investigated in animal studies as well as in large, controlled randomized clinical trials and hold out hope for tissue salvage in acute cerebral ischemia.

Thrombolytic Therapy

The proven efficacy of thrombolytic therapy in acute coronary artery occlusion reactivated interest in thrombolytic therapy for acute cerebral ischemia. Intravenous thrombolytic therapy was previously investigated in several trials since the early 1960s, with generally negative conclusions regarding efficacy and a substantial incidence of adverse effects, particularly cerebral hemorrhage.[12] However, many of these protocols were performed before the advent of CT, and hence some patients with hemorrhage may have been included. In addition, initiation of therapy was often delayed, controls were often lacking, and anticoagulants were sometimes used in combination with thrombolytic agents. Thrombolysis with reperfusion must be performed within a few hours of the onset of ischemia, during the brief period that the ischemic "penumbra" is present. Animal studies demonstrated the efficacy of thrombolysis by both intravenous and intra-arterial routes, with improved functional outcome and reduced infarct size.[12]

A number of clinical studies demonstrated successful recanalization of occluded arteries and improved neurologic outcome, using intra-arterial thrombolysis. One recent study involved the use of intra-arterial streptokinase or urokinase in patients with severe brain stem ischemia and angiographically demonstrated thrombotic vertebrobasilar occlusions.[20] In contradistinction to controls, successful recanalization was achieved in the treated group in a proportion of cases, and this correlated with a significantly improved clinical outcome.

Unlike these exogenous fibrinolytic agents, tissue plasminogen activator (tPA) is an endogenous thrombolytic agent that produces thrombus dissolution by the local generation and release of plasmin.[12] Tissue plasminogen activator is fibrin specific and lacks systemic thrombolytic effects. Nonetheless, arterial recanalization by thrombolytic agents after acute cerebral ischemia is still accompanied by a risk of reperfusion injury and hemorrhagic transformation.

Several large-scale trials are underway to evaluate the safety and efficacy of tPA in acute ischemic stroke.[6,41] Preliminary studies examined recanalization (efficacy) versus the risk of hemorrhagic transformation with clinical deterioration (safety).[41] In the large tPA trials, administration of the thrombolytic agent is performed early, within 90 minutes of the ictus in the National Institutes of Health (NIH) study.[6] These feasibility and safety studies showed a relatively low rate of precipitated cerebral hemorrhage.[6,41]

There remains uncertainty as to whether fibrin-selective agents such as tPA are more effective and less dangerous than the exogenous fibrinolytic agents such as streptokinase. Uncertainty also exists as to whether hemorrhagic transformation of infarcted region of brain tissue actually produces significant clinical deterioration.[12] A large streptokinase trial is being conducted in Australia. The use of these experimental thrombolytic agents should be confined currently to the clinical trial setting.

Hemodilution Therapy

Hematocrit is an important determinant of whole-blood viscosity, particularly at low flow rates in the cerebral microcirculation. Reduction in hematocrit will increase cerebral perfusion, but in the normal brain, oxygen delivery and regional oxygen metabolism remain constant. In contrast, in ischemic brain tissue, there is a favorable inverse correlation between oxygen delivery and hematocrit, although the optimal level of hematocrit reduction remains controversial.[17] Isovolemic and hypervolemic hemodilutional protocols have been described. Hypervolemia is theoretically attractive in patients without impaired cardiac reserve: this therapy increases cardiac output and can thereby increase CBF when brain tissue distal to the site of vascular occlusion is supplied by maximally dilated vessels.[17]

Hypervolemic, hemodilutional therapy is generally regarded as clinically effective in patients with subarachnoid hemorrhage and cerebral vasospasm, although no large, randomized trials have been performed. In ischemic stroke, a number of randomized, controlled human clinical trials of hemodilution therapy have now been reported.[24,26,37] Several studies have used isovolemic hemodilution, combining venesection and infusion of 10% dextran 40 in saline, to achieve a moderate reduction in hematocrit. In some trials, patents have been entered up to 48 hours after stroke onset, although an Italian study enrolled a large number of patients within 12 hours,[26] with a significant number being treated under 6 hours. Overall, the results of these published trials of isovolemic hemodilution have been disappointing, without convincing value in acute ischemic stroke.

An American multicenter trial[24] used a hypervolemic, hemodilution protocol incorporating pentastarch infusion, venesection, and intravenous fluids, with hemodynamic monitoring performed in intensive care units. Graded neurologic and functional scores indicated no overall benefit from this therapy, although some subsets of patients showed improvement compared with controls.

Hemodilution therapy is theoretically attractive and might still have a place in early tissue rescue within the first few hours of cerebral ischemia, although its efficacy has not been established. Future models for acute stroke therapy might include a combination of reperfusion therapy using a protocol of thrombolysis and/or hemodilution therapy in selected cases, combined with other techniques such as calcium channel blockers to "normalize" the environment of the ischemic brain.[18] Hemodilution and hypervolemia may be harmful in certain subgroups of patients with large established cerebral infarction, where edema may be exacerbated and brain herniation possibly precipitated.[24]

Calcium Antagonists

Excessive neuronal calcium entry and liberation of intracellular calcium stores in acute cerebral ischemia are critical factors in determining irreversible neuronal death.[45] The trigger for this calcium ion entry into neurons after ischemia is unknown, but excitatory neurotransmittors such as glutamate may be relevant.[11] The influx of free intracellular neuronal calcium leads to the depletion of high-energy phosphates, activation of phospholipases and proteases, degradation of the neuronal cell membrane, and the production of cytotoxic free radicals, leukotrienes, and prostaglandins.[18,45] Oxidative phosphorylation is disrupted with inhibition of cellular respiration and subsequent neuronal death. Calcium antagonists restrict intracellular entry of calcium and may therefore be protective of cerebral neurons during the acute ischemic insult.[45] In addition, calcium antagonists are vasodilators and platelet antiaggregants, and they improve blood fluidity with increased CBF.[45]

The calcium antagonist nimodipine has an established role in the treatment of vasospasm following subarachnoid hemorrhage. Gelmers and colleagues[16] conducted a multicenter, prospective, double-blind, randomized, controlled trial of oral nimodipine begun within 24 hours of the onset of acute ischemic stroke. They reported a 58% reduction in mortality in men and a significantly better neurologic outcome in the nimodipine treated group. Another large trial using oral nimodipine in acute infarction showed no overall benefit when therapy was begun up to 2 days after the onset of symptoms, but subgroup analysis suggested that early treatment might be effective.[31] Hypotension limits the dosage of calcium antagonists in acute cerebral ischemia and their precise role in acute ischemic stroke is uncertain at the present time, but they are relatively safe and might well be effective in some patients.

Other Experimental Therapies

Pentoxifylline is a hemorheologic agent that increases erythrocyte deformability, inhibits platelet aggregation, and reduces plasma fibrinogen. In a multicenter, double blind, randomized-controlled trial, the safety and efficacy of this agent were assessed in patients with ischemic stroke entered within 12 hours of stroke onset. There was no reduction in mortality or functional impairment in the group treated with the active agent.[25]

GM1 ganglioside[3] is an agent that enhances the cellular response to protective neuronotrophic factors and decreases the effect of the neuronotoxic agent glutamate, an excitatory aminoacid neurotransmittor that potentiates neuronal death after cerebral ischemia. An Italian study[3] showed a higher degree of early neurologic improvement in the GM1-treated patients compared with placebo-treated controls, but no significant differences after four months. Hypoxic neuronal injury has also been modified by glutamate antagonists against N-methyl-D-aspartate (NMDA) receptors in several models of focal brain ischemia.[11] A number of new NMDA antagonists are in the early phases of clinical trial as potential neuroprotective agents.[38]

Prostacyclin is a vasodilator and platelet antiaggregant, but benefits have not been shown by randomized-controlled prospective trials. Reduction of cerebral metabolic needs by the use of barbiturates also has not been shown to be clinically effective.[18]

Conclusions

Many clinical trials in acute ischemic stroke were methodologically flawed by the inclusion of patients with substantial delays after the onset of the ictus. It is now known that the "therapeutic window" after acute ischemia is of the order of a few hours only, before extensive irreversible brain damage occurs. Strategies for effective delivery of acute stroke therapy therefore depend (1) on the identification of specific effective modalities, their precise indications and exclusions, and (2) on strategies for shortening the delays before effective treatment can be given.[5] These include the effective education of patients and their physicians in the community, more rapid transport of stroke sufferers to hospital, with effective triage through emergency departments, and diagnostic imaging. Such mechanisms should be based on the early treatment models developed for patients with acute trauma and myocardial infarction.[3] The development of stroke units or stroke centers with experienced, dedicated, and coordinated staffing is a priority and a natural logistical consequence of the identification of a range of acute, effective stroke therapies.

References

1. Ackerman RH, Albert NM, Correia JA, et al. Positron imaging in ischemic stroke disease. *Ann Neurol.* 1984;15 (suppl): S126-S130.
2. Adams HP, Butler MJ, Biller J. Nonhemorrhagic cerebral infarction in young adults. *Arch Neurol.* 1986;43:793-796.
3. Argentino C, Sacchetti ML, Toni D, et al. GM1 ganglioside therapy in acute ischemic stroke. *Stroke.* 1989;20: 1143-1149.
4. Baker RN, Broward JA,Fang HC, et al. Anticoagulant therapy in cerebral infarction: report on cooperative study. *Neurology.* 1962;12:823-835.
5. Barsan WG, Brott TG, Olinger CP, et al. Early treatment for acute ischemic stroke. *Ann Int Med.* 1989;111:449-451.
6. Brott T, Haley C, Levy D, et al. Safety and potential efficacy of tissue plasminogen activator (tPA) for stroke. *Stroke.* 1990; 21:181. Abstract.
7. Canadian Coopertaive Study Group. A randomized trial of aspirin and sulfinpyrazone in threatened stroke. *N Engl J Med.* 1978;299:53-59.
8. Caplan LR. Vertebrobasilar occlusive disease. In: Barnett HJM, Mohr JP, Stein BM, et al, eds. *Stroke:*

Pathophysiology, Diagnosis, and Management. New York, NY: Churchill Livingstone; 1986:549-619.

9. Cerebral Embolism Task Force. Cardiogenic brain embolism: the second report of the cerebral embolism task force. *Ann Neurol.* 1989;46:727-743.

10. Chancellor AM, Glasgow GL, Ockelford PA, et al. Etiology, prognosis, and hemostatic function after cerebral infarction in young adults. *Stroke.* 1989; 20:477-482.

11. Choi DW. Cerebral hypoxia: some new approaches and unanswered questions. *J Neurosci.* 1990;10: 2493-2501.

12. Del Zoppo GJ. Thrombolytic therapy in cerebrovascular disease. *Current Concepts of Cerebrovascular Disease and Stroke.* 1988;23:7-12.

13. Estol CJ, Pessin MS. Anticoagulation: is there still a role in atherothrombotic stroke? *Current Concepts of Cerebrovascular Disease and Stroke.* 1990;25:1-6.

14. Fisher M. Lacunes: small, deep cerebral infarcts. *Neurology.* 1965;15:774-784.

15. Fisher M. Occlusion of the internal carotid artery. *Arch Neurol Psychiat.* 1951;65: 346-377.

16. Gelmers HJ, Gorter K, De Weerdt CJ, et al. A controlled trial of nimodipine in acute ischemic stroke. *N Engl J Med.* 1988;318: 203-207.

17. Grotta JC. Can raising cerebral blood flow improve outcome after acute cerebral infarction? *Stroke.* 1987;18:264-267.

18. Grotta JC. Current medical and surgical therapy for cerebrovascular disease. *N Engl J Med.* 1987;317: 1505-1516.

19. Hachinski V, Norris JW. Reversibility of Cerebral Ischemia. In: *The Acute Stroke,* Philadelphia, Pa: FA Davis Company; 1985;41-63.

20. Hacke W, Zeumer H, Ferbert A, et al. Intra-arterial thrombolytic therapy improves outcome in patients with acute vertebrobasilar occlusive disease. *Stroke.* 1988;19:1216-1222.

21. Haley EC Jr, Kassell NF, Torner JC. Failure of heparin to prevent progression i n progressing ischemic infarction. *Stroke.* 1988;19:10-14.

22. Hart RG, Kanter MC. Hematologic disorders and ischemic stroke: a selective review. *Stroke.* 1990; 21:1111-1121.

23. Hass WK, Easton JD, Adams HP Jr, et al. A randomized trial comparing ticlopidine hydrochloride with aspirin for the prevention of stroke in high-risk patients. *N Engl J Med.* 1989;321:501-507.

24. Hemodilution in Stroke Study Group. Hypervolemic hemodilution treatment of acute stroke: results of a randomized multicenter trial using pentastarch. *Stroke.* 1989;20:317-323.

25. Hsu CY, Norris JW, Hogan EL, et al. Pentoxifylline in acute nonhemorrhagic stroke: a randomized, placebo controlled double-blind trial. *Stroke.* 1988;19: 716-722.

26. Italian Acute Stroke Study Group. Haemodilution in acute stroke: results of the Italian haemodilution trial. *Lancet.* 1988; 1:318-321.

27. Kilpatrick CJ, Davis SM, Tress BM, et al. Epileptic seizures in acute stroke. *Arch Neurol.* 1990;47: 157-160.

28. Kuller LH. Incidence rates of stroke in the eighties: the end of the decline in stroke? *Stroke.* 1989;20: 841-843.

29. Lassen NA, Astrup J. Ischemic penumbra. In: Wood JH, ed. *Cerebral Blood Flow: Physiologic and Clinical Aspects.* New York, NY: McGraw-Hill Book Company: 1987; 458-466.

30. Millikan C, Futrell N. The fallacy of the lacune hypothesis. *Stroke.* 1990;21:1251-1257.

31. Mohr JP, Dianni M, Muschett JL, et al. Nimodipine in acute ischemic stroke. *Ann Neurol.* 1989;26:124.

32. Norris JW, Hachinski VC. High dose steroid treatment in cerebral infarction. *Br Med J.* [Clin Res] 1986;292:21-23.

33. Norrving B, Cronqvist S. Clinical and radiologic features of lacunar versus nonlacunar minor stroke. *Stroke.* 1989;20:59-64.

34. North American Symptomatic Carotid Endarterectomy Trial Executive Committee. *Clinical Alert.* 1991.

35. Pulsinelli WA, Levy DE, Sigsbee B, et al. Increased damage after ischemic stroke in patients with hyperglycemia with or without established diabetes mellitus. *Am J Med.* 1983;74:540-544.

36. Quest DO. Stroke. A selective history. *Neurosurgery.* 1990;27:440-445.

37. Scandinavian Stroke Study Group. Multicenter trial of hemodilution in acute ischemic stroke, 1: results in the total patient population. *Stroke.* 1987;18: 691-699.

38. Scatton B, Carter C, Benavides J, et al. N-methyl-D-aspartate receptor antagonists: a novel therapeutic perspective for the treatment of ischemic brain injury. *Cerebrovas Dis.* 1991;1:121-135.

39. Scheinberg P. Heparin anticoagulation. *Stroke.* 1989;20:173-174.

40. Stroke Prevention in Atrial Fibrillation Study Group Investigators: Preliminary report of the stroke prevention in atrial fibrillation study. *N Engl J Med.* 1990; 322:863-868.

41. The tPA Acute Stroke Study Group. An open multicenter study of the safety and efficacy of various doses of tPA in patients with acute stroke: a progress report. *Stroke.* 1990;21:181.

42. Toole JF. Transient Ischemic Attacks. In: *Cerebrovascular Disorders.* 3rd Ed. New York, NY: Raven Press; 1984:101-116.

43. WHO Task Force on Stroke and Other Cerebrovascular Disorders. Stroke—1989. Recommendations on stroke prevention, diagnosis, and therapy. *Stroke.* 1989;20:1407-1431.

44. Wise RJS, Bernardi S, Frackowiak RSJ, et al. Serial observations on the pathophysiology of acute stroke: the transition from ischemia to infarction as reflected in regional oxygen extraction. *Brain.* 1983;106:197-222.

45. Wong MCW, Haley EC Jr. Calcium antagonists: stroke therapy coming of age. *Current Concepts of Cerebrovascular Disease and Stroke.* 1989;24:31-36.

46. Zenker G, Erbel R, Krämer G, et al. Transesophageal two-dimensional echocardiography in young patients with cerebral ischemic events. *Stroke.* 1988;19:345-348.

CHAPTER 8

Indications for Surgery in Extracranial Carotid Disease

Christopher M. Loftus MD, FACS

Carotid endarterectomy, first performed for cerebrovascular occlusive disease over 30 years ago, has developed into a procedure that can now be confidently and routinely recommended for patients who, although often presenting with minimal symptoms, are judged to be at high risk for devastating neurologic events. Justification for prophylactic surgical intervention in otherwise healthy patients has been supported by refinements in both surgical and anesthetic techniques. The combined morbidity and mortality rates have fallen below 3% (and as low as 1% in patients without concurrent medical or angiographic risks)[72] through surgical intervention by experienced cerebrovascular surgeons. Improvements in surgical technique have been accompanied by modern, less invasive imaging techniques for the carotid circulation, enhancing the diagnosis and management of cerebrovascular disease. Diagnostic advances have resulted in the identification of a group of patients with radiographically impressive but relatively asymptomatic or minimally symptomatic lesions. Additionally, aggressive medical treatment has improved the survival rate of greater numbers of stroke patients. Consequently, there has been some disagreement over which subgroups of these populations are appropriate surgical candidates. This review examines current indications for both elective and emergency carotid endarterectomy.

Asymptomatic Carotid Disease

Carotid circulation disease can be divided into asymptomatic and symptomatic forms. Asymptomatic carotid disease, which has been the subject of much recent debate, includes patients with (1) asymptomatic carotid bruits, (2) symptoms referable to one carotid territory with radiographic demonstration of clinically silent contralateral carotid stenosis or ulceration, and (3) who, while being prepared for major surgical procedures (most commonly coronary or peripheral vascular surgery), are found to have auscultatory or radiographic evidence of carotid pathology. Symptomatic carotid disease, in which surgical intervention has been more generally accepted, encompasses a spectrum of presentations from transient ischemic attacks (TIAs) to stroke-in-evolution and completed stroke, and includes acute or subacute carotid occlusion as well as the so-called "stump syndromes."

Asymptomatic Bruit

Carotid bruits are heard in 3% to 4% of the asymptomatic U.S. population over 45 years of age and are present in 10% to 23% of patients in referral populations with symptomatic atherosclerosis in other arterial distributions. Two major studies have advocated surgery for asymptomatic carotid bruits.[22,74] Both studies followed a group of unoperated patients with asymptomatic bruits and reported higher rates of neurologic sequelae (with stroke rates of 15% to 17%) as compared to operated controls. Neither report documented the relationship of neurologic events to the territory of the carotid bruit (e.g. ipsilateral or contralateral), nor was it reported which of the patients suffering acute stroke had experienced a warning TIA prior to that event (which would have justified prophylactic endarterectomy in most medical centers). These questions have been addressed, however, in several population studies.[38,86] In one of these studies, carotid bruits were identified in 72 patients, 10 of whom later developed strokes, but in whom the strokes occurred most frequently in different vascular territories.[38] Data from another, The Framingham Study, confirmed that asymptomatic bruit predicted an increased risk of neurologic events, but that the majority of these events were either in other cerebrovascular territories or were etiologically related to noncarotid factors, e.g. aneurysms, lacunar infarcts, or emboli following myocardial infarction.[86] Both studies confirmed that patients with asymptomatic bruit are at increased risk for cerebrovascular and/or cardiac problems, but could not provide justification for prophylactic surgery for the asymptomatic bruit alone.

The question of critical high-grade stenosis remains debatable. Hemodynamic studies have indicated that critical reductions in cerebral blood flow may not be reached until 75% to 84% diameter stenosis has occurred, indicating that stenosis must be of a very high grade to be "hemodynamically significant".[6] Prospective noninvasive studies by one group showed a higher propensity for neurologic events or acute carotid occlusion in lesions that are 80% or more stenotic,[65] and another group's study showed a protective effect from surgical intervention in these patients.[56] Based on these reports, many surgeons feel justified in correcting such severe but otherwise asymptomatic lesions. Chambers and Norris, on the other hand, reported that asymptomatic patients with stenosis of all

degrees were at higher risk of cardiac ischemia than of stroke. In their series, although the risk of cerebral ischemic events was highest in patients with severe carotid artery stenosis, in most instances these patients did not have strokes without some sort of warning event.[20] Many reviews of this subject[21,23,30,55,88] recommend medical management of the patient with asymptomatic carotid bruit or stenosis with antiplatelet aggregating therapy (ASA) and attention to contributing risk factors (notably, hypertension and smoking), with surgical intervention deferred until such time as frank TIAs develop. Yet, other authors emphasize that TIA or minor symptoms may occur during sleep or may be midiagnosed. Major ischemic strokes are not always preceded by recognizable warning.[55]

The continuing controversy over asymptomatic carotid disease has spawned several large clinical trials, most of which are still in progress. The final answers to the asymptomatic question will not be available at the time of this printing but we may summarize briefly some of the results and study designs here. First, in the German CASANOVA Study, no difference could be demonstrated between medical and surgical treatment in a group of 400 patients with asymptomatic stenosis (50% to 99% of the internal carotid artery). Medical treatment in this study consisted of aspirin and dipyridamole. At present this study represents the only available data from a randomized asymptomatic trial.[26] The Veterans Administration Asymptomatic Carotid Stenosis Study randomized 444 patients, all of whom had at least 50% stenosis of the internal carotid artery, into nonoperative and operative groups. Patient intake for this study concluded in October 1987, and patients will continue to be monitored for 5 years before the data is analyzed and released. Medically treated patients in this study received 325 mg of aspirin twice daily. No conclusions can be drawn as yet from this study.[75] Finally, the Asymptomatic Carotid Atherosclerosis Study (ACAS) is currently in the process of patient entry. Patients in this trial must have greater than 60% stenosis of the carotid artery and were randomly assigned to the medically treated group receiving 325 mg of aspirin daily, or a surgically treated group also receiving aspirin. Data collection is continuing, but conclusion data availability dates for this study are not known.[7]

Currently, with few exceptions, there is very little solid evidence to support surgery for asymptomatic carotid stenosis of any degree. Hemodynamically significant lesions (80% or greater) remain an open question and many practioners continue to feel that these represent appropriate surgical lesions. Within the next several years scientific proof in the form of randomized trial data will no doubt help to illuminate this question and hopefully provide more substantial answers.

Contralateral Carotid Stenosis

A number of clinical studies, primarily retrospective, have been performed with the aim of ascertaining the risks of long-term neurologic sequelae in patients with contralateral carotid stenosis managed nonoperatively. The critical point, much as in the followup of asymptomatic bruits, was to determine what percentage of these patients progressed to frank stroke in the appropriate carotid distribution without recognizable warning TIAs. Most studies of this problem have specified 50% stenosis of the contralateral carotid as the criterion for significant disease.[26,40,42,47,48] In three of these reports no patients with contralateral asymptomatic lesions developed strokes without warning TIAs.[42,47,48] In two other reports, a few patients did develop such strokes, but the incidence was invariably less than 3%, and thus less than the accepted risk of surgical morbidity and mortality.[27,40] A single study included all patients with contralateral stenosis from 1% to 99% and reported the incidence of direct stroke in unoperated patients to be 3%; these authors recommended prophylactic surgery on this basis, and also concluded that the percent stenosis did not correlate with the risk of neurologic sequelae.[63] Aside from this group's findings, however, no authors have demonstrated that prophylactic surgery for contralateral lesions of greater than 50% stenosis has any protective effect in the absence of clinical symptoms referable to that lesion.

Carotid Risks in Noncarotid Preoperative Patients

Since carotid surgery is widely available and the consequences of carotid embolization or occlusion have become well recognized, considerable interest has been generated in the proper management of patients who are found to have auscultatory or radiographic evidence of otherwise silent carotid artery disease and who are to undergo other surgical procedures. There are a number of studies addressing this problem, with nearly unequivocal conclusions. One early group performed prophylactic endarterectomies in 34 surgical patients and were able to demonstrate low morbidity and good long-term survival following the procedure.[45] It was not clear, however, that their patients were at increased risk for cerebrovascular events, and thus whether these prophylactic procedures, albeit safe in their hands, were necessary. This point was soon resolved by a series of retrospective studies that followed surgical patients with asymptomatic bruits without carotid surgery.[19,29,76,77] These studies established the incidence of asymptomatic bruits in random preoperative patients to be near 15%. Although they documented a perioperative stroke rate of about 1% in their patient groups, none of the investigators could find a correlation between presence or location of carotid bruits and risk of perioperative stroke. More recent investigations[10,11,15,78] have prospectively examined asymptomatic bruit patients through noninvasive carotid studies in an attempt to correlate percent stenosis with risk of perioperative stroke. Although some of these reports documented higher perioperative mortality in the carotid stenosis groups,[10,11] deaths were primarily attributable to an increased risk of myocardial infarction; and once again no correlation between bruit or stenosis and perioperative stroke risk was demonstrated. In one recent prospective study of preoperative patients with asymptomatic bruits only, the 14% incidence of bruits in this group was confirmed, and all strokes (0.7% of patients) were found in patients having coronary bypass surgery.[66] The concept that increased risk of perioperative stroke in coronary bypass patients arises from femoral arterial cannulation (and consequent retrograde aortic flow during bypass) rather than incidental carotid disease with carotid embolization and/or hypoperfusion, has been supported by a Canadian study that found femoral cannulation to be the only statistically significant common denominator among a group of bypass patients with embolic stroke.[51] In a recent study by Furlan of coronary bypass patients with angiographically documented asymptomatic stenosis greater than 50%, stroke risk was not increased in patients with either < 90% stenosis or with total ICA occlusion. There was an insufficient number of patients in the 90% to 99% group to allow statistical conclusions.[33]

It seems then, that there is little evidence to support prophylactic endarterectomy in preoperative patients with either asymptomatic bruit or stenosis detected by noninvasive carotid studies. Until such data become available it seems unwarranted to attribute perioperative stroke to asymptomatic carotid disease or to perform prophylactic carotid surgery in these patients.

Symptomatic Carotid Disease

Symptomatic disease in the carotid circulation encompasses a spectrum of presentations—from classical carotid TIA to frank embolic or thrombotic stroke—and is at times paradoxical in that the degree of collateral circulation may allow severe carotid pathology to present with only minimal symptomatology (e.g. there is a finite incidence of carotid occlusion presenting with TIAs alone). Whereas the discussion of asymptomatic caro-

tid disease involved primarily a comparison of operated patients versus unoperated control groups, any consideration of surgery for symptomatic carotid disease must be based on objective comparison of surgical morbidity and results with both the natural history of the disease process and the best available medical therapy. The surgical risk in elective carotid endarterectomies performed in major centers approaches 3% as previously mentioned, and this figure should be used for evaluation of therapeutic choices. Guidelines for acceptable surgical morbidity and mortality have recently been developed by both the AHA Stroke Council[13] and the American College of Physicians.[3]

Transient Ischemic Attacks (TIAs)

Three well-accepted studies have documented that the risk of stroke following a first classical carotid TIA approximates 5% per year.[1,8,84] Equally important data shows that 51% of all such strokes occur in the first year following initial TIA and that 21% occur in the first month following such an event.[82] It is only after the first 6 months that the risk of stroke falls to and remains 5% annually. This malignant natural history has prompted several forms of medical therapy. Anticoagulation, although initially effective in stroke prophylaxis following TIA, has proven difficult to control in an outpatient population. Such therapy has also been shown to be associated with a high risk of intracranial hemorrhage which, in patients aged 55 to 74, was eight times greater than in a control group.[83] Furthermore, all studies of anticoagulant therapy in TIAs failed to demonstrate differences in mortality between treated and untreated groups. The consequent decline in use of anticoagulation as primary therapy for TIA has been paralleled by a great interest in antiplatelet-aggregating agents. In the American controlled study of aspirin therapy for cerebral ischemia[32] antiplatelet-aggregating therapy was shown to decrease the incidence of recurrent TIAs but did not significantly decrease the long-term incidence of stroke in treated patients. The Canadian study of aspirin and sulfinpyrazone, however, did show a significant 31% decrease in long-term risk of stroke or death[18]. This risk reduction was sex-dependent, and in males a 48% risk reduction was demonstrated. Dipyridamole has not supplemented aspirin's effect on risk reduction of stroke after TIA.[14] Assuming a 5% annual risk of stroke in untreated patients then, the best medical therapy available reduces this risk by nearly one half—to 2.5% per year.

Much like asymptomatic carotid disease, symptomatic carotid disease became the focus of several randomized cooperative trials in the late 1980's. A European trial of symptomatic patients in all subgroups from 0% to 99% stenosis was paralleled by two trials in North America, the North American Symptomatic Carotid Endarterectomy Trial (NASCET) and the Veterans Administration Cooperative Trial of Symptomatic Carotid Disease. On February 22, 1991, intake of patients with greater than 70% stenosis into the NASCET trial was stopped because an end point was reached in which it was clearly demonstrated that surgical treatment of these patients was unequivocally superior to medical management.[59] The NASCET trial will continue intake and study of patients from 30% to 69% stenosis who are clinically symptomatic. Data from these patients was not available at the time of this publication.

Concurrent with release of data from the NASCET trial, similar data was released by the European group (coincidentally during the same week) that advised a clear surgical benefit for patients with 70% to 99% stenosis.[28] These investigations simultaneously declared that medical therapy was clearly superior for symptomatic patients with stenosis less than 30% (a group not studied by NASCET). The European trial will continue to enter patients between 30% and 70% stenosis, as this subgroup's best treatment has not yet been identified.

More recently, data from the Veterans Administration Cooperative Trial has been analyzed.[52] This study demonstrated a statistically significant surgical benefit for symptomatic patients with greater than 50% stenosis, and thus corroborates the NASCET and European data.

The conclusive results from the NASCET, European, and VA trials shows that surgical treatment is the best option in patients with carotid-territory TIA or minor stroke and greater than 70% ICA stenosis in the appropriate territory demonstrated by arteriography. A clear mandate now exists to proceed with surgical treatment in these patients. However, issues related to patient age, other medical or angiographic risks, and timing for surgery following recent stroke have not been well clarified by these studies. Further analysis of subgroups from these trials will undoubtedly be performed in upcoming months and may shed some light on these questions.

Acute Neurologic Deficit

Surgical intervention is often not a consideration in cases of acute stroke, for several reasons. Many patients presenting with acute neurologic deficits have as their primary problem a noncarotid event such as hypertensive hemorrhage or cardiogenic emboli. Even those patients identified to have carotid embolic disease as the cause of their neurologic deterioration have fared poorly when subjected to emergency carotid surgery. In one early study more than 50% of such patients suffered a fatal intracranial hemorrhage within 72 hours of emergency endarterectomy.[87] Other investigators have reported moderate success, however, with emergency surgery in patients fulfilling strict preoperative criteria. These include crescendo TIAs (attacks abruptly increasing in frequency to at least several per day) in patients with severe stenosis; stroke following angiography; stroke following endarterectomy (if thrombosis is present); and disappearance of a previously auscultated bruit in patients awaiting elective carotid surgery (presumably indicating acute occlusion).[41,54,58] Most recently, encouraging results have been reported by two groups performing emergency surgery for crescendo TIAs and stroke-in-evolution clinically and radiographically localized to one carotid artery.[34,53] In another report by Goldstone and Moore, however, they emphasize that patients with depressed levels of consciousness or acute fixed deficits were excluded from their surgical series, and agree with other authors[54] that such findings must be taken as absolute contraindications for emergency carotid endarterectomy. At present, then, emergency carotid endarterectomy is indicated only in a specific subpopulation of stroke patients, (i.e. those with documented carotid etiology for a progressive but nondebilitating ischemic event, or those in whom evidence of acute carotid thrombosis is present—loss of bruit, stroke following angiography or stroke following endarterectomy—who can be operated upon within several hours of the event and who do not exhibit evidence of distal thromboembolism beyond the circle of Willis).[60]

Complete Carotid Occlusion

Complete carotid occlusion, like many of the carotid syndromes, may present without symptoms, with TIAs or fluctuating neurologic deficit, or with frank stroke. There is some overlap, therefore, in the literature dealing with complete occlusion and addressing emergency endarterectomy for stroke. Aside from the acute nondebilitating neurologic deficits previously discussed, surgery for subacute carotid occlusion has been performed both to restore blood flow to the ipsilateral hemisphere and to prevent emboli originating from the stump of an occluded internal carotid artery from propagating distally. The ability to re-establish flow in such situations depends in large measure on the duration of the occlusion, with several authors reporting 100% success in reopening these arteries within 7 days.[36,39] Delayed surgery has been less promising,[36,73] and successful restoration of flow in late surgical cases (2-5 weeks) appears to be dependent on the degree of collateral filling present from intracavernous and intrapetrous carotid branches.[39,70] One study has documented 58% patency at six

months by follow-up angiography.[43] Surgical intervention for complete carotid occlusion appears to be indicated in a very limited group of patients who present with either acute nondebilitating deficit directly attributable to such occlusion, or with ischemic symptoms referable to embolization from an occluded stump. In these highly selected cases thromboendarterectomy carries a low surgical risk and, depending on the duration of occlusion and degree of collateral filling, has a reasonable chance of achieving long-term patency.

Stump Syndromes

As alluded to previously, in recent years attention has focused on the importance of the often-found "stump" of an occluded internal carotid artery as a possible source for ipsilateral embolic phenomena.[12,24] The presumed mechanism for these TIAs is through embolization of debris from the stump through external carotid—ophthalmic artery collaterals. This mechanism has been documented angiographically.[24,79] Obviously, before the carotid stump can be implicated as the etiologic source, the presence of major collaterals and the absence of other significant atheromatous disease must be documented with four-vessel angiography. In cases where this mechanism seems clear, however, and where reopening of the internal carotid cannot be achieved, surgical ligation of the offending stump, with concurrent endarterectomy of the common and external carotid arteries, appears to be effective therapy for such neurologic phenomena. In our opinion, the treatment of such stumps in appropriate patients appears to be as important to stroke prophylaxis as is treatment of any other symptomatic carotid lesion.

Recent Stroke

Recent stroke is not a contraindication to carotid endarterectomy unless the stroke has been debilitating or involves extensive parenchymal damage.[54] Although many cerebrovascular surgeons empirically recommend a delay of 3-6 weeks prior to performing carotid endarterectomy in patients with fresh but non-debilitating strokes (especially those with significant CT findings and with presumed defective autoregulation[87]), we are unaware of any major studies that have definitively addressed this issue. It should be noted that a number of authors who customarily advocate selective shunting have found intraoperative monitoring to be less reliable in patients having had recent RIND or stroke. These groups recommend empirical shunt placement in all such cases.[57,67] Other surgeons emphasize delayed surgery (in proportion to stroke severity) and subsequent routine carotid endarterectomy with electroencephalographic monitoring and selective shunting.[72,85]

Special Surgical Considerations

We should finally consider several special cases and associated findings in carotid patients, some of which have been considered relative contraindications to successful carotid reconstruction but which have become more acceptable with advances in radiologic, surgical, and anesthetic techniques.

Plaque Morphology

Plaque Ulceration

Correlation of plaque ulceration with ischemic neurologic symptoms and need for surgery is difficult for several reasons. First, studies have shown poor interobserver variability either on ultrasound or arteriographic examinations and poor correlation between pathologic specimens and radiographically demonstrated ulceration. Second, in symptomatic patients deep ulceration is most commonly found in conjunction with significant degrees of carotid stenosis and it becomes difficult to separate clinical symptomatology between these two findings.[35,80]

The significance of intraplaque hemorrhage as a predictor of ischemic symptoms is likewise unclear. Although one recent review suggested that intraplaque hemorrhage was found much more commonly in patients with symptomatic carotid disease[35] other studies suggest that there is a low correlation between ischemic symptoms and plaque hematoma in carotid endarterectomy patients.[46]

Critical Stenosis

The question of critical stenosis has recently been well addressed. As discussed under the topic of asymptomatic bruit, 80% or greater stenosis is felt by many to represent a surgical indication although the scientific foundation for this is at present inconclusive. We reiterate that the NASCET Study has clearly shown surgical benefit in patients with greater than 70% stenosis who are neurologically symptomatic; and surgery is clearly superior in this group of patients.

Intraluminal Thrombus

The problem of surgical timing in patients with angiographically demonstrated propagating intraluminal thrombus remains an open question among cerebrovascular experts. Several authors have addressed this issue and document that an increased risk of perioperative or intraoperative stroke must be accepted when operating on patients who have propagating clot that may extend beyond the area of internal carotid cross clamping or which is more friable and prone to dislodgment than the usual carotid plaque.[14,16,37] Review of the available literature suggests that a period of observation with full heparinization prior to undertaking surgical therapy may reduce the morbidity and mortality in these patients.[14,16] The answer to this question is clearly not yet available. It is equally clear, however, that intraluminal thrombus at the present time should not be considered a surgical emergency but rather should provoke a careful and measured response to the situation. As one author has suggested, heparinization should probably be instituted in every case followed by consideration of endarterectomy in patients who are neurologically stable, and by a delayed surgical plan following a period of expectant observation in neurologically unstable patients or those with serious intercurrent illness or hypercoagulable state.[37]

Contralateral Carotid Occlusion

Early reports of surgery in the face of contralateral carotid occlusion were dismal,[31] but with advances in surgical and anesthetic techniques most surgeons at present have little or no hesitation to approach symptomatic carotid lesions even in the face of such contralateral occlusion. Surgeons who employ selective shunting based on intraoperative monitoring do report a higher incidence of shunt-dependent cases in this group,[17,85] and some groups have reported higher rates of postoperative neurologic deficits in this subgroup when shunts were not used.[9,50] Two series dealing exclusively with this problem have been published, and both reported satisfactory results. Interestingly, both groups employed universal shunting in dealing with contralateral carotid occlusion[5,61]. It has been our policy to approach these cases with EEG monitoring and selective shunting much as the routine carotid procedures are performed, although unquestionably the need for intraluminal shunting has been greater in this subgroup.

Tandem Lesions of the Carotid Siphon

The presence of carotid siphon disease has been proposed as a contraindication to carotid endarterectomy because of inability to pinpoint the symptomatic source and the reputed increased possibilities of postoperative occlusion from decreased carotid flow velocity. Two recent series have repudiated these contentions.[64,69] In both of these no significant association between postoperative complications or recurrent symptoms could be demonstrated in patients undergoing carotid endarterectomy in the face of known "inaccessible" siphon disease. There are several other interesting reports on this problem. Day et al documented two cases of siphon disease resolution following ipsilateral carotid endarterectomy.[25] Little et al described a sim-

ilar entity of angiographic "pseudo-tandem stenosis" that likewise resolved in two cases following endarterectomy.[49] At present, then, the presence of a tandem lesion does not appear to contraindicate successful carotid endarterectomy if the indications and surgical risks are otherwise justified.

Concurrent Carotid Disease and Intracranial Aneurysm

There have been several reports concerning the repair sequencing of symptomatic carotid disease and silent intracranial aneurysm discovered on carotid angiography. Although one report documents rupture of an intracranial aneurysm six months following carotid reconstruction for tight stenosis,[2] most other authors recommend repair of the symptomatic lesion first, which in most cases is the symptomatic carotid artery stenosis.[44,71] These authors conclude that carotid endarterectomy is unlikely to precipitate rupture of intracranial aneurysm during the perioperative period.

Recurrent Carotid Stenosis

There is a small but finite incidence of recurrent carotid stenosis following primary carotid endarterectomy. Most authors quote a symptomatic recurrence rate of approximately 4% to 5%, and in one study of noninvasive followup after carotid surgery, a 4.8% recurrence rate of symptomatic carotid restenosis was documented with an additional 6.6% silent restenosis rate.[68] Piepgras, Sundt, and colleagues have quoted somewhat lower figures with use of patchgraft repair (1% symptomatic, 4% to 5% total at two-year followup).[62]

Aside from technical inadequacies, it has been difficult to identify risk factors associated with recurrent carotid stenosis, although continuation of smoking habits following endarterectomy proved to be a significant risk factor in one study, whereas hypertension, diabetes mellitus, family history, lipid studies, aspirin use, and coronary disease were not found to be significant risk factors by this group.[21]

Reoperation for carotid stenosis is a technically difficult procedure and is reserved for discussion elsewhere. It is associated with significantly higher risks than primary endarterectomy. Sundt documents a risk of complications of 10.5%, four times his customary figure.[62] In our institution, the possibility of reoperation for carotid stenosis is entertained in patients who present with angiographically proven disease and classical neurologic symptoms referable to the appropriate artery. We have been unwilling to assume this surgical risk in asymptomatic patients and because of this have not routinely followed patients with noninvasive studies beyond the first year if they remain clinically stable. Others with great experience in this field, however, do feel that changing bruits or rapidly progressive stenosis justifies surgical intervention.[62]

early < 2 yr — myointimal h ?perplasia
late > 2 yr — atherosclerosis.

Conclusions

Carotid endarterectomy has evolved from a radical procedure involving excision of the diseased segment with end-to-end anastomosis of the parent vessel to a routine and uncomplicated operation recommended for selected patients judged to be at high risk for impending stroke. As has been shown, carotid surgery is not without risks, particularly when one considers the associated diseases present in many of these surgical candidates. Consequently, well-defined criteria must be met before patients can confidently be recommended for surgical therapy.

The literature at present does not support prophylactic carotid endarterectomy for asymptomatic carotid disease, except perhaps for 80% or greater lesion stenosis, despite the low morbidity reported by some authors for such procedures. Strong support now exists for the superiority of surgical therapy in preventing devastating strokes in patients with prior nondebilitating or transient ischemic symptoms and greater than 70% stenosis of the corresponding carotid artery.

This remains the primary and only *proven* indication for carotid endarterectomy. Patients with less than 30% stenosis are best treated medically, and treatment for those in the intermediate (30% to 69%) group remains an open question which is being carefully evaluated at present. Likewise, in some specific types of acute neurologic deficit and some milder forms of complete carotid occlusion, emergency endarterectomy may have an advantage over the best currently available medical therapy. Perhaps the most important factor in recommending carotid surgery is the availability of a skilled cerebrovascular surgeon with a demonstrable morbidity and mortality below 3%. In such hands, and with meticulous attention to intraoperative technical factors and postoperative management of medical problems, carotid endarterectomy has proven a safe and reliable means of long-term stroke prophylaxis. Equally important is that the individual surgeon develop a rational and consistent approach to extracranial vascular diagnosis, indications for surgical intervention, and technical performance of the procedure. It is only with such an intellectually honest approach that various treatment strategies can be effectively compared and true surgical progress made.

References

1. Acheson J, Hutchinson EC. Observations on the natural history of transient cerebral ischaemia. *Lancet.* 1964;2:871-876.
2. Adams HP Jr. Carotid stenosis and coexisting ipsilateral intracranial aneurysm. *Arch Neurol.* 1977; 34:515-516.
3. American College of Physicians. Indications for carotid endarterectomy. *Ann Intern Med.* 1989; 111:675-677.
4. American-Canadian Co-operative Study Group. Persantine Aspirin Trial in cerebral ischemia, II: endpoint result. *Stroke.* 1985;16:406-415.
5. Andersen CA, Rich NM, Collins GJ Jr, et al. Unilateral internal carotid artery occlusion: special considerations. *Stroke.* 1977;8:669-671.
6. Archie JP, Feldtman RW. Critical stenosis of the internal carotid artery. *Surgery.* 1981;89:67-72.
7. Asymptomatic Carotid Atherosclerosis Study Group. Study design for randomized prospective trial of carotid endarterectomy for asymptomatic atherosclerosis. *Stroke.* 1989;20:844-849.
8. Baker RN, Ramseyer JC, Schwartz WS. Prognosis in patients with transient cerebral ischemic attacks. *Neurology.* 1968;18:1157-1165.

9. Baker WH, Dorner DB, Barnes RW. Carotid endarterectomy: is an indwelling shunt necessary? *Surgery.* 1977;82:321-326.

10. Barnes RW, Liebman PR, Marszalek PB. The natural history of asymptomatic carotid disease in patients undergoing cardiovascular surgery. *Surgery.* 1981;90:1075-1083.

11. Barnes RW, Marszalek PB. Asymptomatic carotid disease in the cardiovascular surgical patient: Is prophylactic endarterectomy necessary? *Stroke.* 1981; 12:497-500.

12. Barnett HJM, Peerless SJ, Kaufmann JCE. "Stump" of internal carotid artery—a source for further cerebral embolic ischemia. *Stroke.* 1978;9:448-456.

13. Beebe HG, Clagett GP, DeWeese JA, et al. Assessing risk associated with carotid endarterectomy. A statement for health professionals by an ad hoc committee on carotid surgery standards of the stroke council, American Heart Association. *Stroke.* 1989; 20:314-315.

14. Biller J, Adams HP, Boarini D, et al. Intraluminal clot of the carotid artery. *Surg Neurol.* 1986;25: 467-477.

15. Breslau PJ, Fell G, Ivey TD, et al. Carotid arterial disease in patients undergoing coronary bypass operations. *J Thorac Cardiovasc Surg.* 1981; 82:765-767.

16. Buchan A, Gates P, Pelz D, et al. Intraluminal thrombus in the cerebral circulation: implications for surgical management. *Stroke.* 1988;19:681-687.

17. Callow AD, Matsumoto G, Baker D, et al. Protection of the high risk carotid endarterectomy patient by continuous electroencephalography. *J Cardiovasc Surg (Torino).* 1978;19:55-64.

18. Canadian Cooperative Study Group: A randomized trial of aspirin and sulfinpyrazone in threatened stroke. *N Engl J Med.* 1978;299:53-59.

19. Carney WI Jr, Stewart WB, DePinto DJ, et al. Carotid bruit as a risk factor in aortoiliac reconstruction. *Surgery.* 1977;81:567-570.

20. Chambers BR, Norris JW. Outcome in patients with asymptomatic neck bruits. *N Engl J Med.* 1986;315: 860-865.

21. Clagett GP, Rich NM, McDonald PT, et al. Etiologic factors for recurrent carotid artery stenosis. *Surgery.* 1983;93:313-318.

22. Cooperman M, Martin EW, Evans WE Jr. Significance of asymptomatic carotid bruits. *Arch Surg.* 1978;113:1339-1340.

23. Corman LC. The preoperative patient with an asymptomatic bruit. *Med Clin North Am.* 1979;63: 1335-1340.

24. Countee RW, Vijayanathan T. Intracranial embolization via external carotid artery: report of a case with angiographic documentation. *Stroke.* 1980;11: 465-468.

25. Day AL, Rhoton AL, Quisling RG. Resolving siphon stenosis following endarterectomy. *Stroke.* 1980;11:278-281.

26. Diener H-C, Hamann H, Schäfer H, et al. Carotid surgery versus medical therapy in asymptomatic carotid stenosis. *Neurology.* 1990;40(suppl 1):415.

27. Durward QJ, Ferguson GG, Barr HWK. The natural history of asymptomatic carotid bifurcation plaques. *Stroke.* 1982;13:459-464.

28. European Carotid Surgery Trialists' Collaborative Group. MRC European Carotid Surgery Trial: interim results for symptomatic patients with severe (70-

99%) or mild (0-29%) carotid stenosis. *Lancet.* 1991;337:1235-1243.

29. Evans WE, Cooperman M. The significance of asymptomatic unilateral carotid bruits in preoperative patients. *Surgery.* 1978;83:521-522.

30. Fields WS. The asymptomatic carotid bruit—operate or not? *Stroke.* 1978;9:269-271.

31. Fields WS, Lemak NA. Joint study of extracranial ar5erial occlusion, X: internal carotid artery occlusion. *JAMA.* 1976;235:2734-2738.

32. Fields WS, Lemak NA, Frankowski RF, et al. Controlled trial of aspirin in cerebral ischemia. *Stroke.* 1977;8:301-314.

33. Furlan AJ, Craciun AR. Risk of stroke during coronary artery bypass graft surgery in patients with internal carotid artery disease documented by angiography. *Stroke.* 1985;16:797-799.

34. Goldstone J, Moore WS. A new look at emergency carotid artery operations for the treatment of cerebrovascular insufficiency. *Stroke.* 1978;9:599-602.

35. Gomez, CR: Carotid plaque morphology and risk for stroke. *Stroke.* 1990;21:148-151.

36. Hafner CD, Tew JM. Surgical management of the totally occluded internal carotid artery: a ten-year study. *Surgery.* 1981;89:710-717.

37. Heros RC. Carotid endarterectomy in patients with intraluminal thrombus. *Stroke.* 1990;19:667-668.

38. Heyman A, Wilkinson WE, Heyden S, et al. Risk of stroke in asymptomatic persons with cervical arterial bruits: a population study in Evans County, Georgia. *N Engl J Med.* 1980;302:838-841.

39. Hugenholtz H, Elgie R: Carotid thromboendarterectomy: a reappraisal. *J Neurosurg.* 1980;53:776-783.

40. Humphries AW, Young JR, Santilli PH, et al. Unoperated, asymptomatic significant internal carotid artery stenosis: a review of 182 instances. *Surgery.* 1976;80:695-698.

41. Hunter JA, Julian OC, Dye WS, et al. Emergency operation for acute cerebral ischemia due to carotid artery obstruction: review of 26 cases. *Ann Surg.* 1965;162:901-904.

42. Johnson N, Burnham SJ, Flanigan DP, et al. Carotid endarterectomy: a follow-up study of the contralateral non-operated carotid artery. *Ann Surg.* 1978; 188:748-752.

43. Kusonoki T, Rowed DW, Tator CH, et al. Thromboendarterectomy for total occlusion of the internal carotid artery: a reappraisal of risks, success rate, and potential benefits. *Stroke.* 1978;9:34-38.

44. Ladowski JS, Webster MW, Yonas HO, et al. Carotid endarterectomy in patients with asymptomatic intracranial aneurysm. *Ann Surg.* 1984;200:70-73.

45. Lefrak EA, Guinn GA. Prophylactic carotid artery surgery in patients requiring a second operation. *South Med J.* 1974;67:185-189

46. Lennihan L, Kupsky WJ, Mohr JP, et al. Lack of association between carotid plaque hematoma and ischemic cerebral symptoms. *Stroke.* 1987;18: 879-881.

47. Levin SM, Sondheimer FK. Stenosis of the contralateral asymptomatic carotid artery—to operate or not? *Vasc Surg.* 1973;7:3-13.

48. Levin SM, Sondheimer FK, Levin JM. The contralateral diseased but asymptomatic carotid artery: to operate or not? *Am J. Surg.* 1980;40:203-205.

49. Little JR, Sawhny B, Weinstin M. Pseudo-tandem stenosis of the interal carotid artery. *Neurosurgery.* 1980;7:574-577.

50. Littooy FN, Halstuk KS, Mamdani M, et al. Factors influencing morbidity of carotid endarterectomy without a shunt. *Am Surg.* 1984;50:350-353.

51. Martin WRW, Hashimoto SA. Stroke in coronary bypass surgery. *Can J Neuro Sci.* 1982;9:21-26.

52. Mayberg MR, Wilson SE, Yatsu F, et al. Carotid endarterectomy and prevention of cerebral ischemia in symptomatic carotid stenosis. *JAMA.* 1991;266:3289-3294.

53. Mentzer RM, Finkelmeier BA, Crosby IK, et al. Emergency carotid endarterectomy for fluctuating neurologic deficits. *Surgery.* 1981;89:60-66.

54. Millikan CH, McDowell FH. Treatment of progressing stroke. *Prog Cardiovasc Dis.* 1980;22:397-414.

55. Mohr JP. Asymptomatic carotid artery disease. *Stroke.* 1982;13:431-433.

56. Moneta GL, Taylor DC, Nicholls SC, et al. Operative versus nonoperative management of asymptomatic high-grade internal carotid artery stenosis: improved results with endarterectomy. *Stroke.* 1987;18:1005-1010.

57. Moore WS, Yee JM, Hall AD. Collateral cerebral blood pressure: an index to tolerance to temporary carotid occlusion. *Arch Surg.* 1973;106:520-523.

58. Najafi H, Javid H, Dye WS. Emergency carotid thromboendarterectomy: surgical indications and results. *Arch Surg.* 1971;103:610-614.

59. National Institute of Neurological and Communicative Disorders and Stroke. Benefit of carotid endarterectomy for patients with high-grade stenosis of the internal carotid artery. In: *NASCET Investigators: Clinical Alert.* February 25, 1991.

60. Ojemann RG, Crowell RM, Roberson GH. Surgical treatment of extracranial carotid occlusive disease. *Clin Neurosurg.* 1975;22:214-263.

61. Patterson RH Jr. Risk of carotid surgery with occlusion of the contralateral carotid artery. *Arch Neurol.* 1974;30:188-189.

62. Piepgras DG, Sundt TM Jr, Marsh WR, et al. Recurrent carotid stenosis: results and complications of 57 operations. In: Sundt TM Jr, ed., *Occlusive Cerebrovascular Disease: Diagnosis and Surgical Management.* Philadelphia, Pa: W.B. Saunders; 1987:286-297.

63. Podore PC, DeWeese JA, May AG, et al. Asymptomatic contralateral carotid artery stenosis: a five-year follow-up study following carotid endarterectomy. *Surgery.* 1980;88:748-752.

64. Roederer GO, Langlois YE, Chan ARW, et al. Is siphon disease important in predicting outcome of carotid endarterectomy? *Arch Surg.* 1983;118:1177-1181.

65. Roederer GO, Langlois YE, Jager KA, et al. The natural history of carotid artery disease in asymptomatic patients with cervical bruits. *Stroke.* 1984;15:605-613.

66. Ropper AH, Wechsler LR, Wilson LS. Carotid bruit and risk of stroke in elective surgery. *N Engl J Med.* 1982;307:1388-1390.

67. Rosenthal D, Stanton PE, Lamis PA. Carotid endarterectomy: the unreliability of intraoperative monitoring in patients having had a stroke or reversible ischemic neurological deficit. *Arch Surg.* 1981;116:1569-1575.

68. Salvian A, Baker JD, Machleder HI, et al. Cause and noninvasive detection of restenosis after carotid endarterectomy. *Am J. Surg.* 1983;146:29-34.

69. Schuler JJ, Flanigan DP, Lim LT. The effect of carotid siphon stenosis on stroke rate, death, and relief of symptoms following elective carotid endarterectomy. *Surgery.* 1982;92:1058-1067.

70. Shucart WA, Garrido E. Reopening some occluded carotid arteries: report of four cases. *J Neurosurg.* 1976;45:442-446.

71. Stern J, Whelan M, Brisman R, et al. Management of extracranial carotid stenosis and intracranial aneurysms. *J Neurosurg.* 1979;51:147-150.

72. Sundt TM, Sandok BA, Whisnant JP. Carotid endarterectomy: complications and preoperative assessment of risk. *Mayo Clin Proc.* 1975;50:301-306.

73. Thompson JE, Austin DJ, Patman RD. Endarterectomy of the totally occluded carotid artery for stroke. Results in 100 operations. *Arch Surg.* 1967;95:791-801.

74. Thompson JE, Patman RD, Talkington CM. Asymptomatic carotid bruit: Long-term outcome of patients having endarterectomy compared with unoperated controls. *Ann Surg.* 1978;188:308-315.

75. Towne JB, Weiss GD, Hobson RW. First phase report of cooperative Veterans Administration asymptomatic carotid stenosis study—operative morbidity and mortality. *J Vasc Surg.* 1990;11:252-259.

76. Treiman RL, Foran RF, Cohen JL, et al. Carotid bruit: a follow-up report on its significance in patients undergoing an abdominal aortic operation. *Arch Surg.* 1979;114:1138-1140.

77. Treiman RL, Foran RF, Shore EH, et al. Carotid bruit: significance in patients undergoing an abdominal aortic operation. *Arch Surg.* 1973;106:803-805.

78. Turnipseed WD, Berkoff HA, Belzer FO. Postoperative stroke in cardiac and peripheral vascular disease. *Ann Surg.* 1980;192:365-368.

79. Watts C. External carotid artery embolus from the internal carotid artery "stump" during angiography: case report. *Stroke.* 1982;13:515-517.

80. Wechsler LR: Ulceration and carotid artery disease. *Stroke.* 1988;19:650-653.

81. West H, Burton R, Roon AJ, et al. Comparative risk of operation and expectant management for carotid artery disease. *Stroke.* 1979;10:117-121.

82. Whisnant JP. Epidemiology of stroke: Emphasis on transient cerebral ischemic attacks and hypertension. *Stroke.* 1974;5:68-70.

83. Whisnant JP, Cartlidge NEF, Elveback LR. Carotid and vertebral-basilar transient ischemic attacks: effect of anticoagulants, hypertension, and cardiac disorders on survival and stroke occurrence—a population study. *Ann Neurol* 1978;3:107-115.

84. Whisnant JP, Matsumoto N, Elveback LR. The effect of anticoagulant therapy on the prognosis of patients with transient cerebral ischemic attacks in a community: Rochester, Minnesota, 1955 through 1969. *Mayo Clin Proc.* 1973;48:844-848.

85. Whittemore AD, Kauffman JL, Kohler TR, et al. Routine electroencephalographic (EEG) monitoring during carotid endarterectomy. *Ann Surg.* 1982;197:707-713.

86. Wolf PA, Kannel WB, Sorlie P. Asymptomatic carotid bruit and risk of stroke. The Framingham study. *JAMA.* 1981;245:1442-1445.

87. Wylie EJ, Hein MF, Adams JE. Intracranial hemorrhage following surgical revascularization for treatment of acute strokes. *J Neurosurg.* 1964;21:212-215.

88. Yatsu FM, Hart RG. Asymptomatic carotid bruit and stenosis: a reappraisal. *Stroke.* 1983;14:301-304.

CHAPTER 9

Carotid Endarterectomy: Technical Aspects and Perioperative Management

Daniel L. Barrow, MD, and Junichi Mizuno, MD

Successful carotid endarterectomy is an effective means of reducing the incidence of stroke in selected patients with symptoms of retinal or cerebral ischemia.[8,34,76,77] The benefits of the operation are easily negated if associated morbidity and mortality are excessive.[6] The combined rate of perioperative stroke and death range from 1.5% to more than 20% in various series.[1,19,28,29,31,66,72] Refinements in surgical techniques continue in an effort to reduce the perioperative complication rate.

Significant controversy surrounds a number of technical issues including the use of an indwelling shunt, patch angioplasty, intraoperative monitoring, and type of anesthesia. Excellent results have been reported from various institutions using widely varying surgical protocols. The most important factor contributing to good results appears to be the development of an operative team with a specialized technique, who perform the operation with some frequency.[66,76]

This chapter outlines our technique for carotid endarterectomy, presents alternatives in technique and discusses potential complications.

Indications and Assessment of Risk

Patient selection for endarterectomy plays an important role in the surgical results and all decisions must be individualized.[22] The major factors determining the surgical risk for an individual patient are (1) experience of the operating team, (2) condition of the patient at the time of operation, and (3) postoperative care.[14,68] Important factors to consider in the decision-making process include the patient's symptoms, physiologic state, collateral circulation, and underlying health. Carotid endarterectomy is primarily indicated for patients with clear ischemic neurologic symptoms ipsilateral to a significant carotid stenosis and/or ulceration.

The indications for carotid endarterectomy in large numbers of patients with asymptomatic neck bruits, asymptomatic carotid stenosis, and vertebrobasilar symptoms associated with carotid artery stenosis are quite controversial. We do not recommend further work-up of patients with asymptomatic bruits. Because the natural history of asymptomatic carotid lesions is not well defined, we reserve endarterectomy for only those asymptomatic patients with severe stenosis (<2 mm residual lumen) or deep ulcerations.

Sundt and associates identified medical, neurologic, and angiographically-defined factors that determine the major risks of carotid endarterectomy.[68] They are:

(1) **Medical Risk Factors**
- presence of angina pectoris or myocardial infarction within 6 months
- congestive heart failure
- severe hypertension

- chronic obstructive pulmonary disease
- severe obesity
- > 70 years age

(2) **Neurologic Risk Factors**
- progressing neurologic deficit
- deficit < 24 hours duration
- frequent daily transient ischemic attacks (TIAs)
- neurologic deficits secondary to multiple infarctions

(3) **Angiographically Defined Risk Factors**
- occlusion of the opposite internal carotid artery
- stenosis of the carotid siphon
- extensive involvement of the vessel to be operated on with extension of plaque >3 cm distally in the internal carotid or 5 cm proximally in the common carotid artery
- bifurcation of the carotid artery at the level of C2 in conjunction with a short, thick neck
- evidence of a soft thrombus extending from an ulcerative lesion

Based upon these factors, Sundt et al developed a grading system that is useful in predicting the risks of surgical intervention[68]: (Group 1) Neurologically stable with no major medical or angiographically-defined risks, with unilateral or bilateral ulcerative-stenotic carotid disease; (Group 2) Neurologically stable with no major medical risks but with significant angiographically-defined risks; (Group 3) Neurologically stable with major medical risks, with or without significant angiographically-defined risks; (Group 4) Neurologically unstable, with or without associated major medical or angiographically-defined risks.

Patients in Groups 3 and 4 are at greatest risk for non-neurologic and permanent neurologic complications, respectively.

Preoperative Assessment

Not all cerebral and retinal ischemic events are due to carotid atherosclerotic lesions. The mere presence of an atherosclerotic plaque at the carotid bifurcation does not itself constitute an indication for an endarterectomy.

All patients with cerebrovascular symptoms should be evaluated to determine the cause of the symptoms and to assess the risk of further ischemic events. Those patients with frequent transient ischemic attacks, stroke-in-evolution, or acute onset of a mild deficit are at greatest risk and should be evaluated urgently.

We do not rely heavily on noninvasive tests of the carotid in clinical decision-making. High-quality angiography is essential in the evaluation of patients being considered for carotid endarterectomy. Visualization of the origins of the cerebral vessels in the thorax, and in the extracranial and intracranial distribution are all important. Computed tomography (CT) or magnetic resonance imaging (MRI) is performed to rule out the presence of a mass lesion, such as a tumor, that may cause symptoms mimicking cerebral ischemia. These studies will also reveal old or new infarctions that may alter the timing of surgical intervention, or show a "silent" lesion in the distribution of an otherwise asymptomatic carotid lesion.

The patient's medical condition is investigated to identify any medical risk factors. Prior to surgery, the patient's cardiopulmonary status is carefully evaluated by an internist or cardiologist, as patients with carotid atherosclerosis have a high incidence of coronary and systemic atherosclerosis. In patients with significant cardiac disease, a Swan-Ganz catheter may assist in fluid management in the perioperative period.

Patients with a recent TIA or progressing focal cerebral ischemic event will frequently be placed on heparin while awaiting surgery. If symptoms continue despite adequate anticoagulation, these patients are considered surgical emergencies. Other patients selected for endarterectomy are scheduled for surgery as soon as possible, unless they have had a recent major stroke or recent myocardial infarction that necessitates a delay. There appears to be a higher stroke rate in the first month after the onset of TIA.[78] Therefore, endarterectomy may provide a greater benefit if performed within that time period.[22] Patients awaiting elective endarterectomies are placed on 325 mg aspirin per day before and after surgery. Patients with preocclusive stenosis are fully anticoagulated whenever possible while awaiting surgery, pending medical evaluation or after recent major stroke.

Anesthesia Technique

General endotracheal anesthesia is induced with thiopental sodium (3-5 mg/kg) and paralysis obtained with pancuronium or vecuronium bromide (0.1 mg/kg). Lidocaine (1 mg/kg) or fentanyl (0.05-0.1 mg) is used to diminish the cardiovascular response to intubation. Anesthesia is maintained with a nitrous oxide-oxygen mixture and isoflurane (0.5%-1.5%). Respirations are controlled to maintain an end-tidal CO_2 between 35 and 38 mm Hg. The patient is given glucose-free fluids during and after the operation. Anesthesia monitoring includes urine output, arterial blood pressure measurements, arterial blood gas analysis, end-tidal CO_2 and electrocardiographic monitoring. Monitoring of cerebroelectrical function is carried out with conventional 16-channel electroencephalography (EEG).

During the period of carotid cross-clamping, the patient is given doses of thiopental sodium or etomidate to achieve burst suppression of the EEG. This is discontinued once the artery has been reconstructed.

Operative Positioning

The patient is placed in the supine position with the head on a foam rubber "doughnut" (Figure 1). One or two rolled sheets are placed under the shoulder blades to facilitate extension of the head. Rotation of the head will bring the internal carotid artery lateral to a more accessible position than its normal position behind the external carotid in an anteroposterior plane. The amount of head turning needed for optimal exposure can be determined from the pre-

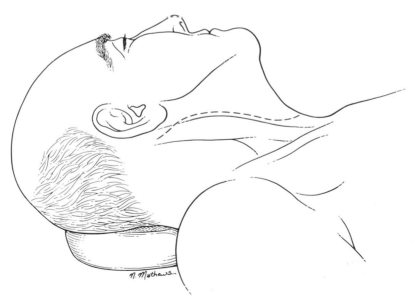

Figure 1. The patient is placed supine with the head on a foam rubber doughnut and turned slightly away from the side of the operation. The skin incision is made along the anterior border of the sternocleidomastoid muscle. It is curved superiorly to facilitate distal exposure without injuring the marginal mandibular branch of the facial nerve. Adapted from Barrow DL. Carotid Endarterectomy. In: Neurosurgical Atlas and Fasicles, Rengachary SS and Wilkins RH, eds. Williams & Wilkins Publishers. 1991.

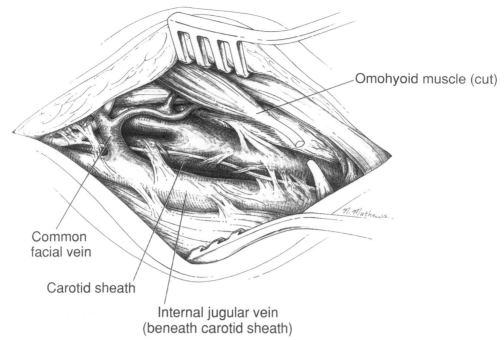

Figure 2. *The loose areolar tissue anterior to the sternocleidomastoid is separated and a self-retaining retractor placed no deeper than the platysma muscle. The omohyoid muscle has been divided to improve proximal exposure.*

operative anteroposterior (AP) angiogram. To diminish the risk of dislodging embolic material from the atherosclerotic plaque, the neck is not scrubbed but only painted with povidone solution. If there is any suggestion from the preoperative angiogram that a venous patch graft will be needed, or if the operation is a repeat procedure, a distal lower extremity is shaved, prepped, and draped for exposure of the saphenous vein for obtaining the graft.

Skin Incision

The skin incision is made along the anterior border of the sternocleidomastoid muscle and curved medially at the lower end to a point just above the sternal notch (Figure 1). The superior limb is curved posteriorly from a point about 1 cm below the angle of the mandible toward the mastoid process to avoid injury to the marginal mandibular branch of the facial nerve. The

exact length of the incision is dictated by the position of the carotid bifurcation and pathology of the plaque as demonstrated on the angiogram. The skin incision is carried down to the platysma muscle, dividing the transverse cervical nerve. Division of the nerve results in unavoidable numbness anterior to the skin incision, but patients seldom complain of this symptom.

Operative Procedure

Meticulous hemostasis is maintained throughout the operation. The platysma is divided sharply and a self-retaining retractor is placed into the wound with the medial side more superficial to avoid injury to the laryngeal nerves (Figure 2). Loose areolar tissue is dissected along the anterior border of the sternocleidomastoid to separate this muscle from the strap muscles overlying the trachea. The plane of dissection is followed down to the internal jugu-

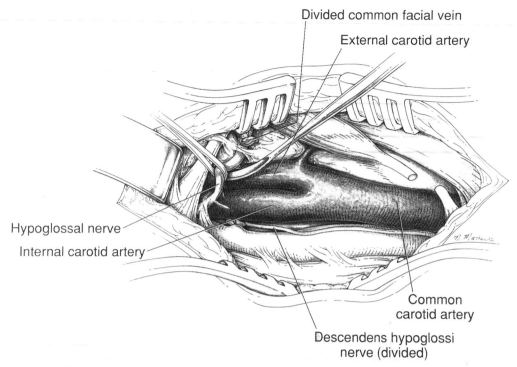

Divided common facial vein

External carotid artery

Hypoglossal nerve

Internal carotid artery

Common carotid artery

Descendens hypoglossi nerve (divided)

Figure 3. The common facial vein has been doubly ligated and divided, and the carotid sheath has been opened. Division of the descendens hypoglossi allows greater mobilization of the hypoglossal nerve and reduces the risk of traction injury to the latter.

lar vein. This vein is a key landmark for the exposure and lies lateral, parallel, and slightly anterior to the internal and common carotid arteries. Extreme care is taken to avoid manipulation of the carotid bifurcation and proximal internal carotid artery to minimize the risk of dislodging embolic material from the plaque. If the artery must be palpated during exposure, as in patients with thick necks, it should be performed only on the common carotid artery and far away from the bifurcation.

Once the jugular vein is identified, dissection is along the medial border of the vein (Figure 3). The common facial vein, which crosses the carotid at the level of the bifurcation, is doubly ligated with 2-0 silk sutures and divided. It is often necessary to divide the omohyoid muscle to obtain adequate proximal exposure. The carotid sheath is incised over the common carotid artery. Tacking the sheath up to the exter-

nal cervical fascia with 3-0 Vicryl sutures helps elevate the carotid in the wound. Two self-retaining retractors are placed into the external fascia, further elevating the carotid.

As dissection is carried superiorly, the descending hypoglossal nerve may be divided as it joins the hypoglossal nerve proper to prevent undue traction on the latter structure and to mobilize it for distal dissection of the internal carotid artery. The superior thyroid artery is identified and dissected circumferentially. It is mandatory to gain access to the distal internal carotid artery. To do so, it may be necessary to divide the digastric muscle and mobilize the hypoglossal nerve. Injection of local anesthetic into the carotid body and sinus is not routinely performed. However, if the anesthesiologist notes any change in vital signs during dissection of the bifurcation, 2-3 cc of 1% lidocaine are used to temporarily block the

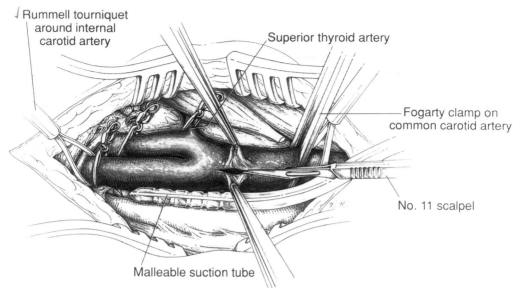

Figure 4. *The common and external carotid arteries have been dissected free from their underlying beds, where clamps are placed around them. Rummell tourniquets have been fashioned for the common and internal carotid arteries in the event a shunt is necessary. Once heparin and barbiturates have circulated, the internal carotid artery is occluded first with an aneurysm clip. Next, the common carotid artery is occluded with a Fogarty clamp and aneurysm clips are placed on the external carotid and superior thyroid arteries. The arteriotomy is initiated with a #11 scalpel.*

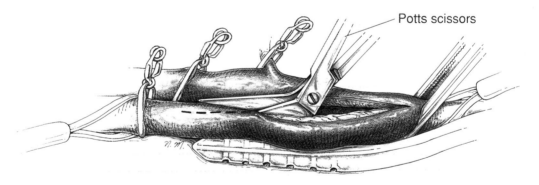

Figure 5. *The arteriotomy is extended distally with Potts arterial scissors. The opening should extend up the midline of the vessel and within the true lumen of the artery. The arteriotomy is extended distally until the limit of the plaque on the posterior wall of the internal carotid artery is identified. The arteriotomy into the common carotid is continued until the plaque ceases to be ulcerated and the wall of the vessel becomes more normal in texture.*

effects of carotid sinus stimulation.

The common and external carotid arteries are dissected free from their underlying beds only in those areas where umbilical tapes or clamps are placed around them. The umbilical tape placed around the

common carotid artery is threaded through a rubber tubing to fashion a Rummell tourniquet. This should be placed well proximal to the plaque as determined by the angiogram.

A #9 French malleable multiperforated

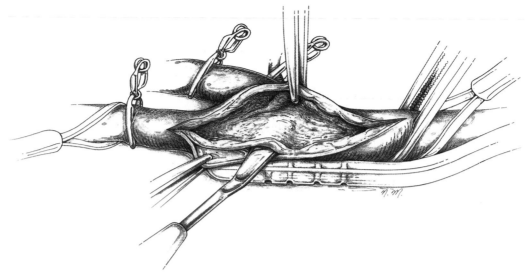

Figure 6. The plaque is removed by developing and following the pathologic cleavage plane created by the atherosclerosis between the intima and media.

suction tube (Microvac™, [PMT Inc., Hopkins, Minnesota]) is placed adjacent to the common and internal carotid arteries and fixed into position by stapling it to the surgical drapes. This constant suction will clear irrigation during the procedure and free one hand of the assistant.

Prior to carotid artery clamping, 100 U/kg heparin is given intravenously. Bolus doses of thiopental sodium (150-250 mg) are given until 15- to 30-second burst suppression is seen on the EEG recording. Barbiturate is continued by bolus injections or constant infusion to maintain burst suppression until internal carotid artery flow is re-established. Phenylephrine infusion is occasionally required to maintain systemic blood pressure in the normal range. Hypotension must be avoided. More recently, we have used etomidate rather than thiopental for cerebral protection in some patients.[47,56] As noted by Batjer et al,[10] this agent has less deleterious effects on the blood pressure and level of consciousness than barbiturates.

Once the heparin and barbiturates (or etomidate) have circulated, the internal carotid artery is occluded first with an aneurysm clip. The common carotid artery is then occluded with a Fogarty vascular clamp and temporary aneurysm clips placed on the external carotid and superior thyroid arteries (Figure 4).

The arteriotomy is initiated in the common carotid artery with a #11 scalpel and extended distally beyond the termination of the plaque in the internal carotid artery with Potts arterial scissors (Figure 5). The true lumen of the vessel is entered, and no attempt is made to perform an extraluminal dissection of the plaque from the artery. Great care must be taken to insure that the back wall of the carotid is not damaged. The arteriotomy incision should extend up the midline of the vessel to facilitate later closure of the arteriotomy.

The arteriotomy into the common carotid artery is continued until the plaque ceases to be ulcerated and the wall of the vessel becomes more normal in texture. The atherosclerotic plaque is first removed from the distal internal carotid artery by careful dissection with a microdissector or small spatula (Figure 6). The plaque is removed by following the pathologic cleavage plane created by the atherosclerosis between the

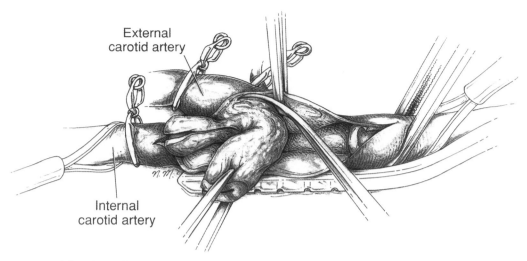

Figure 7. *The plaque has been removed from the intimal carotid artery initially so that a shunt may be more safely placed if necessary. The plaque has been sharply excised from the wall of the common carotid artery with Potts scissors. Next, the plaque is elevated and dissected from the external carotid artery by working through its orifice with a spatula. Once the plaque becomes thin, it is grasped with a hemostat and pulled inferiorly.*

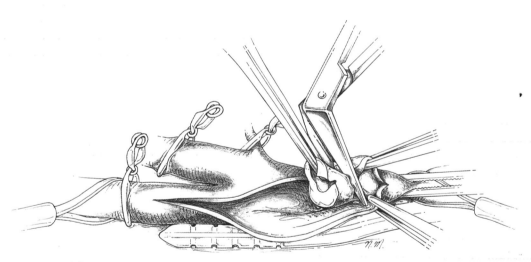

Figure 8. *The proximal end of the common carotid artery is inverted and the plaque cut circumferentially 1.0 to 2.0 cm below the end of the arteriotomy. This maneuver makes closure of the proximal arteriotomy easier and avoids stenosis by removing plaque below the end of the arteriotomy incision.*

intima and the fine layer of media.

During the dissection, a vascular pick-up is used to hold the wall of the artery as the assistant holds the edge of the plaque. The spatula is moved from side to side, developing the plane described above, which is usually readily separated. Dissection proceeds halfway around the wall before repeating the separation from the other side. A clean feathering away of the plaque is usually possible in the distal internal carotid artery, but not in the common carotid artery.

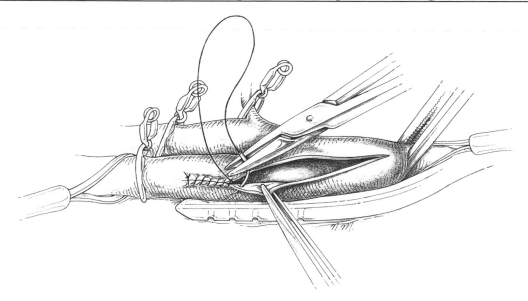

Figure 9. The arteriotomy is closed under the operating microscope with running 6-0 Prolene™ sutures.

In removal from the external carotid artery, the plaque is elevated from the wall through the orifice of the vessel (Figure 7). As it thins, the vessel is everted, and the plaque is grasped with a small hemostat and pulled inferiorly. Although this is a blind procedure, the plaque usually breaks cleanly from the wall of the external carotid artery. Patency of this artery may be determined by intraoperative angiography or by palpation of the superficial temporal artery pulse following restoration of blood flow.

The proximal end of the common carotid artery is inverted, and the plaque is cut circumferentially 1-2 cm below the end of the arteriotomy (Figure 8). This allows plaque removal below the end of the arteriotomy incision, making closure of the vessel easier and avoiding proximal stenosis.

Once the plaque has been removed, the operating microscope is positioned to allow both the surgeon and assistant to have clear binocular vision. Loose fragments of atherosclerotic material and abnormal intima are meticulously removed under continuous heparinized saline irrigation. The irrigation fluid and blood are cleared from the wound by the Microvac™ suction tube. With the operating microscope, the distal internal carotid artery is carefully inspected, and any elevation of the intima beyond the end of the plaque is carefully trimmed with microscissors. If there is an abrupt step-off, or if the intima loosely adheres to the media, double-armed 7-0 Prolene™ sutures are placed vertically from the inside of the vessel outward so they traverse the intimal edge and are tied outside the adventitial layer. The arteriotomy is closed using a running 6-0 Prolene™ suture, starting at the distal end of the incision (Figure 9). The use of the operating microscope to place small, closely spaced stitches results in a tight, nonleaking suture line without compromising the lumen of the vessel.

Prior to final closure, back-bleeding from all the vessels is performed to expel air and debris from the lumen of the repaired segment. Following final closure of the arteriotomy, the arteries are reopened in a specific order. The external carotid artery is opened initially, followed by the common carotid artery. The common carotid artery is briefly reclosed while the internal carotid artery is opened to allow any embolic

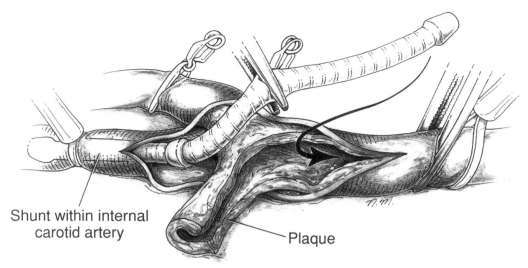

Shunt within internal
carotid artery

Plaque

Figure 10. In the event that a shunt is required, the plaque is initially removed from the distal internal carotid artery. The shunt is grasped in the center with hemostats and placed into the internal carotid artery. The hemostats are temporarily opened to allow back-bleeding to fill the shunt with blood. The proximal end is then placed into the common carotid artery and secured with the Rummell tourniquet.

material to be washed into the external carotid artery. The common carotid artery is then unclamped.

Placement of a Shunt

A shunt is used when there are changes in the EEG that do not immediately respond to a trial of induced hypertension. We prefer the Sundt internal shunt. A shunt is placed after the plaque has been carefully removed from the distal internal carotid artery (Figure 10). A 2-0 silk suture is loosely placed around the shunt to facilitate its removal. The distal end of the shunt is first placed into the internal carotid artery. Back-bleeding from the internal carotid artery will fill the shunt with blood. The proximal end is then placed into the common carotid artery and secured with the Rummell tourniquet. The shunt should easily thread up the internal carotid artery; no force should be used to advance the shunt if intimal damage and dissection are to be avoided. Plaque removal is completed by working around the shunt.

Prior to completely closing the arteriotomy, the shunt is withdrawn through a small open segment of the arteriotomy by the suture previously placed around the shunt. The arteriotomy closure is then completed in a routine fashion.

Wound Closure

The retractors are removed and sufficient time is spent obtaining excellent hemostasis, as the heparin is not reversed. The platysma and subcutaneous tissue are reapproximated and the skin closed with a 4-0 Vicryl™ subcuticular suture and Steri-strips™. Wound drainage is not always necessary under these circumstances.

Postoperative Care

With the use of barbiturates, many patients are obtunded for a short period of time following recovery from anesthesia, and may require continued intubation until they are alert. These patients may be examined, however, as brain stem function is readily tested, and the patients will move their extremities in response to noxious stimulation.

Blood pressure is carefully monitored both in the recovery room and in the intensive care unit, and both hypotension and hypertension are avoided. Patients generally spend 24 to 48 hours in the intensive care unit following surgery. Once the patient tolerates liquids, aspirin is restarted and continued indefinitely.

Alternatives in Surgical Technique

A number of technical variations in performing a carotid endarterectomy are quite acceptable. Excellent surgical teams have advocated the routine use of venous patch grafts, routine shunting, local anesthesia, and many other personal preferences. It is important that the surgical team become comfortable with their method and frequently assess their results.

Venous Patch Angioplasty

Patch angioplasty has been advocated as a technical means of lowering the incidence of acute complications, primarily carotid occlusion, and preventing or delaying restenosis following carotid endarterectomy.[3,6,24,38,46,51,68] There are theoretical, experimental, and clinical data to support the use of patch angioplasty. Patch angioplasty has a significantly favorable impact on the hemodynamics of the reconstructed artery.[3,24,81]

By increasing the vessel diameter at the distal end of the arteriotomy from a mean of 4.5-7.4 mm, there is a three-fold increase in the cross-sectional area at the distal end, the critical end where most technical complications occur.[6] The patch makes the transition in lumen diameter from the common carotid to the internal carotid artery more gradual, and has the net effect of moving the carotid bulb more

cephalad. It has been estimated that the hemodynamic effects of these changes result in a five-fold reduction in shear stress at the origin of the internal carotid artery.[81] This shear stress and associated changes in peak velocity may play roles in early thrombosis and lead to recurrent atherosclerosis in the wall of the reconstructed artery.[41]

Experimental studies have elucidated the favorable biologic behavior of the graft, which results in smooth incorporation of the graft into the reconstructed vessel wall.[11,12,24,41,42,44,73]

Furthermore, a number of clinical studies have supported the contention that patch angioplasty reduces the incidence of acute carotid occlusion and delays or prevents recurrent stenosis.[3,6,38,46,51]

There are a number of potential drawbacks to the routine use of patch angioplasty, including increased cross-clamp time required for reconstruction,[6] suture line or graft disruption due to the longer suture line or weakness of graft wall, respectively,[17,37,46] and risk of an accelerated form of atherosclerosis in venous structures exposed to arterial pressures.[11,73,81]

Concern regarding vein graft rupture led surgeons to recommend the use of the thigh vein and decry the use of the ankle saphenous vein.[61] Archie and Green measured diameter and rupture pressure in fresh saphenous vein segments from the ankle, knee, or thigh of 157 patients.[4] Circumferential hoop rupture stress was calculated, and the results applied to carotid endarterectomy reconstructions. Small-diameter veins were more prone to rupture than large-diameter veins. Saphenous veins harvested from the thigh or knee were larger than those from the ankle, and generally females had smaller diameter veins than males.

Vein rupture pressure and diameter data were applied to carotid reconstructions at varying degrees of pressure. From their study, the authors predicted that 1.8% of females and 0% males might have experienced patch rupture at blood pressures up

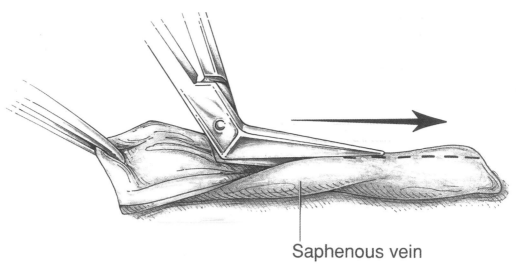

Saphenous vein

Figure 11. To prepare a saphenous vein graft, the vein is opened with Potts scissors. The inferior margin of the vein is grasped with forceps and the partially opened Potts scissors are advanced to produce a truly linear incision.

to 200 mm Hg.[4] All ruptures occurred in small-diameter veins. No veins greater than 4 mm in diameter would have ruptured under these conditions, regardless of the site of harvest or gender. Parallel experiments showed that external jugular and accessory ankle veins had greatly reduced pressures.[4]

Concern has also been raised regarding the use of a saphenous vein graft in a patient who may later require a vein graft for a subsequent operation such as coronary bypass or femoropopliteal bypass.[25,40] We make liberal use of a venous patch angioplasty in the closure of an endarterectomy, although it is not employed routinely. A venous patch graft is used in all reoperative cases, or if there is a suggestion from the arteriogram that the internal carotid artery is small in diameter. Use of the operating microscope allows for closure of the arteriotomy with small bites and little compromise of the vessel lumen, thus reducing the need for routine patch angioplasty.

The venous graft is harvested from the saphenous vein just anterior to the medial malleolus at the ankle. A segment of vein 6.0 to 8.0 cm in length is removed, and the direction of flow is maintained. The vein is opened by initially creating a small incision with the Potts scissors and advancing the partially opened scissors along the vein (Figure 11). The distal end of the patch graft is preshaped and the vein stored in heparinized saline until ready for use.

The saphenous vein patch graft is sewn into place under the operating microscope with a 6-0 running double-armed Prolene™ suture (Figure 12). The initial suture is placed through the apex of the graft and most distal point of the arteriotomy. This suture should be placed from the exterior of the graft to the interior and from the intimal surface of the internal carotid artery to the adventitial surface. Once the distal half of the graft has been sewn into place on both sides, the proximal end of the graft is shaped to conform to the proximal portion of the arteriotomy and the angioplasty completed.

Shunting

Opinions regarding the use of internal shunts during carotid endarterectomy vary widely among surgeons performing the

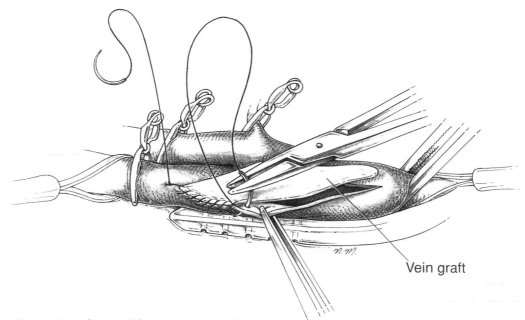

Vein graft

Figure 12. In closure of the arteriotomy with a saphenous vein patch graft, the distal end of the graft has been preshaped and is sewn into place under the operating microscope with a 6-0 running double-armed Prolene™ suture. Sutures should be placed from the exterior of the graft to the interior, and from the intimal surface of the internal carotid artery to the adventitial surface.

operation. There are three different schools of thought: (1) to routinely shunt, (2) to never or very rarely shunt, and (3) to shunt selectively, with that decision based on some form of intraoperative monitoring to detect cerebral ischemia.[30]

Among those surgeons who monitor during surgery, opinions differ regarding the most appropriate method. Suggested monitoring techniques include EEG, measurements of carotid stump pressure, determinations of cerebral blood flow, somatosensory evoked potentials, transcranial Doppler, and serial neurologic examinations performed with the patient awake during surgery.[30,33,48,53,58,60,70,72,83]

Controversy over the use of shunts centers on a fundamental disagreement as to whether intraoperative strokes are a result of hemodynamic insufficiency or embolization. Proponents of routine shunting believe that the risk of temporary carotid occlusion is significant.[36,74] Those surgeons reporting

a technique without the use of shunts believe that the hemodynamic risk of temporary carotid cross-clamping is exaggerated. Rather, it is their opinion that most intraoperative strokes are the result of embolization, a risk that is increased with the use of a shunt.[1,7,15,32,79] Excellent results have been reported by a number of groups adhering to each of these schools of thought. In an attempt to reduce perioperative risk to a minimum, we prefer to monitor patients with EEG, use barbiturates or etomidate to increase the brain's tolerance for ischemia, and selectively employ shunts in those patients who develop asymmetry on the EEG after cross-clamping.

The EEG is a highly reliable monitor for assessment of cerebral function during endarterectomy.[16,59,65,71] In comparing EEG changes to measured cerebral blood flow, Sundt et al found a very close correlation.[71] Furthermore, the EEG is able to detect the occurrence of microembolization.[71]

Barbiturate Anesthesia

Carotid endarterectomy has been performed with excellent results under either local anesthesia or general anesthesia without the use of barbiturates. The advantage of local anesthesia is the ability to neurologically monitor the patient during surgery. Barbiturates reduce the metabolic requirements of neural tissue and have been shown to modify or prevent cerebral injury from focal, reversible ischemia.[39,55,57,62,64,67,69,80] They are most effective if given prior to the period of temporary focal ischemia, at a dosage that achieves burst suppression of the EEG.[62,63] For these reasons, we routinely administer thiopental sodium prior to carotid cross-clamping and maintain burst suppression of the EEG with thiopental until the flow is re-established. Spetzler and associates have advocated the routine use of barbiturates for carotid endarterectomy and reported a 1.5% morbidity and mortality in a series of 200 consecutive endarterectomies.[66]

Despite barbiturate-induced burst suppression of the EEG, asymmetry of the recordings between the two hemispheres can be readily appreciated. This allows for the placement of a shunt if a trial of induced hypertension does not correct the asymmetry.

More recently we have used etomidate for cerebral protection in some cases. Like barbiturates, etomidate reduces metabolic requirements of neural tissue, but does not produce the hypotension often seen with barbiturates.[10,47,56] In our opinion, the added cerebral protection of barbiturates or etomidate may provide the time necessary for a safe, meticulous, unhurried endarterectomy. Other options for cerebral protection during cross-clamping (to be used in conjunction with or in lieu of the above measures) include intravenous mannitol (1 g/kg) and phenytoin (15 mg/kg).

Operating Microscope

Carotid endarterectomies can be performed using only loupe magnification and headlight illumination. We have found that the superior illumination and magnification afforded by a microscope provide exceptional visualization of the operative field, especially the distal internal carotid artery. After removing the atherosclerotic plaque, the microscope is brought into the field to complete a meticulous endarterectomy by removing small fragments of plaque and diseased intima. With the microscope one can inspect the critical region of the distal internal carotid to be certain there is a smooth internal surface. During closure of the arteriotomy, the sutures are placed with small, close bites of a precise thickness of the vessel wall. Such a closure avoids stenosis of the internal carotid, reduces the need for patch angioplasty, and invariably results in a completely dry arteriotomy closure.

Intraoperative Angiography

Technical complications of carotid endarterectomy include residual plaque, intimal flaps, stenosis, and thrombosis. Such defects may cause perioperative stroke through occlusion of the carotid, distal embolization, or delayed recurrent stenosis.[18,21,82] Some surgeons elect to perform postoperative digital or conventional angiography to detect such defects. Others use noninvasive carotid testing to determine the presence of technical deficiencies.

With the availability of compact, portable, digital intraoperative angiography equipment, we have found intraoperative angiography to be simple and quite helpful.[9] Intraoperative assessment of technical results prior to wound closure allows for recognition and correction of technical defects, reducing the need for reoperation and potentially lowering operative and postoperative complications. Once the arteriotomy is closed and flow re-established, a 19-gauge butterfly needle is placed into the common carotid artery proximal to the endarterectomy site. After the fluoroscope is put into place, about 5 ml of 60% meglumine iothalamate is manually injected as rapidly as possible. If intraoperative angiography equipment is not available, a standard, single-shot conventional x-ray done during contrast injection will provide adequate detail. If a large x-ray plate is positioned under the neck and head, an adequate film of the cervical and intracranial vessels can be obtained.

Complications of Carotid Endarterectomy

Any therapeutic advantage of a carotid endarterectomy is easily negated if morbidity and mortality are excessive. Although many centers have reported large series of operations with very low morbidity and mortality, the incidence of complications varies widely. In an effort to analyze the results of endarterectomy in North America, a retrospective multicenter audit of carotid endarterectomy was conducted in 1981.[35] In the 3,328 cases reported, there were 82 postoperative TIAs or reversible ischemic deficits (2.5%), 44 minor strokes (1.3% incidence), and 96 major strokes (2.9%), for an overall incidence for transient deficits of 2.5% and for permanent deficits of 4.0%. There were 26 deaths from myocardial infarction (over 1% incidence) and 40 deaths due to stroke (1.2%) Thus, there was a 2.5% risk of transient neurologic dysfunction following surgery and a 6% risk of death from endarterectomy in the group. The intrainstitutional combined morbidity and mortality varied from 21% to 0%.[35]

Complications may result from technical errors in performing the operation, or may be related to underlying systemic and coronary atherosclerosis. Unfortunate consequences of carotid endarterectomy may be divided into non-neurologic and neurologic complications.

Non-Neurologic Complications
Cardiac Ischemia

The atherosclerosis necessitating carotid endarterectomy generally reflects systemic vascular disease, and these patients have a high incidence of coronary artery disease. Myocardial infarction is the most serious systemic complication following carotid endarterectomy, and accounts for the majority of postoperative deaths. Proper selection of patients for surgery is necessary in those with a significant cardiac history. They require close perioperative monitoring of cardiac function, including pulmonary artery catheterization as well as strict avoidance of severe hypertension or hypotension.

Wound Infection

Wound infection following endarterectomy is fortunately uncommon. Staphylococci are usually the causative organisms. This complication usually responds to the re-exploration of the wound with irrigation and debridement. If the infection appears to involve deeper fascial layers, an arteriogram should be performed to exclude the possibility of a false aneurysm. We routinely use an antistaphylococcal antibiotic prophylactically in the perioperative period to decrease the risk of infection.

False Aneurysm

This rare complication should be considered whenever there is a persistent hematoma or an infection. The diagnosis is made by arteriography. Treatment consists of excision of the aneurysm wall with repair of the artery, using a saphenous vein patch graft. This complication is more common when synthetic patch grafts are used to close the arteriotomy, especially if a deep wound infection occurs.

Wound Hematoma

Postoperative swelling of the wound due to hematoma is not uncommon with the perioperative use of aspirin and intraoperative heparin without reversal. This is usually a self-limiting process that will resolve in a few weeks. However, if airway compromise is present, the wound should be immediately re-explored, the hematoma evacuated, and the source of bleeding controlled.

Neurologic Complications

Embolization or Thrombosis

Distal embolization may occur at any time during or after the operative procedure. The highest risk for this complication is during dissection and manipulation of the artery and placement of a shunt. Meticulous technique with minimal manipulation and dissection in the region of the plaque will reduce the risks of embolization. Placing the clip on the internal carotid artery prior to occluding the common and external carotid arteries also reduces the chance of distal embolization, as does appropriate back-bleeding prior to completion of the arteriotomy closure.

Another potential source of intraoperative or postoperative emboli or thrombosis is the newly exposed media of the artery, which is quite thrombogenic. Avoiding reversal of the heparinization may allow the formation of a platelet "pseudoendothelium" and may decrease the incidence of this problem.[26] Perioperative treatment with aspirin may also reduce the incidence of embolic and thrombotic complications.[66]

Ischemia During Carotid Occlusion

Most patients are able to tolerate the temporary carotid occlusion necessary for performing an endarterectomy. In the Mayo Clinic series, where cerebral blood flow was measured during carotid endarterectomy, 8.0% of patients had levels below 10 ml/100 g/min.[72] This level of cerebral blood flow is below the threshold necessary for maintenance of cellular integrity, and ischemia of this magnitude for more than a few minutes will result in cerebral infarction.[5,20,54]

We employ barbiturates or etomidate dur-

ing the period of time the carotid is occluded to protect the brain from ischemia. If there is EEG evidence of ischemia, a shunt is placed to provide collateral blood flow during the operation.

Postoperative Hemorrhage

This complication, occurring rarely, may result from poorly controlled postoperative hypertension, especially in the setting of a completed infarction in hypertensive patients and patients receiving anticoagulants.[13,23,27,72,75] An unusually high incidence of this complication is seen in Sundt Grade IV patients with a high-grade carotid stenosis and marked hyperperfusion following endarterectomy.[72] Sundt et al suggested that a normal perfusion pressure breakthrough phenomenon, similar to that observed in some patients undergoing resection of arteriovenous malformations, may be a mechanism of postoperative hemorrhage.[67] It is postulated that patients with a high-grade carotid stenosis are chronically hypoperfused, and the intracranial vessels become dilated to maintain perfusion and lose the ability to autoregulate. These chronically dilated vessels are then unable to handle the restored perfusion pressure after endarterectomy.

Seizures

Seizures rarely complicate carotid endarterectomy, usually appearing within 1 to 2 weeks of surgery. Edema secondary to relative hyperperfusion of the hemisphere is the postulated cause. The complication is more common in patients who have had a preoperative stroke.

Cranial Nerve Injuries

A variety of cranial nerves are exposed to potential injury during a carotid endarterectomy, including the greater auricular, facial, hypoglossal nerves, as well as the vagus nerve and its branches.[2] The incidence of cranial nerve injuries ranges from 12% to 27% in reported series.[43,49,50,52] Cranial nerve injuries are related to surgical technique and can usually be avoided. The mechanism is usually traction; unless the nerve is inadvertently severed, it will usually recover. If bilateral endarterectomies are planned, it is advisable to assess the function of the vocal cords prior to the second operation, as bilateral vocal cord paralysis due to bilateral recurrent laryngeal nerve injury is a serious complication that may necessitate a tracheostomy.[50]

References

1. Allen GS, Preziosi TJ. Carotid endarterectomy: a prospective study of its efficacy and safety. *Medicine.* 1981;60:298-309.
2. Alexander LF, Smith RR. Cranial nerve injuries during carotid endarterectomy. In: Barrow DL, ed. *Perspectives in Neurological Surgery,* Vol. 1, No. 1, St Louis, Mo: Quality Medical Publishing, Inc. 1990:79-83.
3. Archie JR Jr. Prevention of early restenosis and thrombosis-occlusion after carotid endarterectomy by saphenous vein patch angioplasty. *Stroke.* 1986;17:901-905.
4. Archie JP Jr, Green JJ Jr. Saphenous vein rupture pressure, rupture stress, and carotid endarterectomy vein patch reconstruction. *Surgery.* 1990;107:389-396
5. Astrup J, Siesjo BK, Symon L. Thresholds in cerebral ischemia—the ischemic penumbra. *Stroke.* 1981;12:723-725.
6. Awad IA, Little JR. Patch angioplasty in carotid endarterectomy. Advantages, concerns, and controversies. *Stroke.* 1989;20:417-422.
7. Baker WH, Dorner DB, Barnes RW. Carotid endarterectomy: Is an indwelling shunt necessary? *Surgery.* 1977;82:321-326.
8. Baker WH, Hayes AC, Mahler D, et al. Durability of carotid endarterectomy. *Surgery.* 1983;94:112-115.
9. Barrow DL, Boyer KL, Joseph GJ. Intraoperative angiography in the management of neurovascular disorders. *Neurosurgery.* 1992;30:153-159
10. Batjer HH, Frankfurt AI, Purdy RD, et al. Use of etomidate, temporary arterial occlusion, and intraoperative angiography in surgical treatment of large and giant cerebral aneurysms. *J Neurosurg.* 1988;68:234-240.
11. Baumann FG, Imparato AM, Kim G. A study of the evolution of early fibromuscular intimal lesions hemodynamically induced in the dog. I. Light and transmission electron microscopy. *Circ Res.* 1986;39:809-827.
12. Baumann FG, Imparato AM, Kim G, et al. A study of the early evolution of fibromuscular lesions hemodynamically induced in the dog renal artery: Scanning and correlative transmission electron microscopy. *Artery.* 1987;4:67-99.
13. Bernstein M, Fleming JFR, Deck JHN. Cerebral hyperperfusion after carotid endarterectomy: a cause of cerebral hemorrhage. *Neurosurgery.* 1984;15:50-56.
14. Blaisdell WF, Clauss RH, Galbraith JG, et al. Joint study of extracranial arterial occlusion. IV. A review of surgical considerations. *JAMA.* 1969;209:1889-1895.
15. Bland JE, Lazar ML. Carotid endarterectomy without a shunt. *Neurosurgery.* 1981;8:153-157.
16. Boysen G. Cerebral hemodynamics in carotid surgery. *Acta Neurol Scand.* 1973;49(suppl 52):1-84.
17. Branch CL, Davis CH. False aneurysm complicating carotid endarterectomy. *Neurosurgery.* 1986;19:421-425.
18. Bredenberg CE, Iannettoni M, Rosenbloom M, et al. Operative angiography by intra-arterial digital subtraction angiography: a new technique for quality control of carotid endarterectomy. *J Vasc Surg.* 1989;9:530-534.
19. Brott T, Thalinger K. The practice of carotid endarterectomy in a large metropolitan area. *Stroke.* 1984;15:950-955.
20. Carter LP, Yamagata S, Erspamer R. Time limits of reversible ischemia. *Neurosurgery.* 1983;12:620-623.
21. Chino ES, Gwinn BC. The impact of completion arteriography on results and technique of carotid surgery. *Ann Vasc Surg.* 1988;2:326-331.
22. Committee on Health Care Issues, American Neurological Association: Does carotid endarterectomy decrease stroke and death in patients with transient ischemic attacks? *Ann Neurol.* 1987;22:72-76.
23. Crowell RM, Ojemann RG. Results and complications of carotid endarterectomy. In: Smith RR, ed. *Stroke and the Extracranial Vessels.* New York: Raven Press; 1984:203-212.
24. Derin G, Ballotta E, Bonavina L, et al. The rationale for patch-graft angioplasty after carotid endarterectomy: early and long-term follow-up. *Stroke.* 1984;15:972-979.
25. DeVries AL, Riles TS, Lamparello PJ, et al. Should proximal saphenous vein be used for carotid patch angioplasty: a clinical study of the need for vein in subsequent operations. *Eur J Vasc Surg.* 1990;4:301-304.
26. Dirrenberger RA, Deer GH Jr, Sundt TM Jr. Temporal profile of the healing process following endarterectomy. In: Sundt TM Jr, ed. *Occlusive Cerebrovascular Disease: Diagnosis and Surgical Management.* Philadelphia: WB Saunders; 1987:232-242.
27. Dunsker SB. Complications of carotid endarterectomy. *Clin Neurosurg.* 1976;23:336-341.
28. Easton JD, Sherman DG. Stroke and mortality rate in carotid endarterectomy: 228 consecutive operations. *Stroke.* 1977;8:565-568.
29. Ennix CL Jr, Lawrie GM, Morris GC Jr, et al. Improved results of carotid endarterectomy in patients with symptomatic coronary disease: an analysis of 1,546 consecutive carotid operations. *Stroke.* 1979;10:122-125.
30. Ferguson GG. Carotid endarterectomy. To shunt or not to shunt? *Arch Neurol.* 1986;43:615-618.
31. Ferguson GG. Extracranial carotid artery surgery. *Clin Neurosurg.* 1982;29:543-574.
32. Ferguson GG, Blume WT, Farrar JK. Carotid endarterectomy: An evaluation of results in 282

consecutive cases in relationship to intraoperative monitoring. Abstract No. 54. Program of the Annual Meeting of the American Association of Neurological Surgeons, Atlanta, April 23, 1985.

33. Ferguson GG, Gamache FW. Cerebral protection during carotid endarterectomy: intraoperative monitoring, anesthetic techniques, and temporary shunts. In: Smith RR, ed. *Stroke and the Extracranial Vessels.* New York: Raven Press; 1984:187-201.

34. Fields WS, Maslenikov V, Meyer JS, et al. Joint study of extracranial artery occlusion. V. Progress report of prognosis following surgery or nonsurgical treatment for transient cerebral ischemic attacks and cervical carotid artery lesions. *JAMA.* 1970; 211:1993-2003.

35. Fode NC, Sundt TM Jr, Robertson JT, et al. Multicenter retrospective review of results and complications of carotid endarterectomy in 1981. *Stroke.* 1986;17:370-376.

36. Giannotta SL, Dicks RE, Kindt GW. Carotid endarterectomy: technical improvements. *Neurosurgery.* 1980;7:309-312.

37. Grauer ML, Mulcare RJ. Pseudoaneurysm after carotid endarterectomy. *J Cardiovasc Surg.* 1986; 27:294-297.

38. Hertzer NR, Beven EG, O'Hara PJ, et al. A prospective study of vein patch angioplasty during carotid endarterectomy. *Ann Surg.* 1987; 206: 628-635.

39 Hoff JT, Smith AL, Hankinson HL, et al. Barbiturate protection from cerebral infarction in primates. *Stroke.* 1975;6:28-33.

40. Houser SL, Hashimi FH, Jaeger VJ, et al. Should the greater saphenous vein be preserved in patients requiring arterial outflow reconstruction in the lower extremity? *Surgery.* 1984;95:467.

41. Imparato AM, Baumann FG. Consequences of hemodynamic alterations on the vessel wall after revascularization. In: Bernhard VM, Towne JB, eds. *Complications in Vascular Surgery.* New York: Grune & Stratton, Inc.; 1980:107-131.

42. Imparato AM, Baumann FG, Pearson J, et al. Electron microscopic studies of experimentally produced fibromuscular arterial lesions. *Surg Gynecol Obstet.* 1974;139:497-504.

43. Imparato AM, Bracco A, Kim GE, et al. The hypoglossal nerve in carotid arterial reconstructions. *Stroke.* 1972;3:576-578.

44. Imparato AM, Weinstein GS. Clinicopathologic correlation in postendarterectomy recurrent stenosis. *J Vasc Surg.* 1986;3:657-662.

45. Jonas S, Hass WK. An approach to the maximal acceptable stroke complication rate after surgery for transient cerebral ischemia (TIA). *Stroke.* 1979; 10:104. Abstract.

46. Katz MM, Jones T, Degenhardt J, et al. The use of patch angioplasty to alter the incidence of carotid restenosis following thromboendarterectomy. *J Cardiovasc Surg.* 1987;28:2-8.

47. Kugler J, Doenicke A, Lamb M. The EEG after etomidate. In: *Anaesthesiology and Intensive Care Medicine 106.* Berlin: Springer-Verlag; 1977:31-48.

48. Lee KS, Davis CH, McWhorter JM. Low morbidity and mortality of carotid endarterectomy performed with regional anesthesia. *J Neurosurg.* 1988; 69:483-487.

49. Lehv MS, Salzman EW, Silen W. Hypertension

complicating carotid endarterectomy. *Stroke.* 1970;1:307-313.

50. Liapsis CD, Satiani B, Florance CL, et al. Motor speech malfunction following carotid endarterectomy. *Surgery.* 1981;89:56-59.

51. Little JR, Bryerton BS, Furlan AJ. Saphenous vein patch grafts in carotid endarterectomy. *J Neurosurg.* 1984;61:743-747.

52. Lyons C, Galbraith G. Surgical treatment of atherosclerotic occlusion of the internal carotid artery. *Ann Surg.* 1957;146:487-496.

53. Markand ON, Dilley RS, Moorthy SS, et al. Monitoring of somatosensory evoked responses during carotid endarterectomy. *Arch Neurol.* 1984;41: 375-378.

54. Meyer FB. Ischemic neuronal protection. In: Barrow DL, ed. *Perspectives in Neurological Surgery.* 1990;1(1):57-78.

55. Michenfelder JD, Milde JH, Sundt TM Jr. Cerebral protection by barbiturate anesthesia: Use after middle cerebral artery occlusion in Java monkeys. *Arch Neurol.* 1976;33:345-350.

56. Milde LN, Milde JH. Preservation of cerebral metabolites by etomic date during incomplete cerebral ischemia in dogs. *Anesthesiology.* 1985;63: 371-377.

57. Moseley JI, Laurent JP, Molinari GF. Barbiturate attenuation of the clinical course and pathologic lesions in a primate stroke model. *Neurology.* 1975;25:870-874.

58. Ojemann RG. Extracranial carotid artery atherosclerosis. In: Wilkins RH, Rengachary SS, eds. *Neurosurgery.* New York: McGraw-Hill; 1985: 1236-1247.

59. Perez-Borja C, Meyer JS. Electroencephalographic monitoring during reconstructive surgery of the neck vessels. *Electroencephalogr Clin Neurophysiol.* 1965;18:162-169.

60. Powers AD, Smith RR, Graeber MC. Transcranial Doppler monitoring of cerebral flow velocities during surgical occlusion of the carotid artery. *Neurosurgery.* 1989;25:383-389.

61. Riles TS, Lamparello PJ, Giangola G, et al. Rupture of the vein patch: a rare complication of carotid endarterectomy. *Surgery.* 1990;107:10-12.

62. Selman WR, Spetzler RF, Roessmann UR, et al. Barbiturate-induced coma therapy for focal cerebral ischemia. Effect after temporary and permanent MCA occlusion. *J Neurosurg.* 1981;55:220-226.

63. Selman WR, Spetzler RF, Roski RA, et al. Regional cerebral blood flow following middle cerebral artery occlusion and barbiturate therapy in baboons. *J Cereb Blood Flow Metab.* 1981;1:214-215.

64. Shapiro HM. Barbiturates in brain ischaemia. *Br J Anesth.* 1985;57:82-95.

65. Sharbrough FW, Messick JM Jr, Sundt TM Jr. Correlation of continuous electroencephalograms with cerebral blood flow measurements during carotid endarterectomy. *Stroke.* 1973;4:674-683.

66. Spetzler RF, Martin NA, Hadley MN, et al. Microsurgical endarterectomy under barbiturate protection: a prospective study. *J Neurosurg.* 1986;65: 63-73.

67. Spetzler RF, Wilson CB, Weinstein P, et al. Normal perfusion pressure breakthrough theory. *Clin Neurosurg.* 1978;25:651-672.

68. Sundt TM Jr, Sandok BA, Whisnant JP. Carotid

endarterectomy: Complications and preoperative assessment of risk. *Mayo Clin Proc.* 1975;50: 301-306.

69. Sundt TM Jr, Anderson RE, Michenfelder JD. Intracellular redox states under halothane and barbiturate anesthesia in normal, ischemic, and anoxic monkey brain. *Ann Neurol.* 1979;5:575-579.

70. Sundt TM Jr, Sharbrough FW, Anderson RE, et al. Intraoperative monitoring techniques. In: Sundt TM Jr, ed. *Occlusive Cerebrovascular Disease. Diagnosis and Surgical Management.* Philadelphia, Pa: WB Saunders; 1987:182-190.

71. Sundt TM Jr, Sharbrough FW, Anderson RE, et al. Cerebral blood flow measurements and electroencephalograms during carotid endarterectomy. *J Neurosurg.* 1974;41:310-320.

72. Sundt TM Jr, Sharbrough FW, Piepgras DG, et al. Correlation of cerebral blood flow and electroencephalographic changes during carotid endarterectomy, with results of surgery and hemodynamics of cerebral ischemia. *Mayo Clin Proc.* 1981;56:533-543.

73. Texon M, Imparato AM, Lord JW, et al. Experimental production of arterial lesions. *Arch Int Med.* 1962;110:50-52.

74. Thompson JE. Complications of endarterectomy and their protection. *World J Surg.* 1979;3:155-165.

75. Towne JB, Bernhard VM. The relationship of postoperative hypertension to complications following carotid endarterectomy. *Surgery.* 1980;88:575-580.

76. Whisnant JP, Sandok BA, Sundt TM Jr. Carotid endarterectomy for unilateral carotid system transient cerebral ischemia. *Mayo Clin Proc.* 1983; 58:171-175.

77. Whisnant JP, Sandok BA, Sundt TM Jr. Endarterectomy for transient cerebral ischemia: long term survival and stroke probability. *Stroke.* 1982;13:113. Abstract.

78. Whisnant JP, Wiebers DO. Clinical epidemiology of transient cerebral ischemic attacks (TIA) in the anterior and posterior cerebral circulation. In: Sundt TM Jr., ed. *Occlusive Cerebrovascular Disease. Diagnosis and Surgical Management.* Philadelphia: WB Saunders; 1987:60-65.

79. Whitney DG, Kahn EM, Estes JW, et al. Carotid artery surgery without a temporary indwelling shunt: One thousand nine hundred seventeen consecutive procedures. *Arch Surg.* 1980;115:1393-1399.

80. Yatsu FM. Pharmacologic protection against ischemic brain damage. *Neurol Clin.* 1983;1:37-53.

81. Zarins CK, Giddens DP, Glagov S. Atherosclerotic plaque distribution and flow velocity profiles in the carotid bifurcation. In: Bergan JJ, Yao JST, eds. *Cerebrovascular Insufficiency.* New York: Grune & Stratton, Inc.; 1983:19-30.

82. Zeirler RE, Bandyk DF, Thiele BL. Intraoperative assessment of carotid endarterectomy. *J Vasc Surg.* 1984;1:73-81.

83. Zuccarello M, Yeh H, Tew JM. Morbidity and mortality of carotid endarterectomy under local anesthesia: a retrospective study. *Neurosurgery.* 1988;23:445-449.

CHAPTER 10

Arterial Trauma and Dissection

Cathy A. Sila, MD, and Issam A. Awad, MD, MS, FACS

Cervical and cerebral arterial dissections remain an uncommon cause of brain ischemia since Jentzer's original description four decades ago.[33] Since then, a multitude of case reports and small series of patients have led to a growing recognition of the disorder with its myriad neurologic manifestations, etiologic association, and variable and often benign clinical course.[3,9,18] Often contradicting information and recommendations seem to be presented in the medical and surgical literature. The role of trauma seems to be well documented, but the pathophysiology of spontaneous arterial dissections and the role of predisposing and compounding factors are not well understood. In this chapter, we synthesize available information regarding arterial trauma and dissection and include a consensus perspective of current strategies of clinical management.

Spectrum of Arterial Trauma

The spectrum of arterial traumatic injuries includes cases with frank arterial laceration, exsanguination, or false aneurysm formation[4,36] and cases with less than total disruption of the arterial wall from blunt or indirect trauma.[1-3,5-7,10,23,30,32,59,61] Nonpenetrating arterial injuries frequently involve disruption of one or more layers of the arterial wall and dissecting intramural hematomas, luminal thrombosis, or aneurysm formation.

The most frequently disrupted layer is the arterial media. When associated with an intimal tear, subintimal dissection may result in narrowing of the arterial lumen and varying degrees of luminal stenosis including what may appear as a "string sign" on angiography.[3,18] Total luminal compromise will result in a tapered arterial occlusion, which with time may resolve or accumulate antegrade and retrograde propagating thrombosis. Subadventitial dissection may result in outpouching, frank aneurysm formation, or circumferential vascular expansion with or without secondary luminal constriction.[3,9,18] The clinical sequelae of arterial dissection may rarely be due to hemodynamic compromise; more likely they are due to thromboembolism or propagating thrombosis. It is not known to what degree arterial dissection may occur asymptomatically following various degrees of trauma. In this clinical setting, it is rarely diagnosed unless it has already resulted in significant neurologic deficits, usually from cerebral thromboembolism. Among lethal traumatic injuries, there is a very high prevalence of multifocal disruptions in all cervicocephalic vessels.[50,69]

Penetrating Arterial Injury

Penetrating stab wounds or missiles may result in direct arterial injury, commonly disrupting all layers of the artery and resulting in frank exsanguination or contained false aneurysms within fascial planes.[4,36] Arterial injury should be suspected in all instances of penetrating neck or base of skull wounds. There is a high incidence of associated injuries to adjacent tracheoesophageal structures, nerves, and major veins. Penetrating injuries to the orbit and the base of the skull may result in carotid-cavernous fistulae.

The treatment of penetrating injuries to craniocephalic vessels is usually emergent. Prompt securing of the airway is paramount. In instances of exsanguination, immediate control of the hemorrhage is essential. In neck injuries, compression may be sufficient to arrest bleeding and should be followed by prompt wound exploration in conjunction with preparations for primary vascular repair or ligation, and exploration and repair of adjacent structures.[36] Ligation of a disrupted artery may be considered if stump pressures or intraoperative electroencephalography indicate probable host tolerance, if there is no back bleeding after attempts at thrombectomy, or in cases of intracranial extension of arterial disruption.

In instances of penetrating cervical wounds without frank exsanguination, there may or may not be a palpable pulsatile neck mass. Angiography should be performed emergently to assess the extent of any vascular injury. Further treatment is dictated by the angiographic findings. The presence of a false aneurysm may dictate immediate surgical exploration and repair,[4] whereas total arterial occlusion may dictate the use of anticoagulant therapy (unless otherwise contraindicated).

Cranial injuries with suspected direct arterial disruption are managed by prompt securing of an airway, and tamponade of any nasopharyngeal hemorrhage by packing or balloon catheters. Prompt angiography should be performed to assess the extent of arterial injury and to allow interventional luminal balloon occlusion of disrupted arterial segments. Intracranial traumatic aneurysms resulting from missile injury should be treated by direct repair.

Nonpenetrating Arterial Injury

Nonpenetrating arterial injury may result from blunt trauma to an artery or from the indirect impact of adjacent sharp trauma. A missile may result in arterial dissection via indirect transmission of energy without direct puncture of the vessel (Figure 1). The pathophysiology of nonpenetrating arterial injury consists of various degrees of dissections. Subintimal dissections result in arterial stenosis, thrombosis, or thromboembolism, or a combination of these, whereas subadventitial dissections result in outpouching and aneurysm formation. Extracranial dissecting aneurysms (outside the subarachnoid space) have rarely been reported to rupture. The exception is false aneurysms related to direct penetrating arterial injury (see previous section). In contrast, dissecting intracranial aneurysms (within the subarachnoid space) have a greater propensity to hemorrhage in view of the weaker outer layers of subarachnoid arteries.[20]

Most clinical manifestations of nonpenetrating arterial injury occur in a delayed fashion, usually after initial stabilization of the traumatized patient. Symptoms typically consist of ipsilateral brain ischemia prompting diagnostic investigations (usually angiography) and identification of the arterial dissection. The spectrum of angiographic findings parallels the possibilities of degrees of arterial wall dissection and associated thrombosis. The angiographic appearance may be normal.[18,66] Normal angiographic appearance may be due to a healing of a previous intimal flap or to subadventitial dissection without luminal outpouching or compromise; however, in most instances of dissection, angiography will reveal focal stenosis, focal aneurysmal dilation, elongated stenosis, string sign (due to sluggish antegrade flow, luminal thrombosis, or long segment of dissection), arterial occlusion (typically a tapered occlusion), and/or various degrees of intimal flaps and luminal densities. Cases presenting with massive stroke usually have a dismal prognosis related to brain infarction or multiple associated

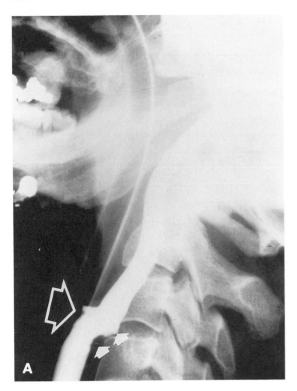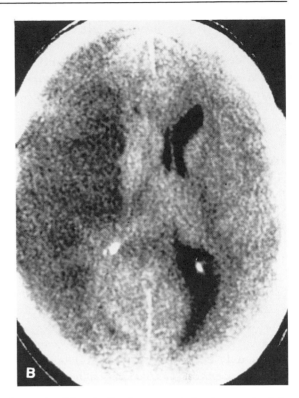

Figure 1. *This patient sustained a gunshot wound to the neck with a bullet fragment lodged near the left mandible. The patient had dense right hemiplegia on arrival to the emergency room. There was diffuse neck swelling but no evidence of exsanguination or pulsatile mass. (A) After emergency intubation, carotid angiography revealed total occlusion of the external carotid artery at its origin (open arrow) and luminal irregularity at the distal common carotid artery (double arrows). The internal carotid artery was widely patent. (B) Computed tomographic scan 2 days later revealed a massive infarction in the territory of the left middle cerebral artery. The infarction was presumed secondary to thromboembolism from the stump of the occluded external carotid artery, or from a mural thrombus in the region of common carotid artery dissection. A missile may cause disruption to the cervicocephalic arteries without frank vessel transection. Severe neurologic deficit may occur in the face of a widely patent internal carotid artery and is presumed due to thromboembolism.*

injuries, or both. Cases with minor stroke or with reversible brain ischemia usually have a benign prognosis with expectant therapy, anticoagulation, or direct arterial repair.

The literature on the most optimal treatment of traumatic arterial dissection is heavily biased, with most surgical series recommending surgical repair whenever possible.[31,34,37,46,57,72,77] These surgical reports often invoke therapeutic attitudes used in thoracic and abdominal arterial dissection that may or may not be applicable to the situation of craniocerebral dissection. Other reports urge heroic arterial repairs, even in instances where the dissection reaches quite far distally.[56]

A critical analysis of these surgical reports does not support an aggressive surgical attitude toward all cases of blunt arterial trauma. The reports frequently consist of anecdotal cases, with no series exceeding a handful of patients managed in a uniform fashion. They all mention the same rationale for surgical intervention: the high mortality of cases with major stroke and arterial dissection; however, these reports ignore the obvious selection bias whereby cases without major cerebral infarction, and usually with less extensive dissection, are selected for surgical repair with good results. These cases may have an inherently more benign prognosis regardless

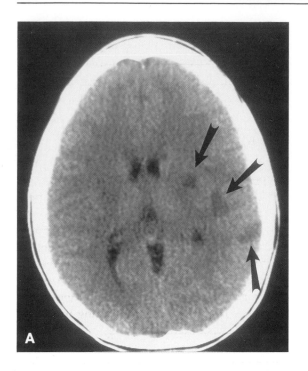

Figure 2. A young female who was a passenger in a head-on motor vehicle collision and was wearing a seat belt with shoulder harness. Several hours after the accident, she developed mild right hemiparesis, dysphasia and left Horner's syndrome. (A) Initial CT scans were negative; the scan performed 2 days after the onset of neurologic deficits revealed patchy multifocal infarctions in the left cerebral hemisphere, consistent with embolism. (B) Carotid angiography revealed subtle luminal densities and irregularities in the distal cervical internal carotid artery. The patient was anticoagulated. (C) Repeat carotid angiography 10 days later revealed a small aneurysmal dilatation at the level of C2 (closed arrow) and a luminal dilatation with a ledge in the proximal intrapetrous segment of the vessel (open arrow). The patient was maintained on anticoagulant therapy for 3 months and on antiplatelet therapy thereafter. (D) Repeat carotid angiography 1 year later revealed total healing of the aneurysm (closed arrow) and persistent subtle intimal ledge distally (open arrow). The patient has remained asymptomatic on antiplatelet therapy for 4 years.

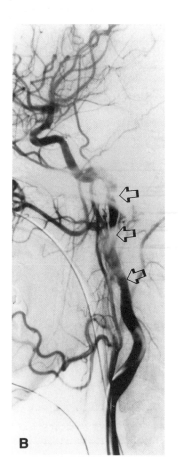

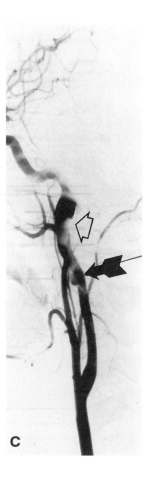

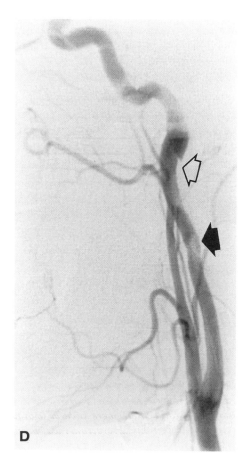

of therapeutic intervention. More recently, expectant therapy has been advocated for cases of traumatic carotid dissection.[37,38] There are few cases of well-documented symptom progression from carotid dissection following anticoagulant therapy, prompting the recommendation of anticoagulation (unless contraindicated). Anticoagulation decreases the likelihood of propagating thrombosis and thromboembolism, which are the most likely causes of neurologic sequelae following blunt arterial injury.[3,7,74]

Anticoagulation may not be possible in the setting of acute trauma, in view of multiple hemorrhagic tendencies in other injured organs. The presence of massive brain infarction or cerebral hemorrhage, or both, also represents contraindications to anticoagulation. In these instances, and in cases where the dissected segment is accessible, surgical repair may be entertained with excellent results.

There is no evidence that more heroic surgical interventions including extensive ex-cisions of vascular segments or arterial ligations provide a better prognosis than expectant therapy alone and anticoagulation.[3]

The delayed sequelae of arterial dissection may involve complete or near complete spontaneous healing of the dissected segment (Figure 2). Even luminal outpouching and aneurysms may heal spontaneously on serial angiography. In other situations, there may be persistent luminal webs with significant hemodynamic compromise (Figure 3) or persistent or expanding aneurysmal abnormalities (Figure 4). When accessible, these delayed pathoanatomic sequelae or dissection may be treated surgically after careful consideration of risks and benefits in the individual case. It is our policy to repair residual luminal flaps and webs if accessible and resulting in preocclusive luminal stenosis. Distal cervical aneurysms associated with carotid dissection have never been documented to rupture (these are not to be confused with false aneurysms arising from direct penetrating arterial injury that may rupture with disastrous consequen-

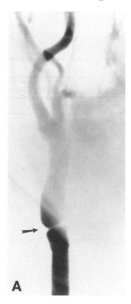 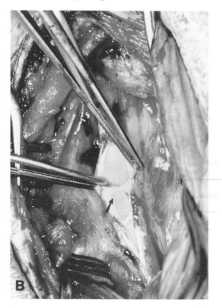

Figure 3. A young man with a history of left hemispheric TIAs and left ocular transient amaurosis 5 years following a motorcycle accident during which he had sustained a closed head injury. **(A)** Carotid angiography revealed a focal web in the left common carotid artery resulting in near total occlusion of the artery at that level (arrow). There was excellent antigrade flow and the artery was normal distally. **(B)** At exploration of the common carotid, there were several web-like defects within the lumen of the vessel, resulting in near total arterial occlusion. Endarterectomy was performed and the artery was repaired primarily. It is presumed that the web-like lesion in the common carotid artery is the delayed pathoanatomic residuum of a blunt arterial trauma.

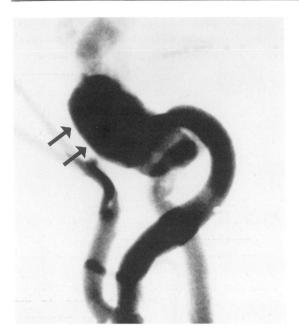
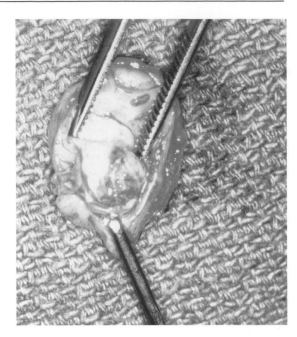

Figure 4. *This patient presented with recurrent spells of right hemispheric transient ischemic attacks despite antiplatelet therapy. Over the previous 5 years, she had undergone regular chiropractic manipulations. Following one chiropractic neck manipulation a year earlier, the patient suffered severe neck and head pain and a transient syncope. (A) Carotid angiography revealed a large dissecting aneurysm involving the distal cervical internal carotid. (B) At surgical exploration, the aneurysmal arterial segment was resected and the artery was reconstructed using a segment of saphenous vein; the aneurysmal dome contained multiple webs, friable atherosclerotic material, and fresh thrombus.*

ces). Extracranial dissecting aneurysms may expand and serve as embolic sources. If symptomatic, they are treated by direct excision or balloon obliteration.

Intracranial traumatic dissecting aneurysms have an unfavorable prognosis and are frequently associated with subarachnoid or cerebral hemorrhage.[20,75] These aneurysms should be excised without delay, and this is usually performed via direct surgical approach.

In summary, a high index of suspicion is necessary for the prompt diagnosis and timely therapeutic intervention in cases of nonpenetrating arterial injury. Diagnosis is often delayed because of subacute clinical manifestations (usually from thromboembolism) or because of a low index of suspicion. In the acute and subacute phases, treatment should be directed toward the prevention of thromboembolism, with the use of anticoagulation whenever possible. Surgery is reserved for cases where the disrupted vascular segment is easily accessible or where delayed anatomic sequelae may be progressive or symptomatic. The natural history is usually benign, and the overall prognosis is determined by the extent of cerebral ischemic damage prior to diagnosis. The bad outcome of certain untreated cases with severe brain infarction is not necessarily a justification for surgical repair of cases with arterial dissection and little or no brain ischemia. Expectant therapy of such cases is usually successful, especially with the use of anticoagulation to prevent propagating thromboembolism.

Traumatic Versus Spontaneous Arterial Dissection

The role of major trauma in the pathogenesis of arterial dissection is well documented.[1,2,5-7,10,12,23,31,34,37,46,50,53,57,59,61,69,72,77] The spectrum of offending trauma is highly diverse. Craniocephalic arterial dissection has been reported following prolonged neck turning during a parade, chiropractic manipulation, motor vehicle trauma with shoulder seat belt tethering, mandibular fractures, and missile injuries to the head and neck. Traumatic association is easy to establish in such situations, especially when the onset of symptoms is not delayed by more than a few days from a well-defined traumatic incident.

In other situations, the trauma may be more subtle or the symptoms of arterial dissection may be quite delayed. An example of this would be a patient who underwent a neck massage approximately 2 weeks prior to a cerebral embolic event. Another example would be the case of a patient who sustained severe craniocervical trauma in a motor vehicle accident and presents with cerebral ischemic spells several months following the accident. Late anatomic residua of arterial dissection may be discovered on angiography, such as a luminal web or a dissecting aneurysm. In such situations, the causative role of trauma is presumptive but difficult to prove with complete certainty.

In yet other situations, the history of trauma may be so subtle or so remote that it cannot be established. It is not known to what extent such subtle, remote, or repetitive minor trauma may contribute to the genesis of so-called spontaneous cervicocephalic arterial dissections.

Host-related factors other than trauma may be associated with arterial dissection. These include primary vasculopathies such as fibromuscular dysplasia, Marfan's syndrome, syphilis, atherosclerosis, and polyarteritis nodosa.[3,17,42,43,64,76] It is not known to what extent such predisposing arteriopathy can precipitate an arterial dissection without inciting trauma. There have been instances of minor or trivial trauma precipitating an arterial dissection in patients with known fibromuscular dysplasia.[76]

There remain many situations of overt arterial dissection with neither a well-documented traumatic inciting event nor an underlying vasculopathy. Such spontaneous idiopathic dissections almost invariably involve the distal carotid arteries at the level of the C2 lateral masses, or the distal vertebral arteries at the level of the arch of the atlas. There may be focal histologic vulnerabilities of the arteries at these particular levels (changes in the cytoarchitecture of the medial layer) in addition to traumatic vulnerability (tethering of the arterial wall against bony structures) that predispose to dissection of that particular segment.[3,43]

In summary, a spectrum of traumatic injuries has been implicated in the etiology of craniocephalic arterial dissections. An underlying host-related vasculopathy or a history of chronic repetitive minor trauma may also predispose to arterial dissection. In some cases, one or more of these factors may be operative alone or in combination. In yet other instances, arterial dissection may occur without any association with known vasculopathy or documented trauma. It is not known if the natural history and prognosis of arterial dissections with or without trauma, and with or without overt vasculopathy, are significantly different. Underlying vasculopathy may certainly predispose to multifocal arterial dissections and recurrence of arterial dissection in the same patient. Other aspects of the natural course and clinical management of this entity are discussed in the following sections according to the anatomic location of the arterial dissection.

Extracranial Carotid Artery Dissection

Clinical Spectrum

The extracranial carotid artery is the most commonly recognized site of cervicocephalic arterial dissection.[3] Although its incidence remains unknown, angiographic documentation of an extracranial carotid artery dissection occurred in 11 (0.24%) of 4,530 patients with acute cerebrovascular symptoms, mostly cerebral infarction, and 30 (2.5%) of 1,200 consecutive patients with a first stroke.[8,9] Aggregate data of case reports describe dissections in patients from the second to the eighth decade, but 75% are between the ages of 35 and 50 with a mean age of 45 years.[27]

Transient ischemia or infarction of the brain or retina is the predominant clinical presentation, occurring in up to 50% of patients; however, this is undoubtedly over-represented as these patients are more likely to undergo extensive evaluations such as angiography and also more likely to be reported. Ipsilateral pain involving the head or neck is present in up to 75% of patients. The pain may have vascular features of throbbing or nonthrobbing pain, nausea, and photophobia. The typical pain locations are frontal, retro-orbital, and anterior cervical in the region of the mandible and may precede the onset of other neurologic symptoms by hours or days. The pain syndrome may be confusing in the setting of previous trauma and associated head and neck injury.[59]

Ipsilateral oculosympathetic paresis is present in 20% to 40% of patients with ptosis, miosis, and variable anhidrosis in the supra-orbital region indicating disruption of the pericarotid sympathetic postganglionic fibers from the internal carotid plexus.[70] Pulsatile tinnitus, an uncommon manifestation of carotid occlusive disease, is a prominent complaint in up to one-third of patients and usually spontaneously resolves within days or weeks. It has been suggested that the bruit may more accurately signal the onset of the dissection.[18,65] Cranial nerve palsies have been reported in less than 5%. Compression of the glossopharyngeal, vagal, accessory, and hypoglossal nerves, alone or in combination, occurs with focal enlargement of the dissecting mural hematoma within the tight confines of the carotid sheath at or about the jugular foramen, whereas intracranial extension into the inferior cavernous sinus can compress the trigeminal and abducens nerves.[16,19,40,44,55,71]

The clinical course of extracranial carotid artery dissection is variable. Patients with single or multiple transient ischemic events or minor stroke on presentation generally have a good outcome whether treated with anticoagulant, antiplatelet, or no therapy;

however, descriptions of delayed ischemic events due to embolism or stenosis progressing to occlusion have prompted many authors to recommend a course of anticoagulant or antiplatelet therapy until repeat angiographic studies can document resolution of the dissection. Of patients presenting with a stroke in a setting of an internal carotid artery occlusion, nearly two-thirds have a progressive or fluctuating course. Although 40% of such patients in a recent series made a good recovery associated with recanalization of the internal carotid artery, 23% died within 1 week, and the remainder had a permanent disabling deficit related to significant infarction incurred at the onset of the dissection or failure of recanalization.[9] Dissecting aneurysms in the extracranial location have not been described to rupture, although carotid-cavernous fistula formation has rarely occurred with intracranial extension.[52,68]

Angiographic Course

Angiographic studies show an eccentric tapered stenosis in the internal carotid artery usually several centimeters distal to a normal cervical carotid bifurcation in 75% of cases (Figure 5), with one-third also manifesting an aneurysmal pouch (see Figure 2C). Rarely, spontaneous dissection may involve the common carotid artery,[24] although this is more prevalent among traumatic dissections. Subadventitial dissection documented by magnetic resonance (MR) has been described with a normal angiogram.[66] Approximately 18% of cases are occluded at onset (classically a "tapered occlusion" beyond a normal cervical carotid bifurcation), and less than 10% present with an aneurysm alone. Aneurysms are present in 35% to 40% of extracranial internal carotid artery dissections. Two-thirds of these are located in the upper cervical region, usually at the C2 level, and one-third are in the midcervical region.

The high cervical location occurs at a transition from large elastic to medium-size muscular architecture and is also a site of a

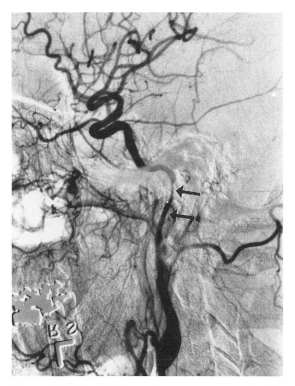

Figure 5. This middle-aged woman presented with spontaneous oculocephalic and cervical pain accompanied by left Horner's syndrome. Carotid angiography revealed a typical appearance of internal carotid artery dissection consisting of tapered irregularity of the distal internal carotid with an abrupt distal ledge (arrows). Note the normal appearance of the proximal internal carotid artery.

relatively fixed position of the vessel where it enters the carotid canal. These observations have led to the theory that some form of trauma coupled with an underlying defect in vessel architecture at a specific anatomic site is the cause of most "spontaneous" carotid dissections.[43]

Follow-up angiographic studies, usually performed at least 3-6 months after the initial study, document improvement or resolution in 75% to 80% of cases, progression of stenosis or aneurysmal enlargement in 15% to 20%, and angiographic residual in 25%. The exact time course of resolution is not clear. Early angiographic studies have demonstrated resolution as early as 3-6 weeks, but a delayed spontaneous resolution of an extracranial carotid aneurysm has been de-

scribed where an aneurysm at the C2 level was present on angiography 2 months after documented dissection and had resolved on repeat study 16 months later.[11,45,47,48] There is no reliable information about the impact of medical therapy (including anticoagulation) on the resolution of stenoses or aneurysms associated with dissection. Also, there are no data on factors predisposing to vascular healing or persistent anatomic anomalies.

Multiple dissections occur in 5% to 10% of cases, although this incidence increases to 23% to 33% in patients who present with vertebrobasilar symptoms. This is probably due to the increased likelihood of performing four-vessel angiographic studies in patients presenting with symptoms in the vertebrobasilar rather than carotid territory.[45,51] Multiple dissections are common at autopsy following lethal trauma.[50] Recurrent dissections, either ipsilateral or within another vascular territory, have also been described.[9,15]

Noninvasive Evaluation

Noninvasive studies such as Doppler ultrasonography and oculoplethysmography suggest significant improvements in flow as early as 1-4 weeks following documented dissection.[9,21] Doppler ultrasound examination can have as high as a 25% false-positive rate wherein reduced internal carotid flow can be present without other abnormalities of the cervical carotid artery in the presence of multiple intracranial vascular occlusions of the distal branches of the middle and anterior cerebral arteries or the distal segments of the internal carotid artery. A characteristic high-resistance Doppler flow pattern in extracranial internal carotid artery dissection has been described in 76% of patients consisting of an often high-amplitude Doppler signal with markedly reduced systolic Doppler frequencies and alternating flow direction. The alternating Doppler signal has a small early systolic component and a secondary component directed toward the brain on which another component becomes superimposed in a ret-

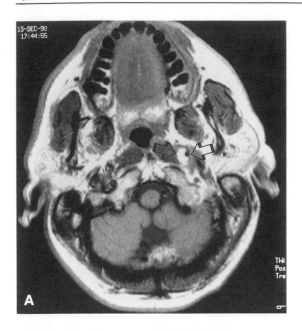

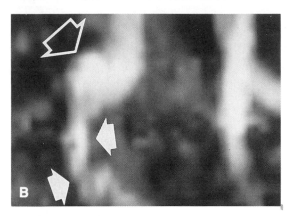

Figure 6. Middle-aged man with sudden onset of right hemispheric neurologic deficit 3 days after a football tackling injury. (A) MRI (T1-weighted axial scan) of the skull base revealed an eccentric mural hematoma consistent with dissection of the right internal carotid artery at the skull base (arrows). (B) MRA revealed luminal irregularities of the distal cervical internal carotid artery (solid arrows) and an aneurysmal dilatation of the proximal intrapetrous segment (open arrows). Such MRA appearance is typical of carotid dissection; however, no accurate estimate of true luminal size can be made from the MR angiographic picture alone, since flow disturbances and mural thrombosis are known to cause artifactual appearance of the vascular lumen. At present, MRA is used in conjunction with conventional axial MRI of the carotid artery. MR is an excellent modality for the diagnosis and serial followup of cervicocephalic arterial dissections.

rograde fashion. This is thought to result from low bidirectional movements of the blood column and abnormal vessel wall pulsations in the presence of a long tapering occlusion or a severe stenosis in the carotid artery at its entrance into the carotid canal.[29] Serial transcranial Doppler ultrasound studies may also be useful in guiding the acute hemodynamic management of patients with intracranial pressure-dependent stenoses.[35] Dynamic thin-section computed tomography scanning of the neck has been useful in demonstrating a pseudoaneurysm that may not be apparent on initial angiography or where angiography underestimates its true extent.[58]

MR imaging can provide cross-sectional images for evaluation of the lumen, vessel wall, and surrounding structures without requiring intravenous contrast (Figure 6).[22,25,62] MR angiography is potentially useful as a screening modality for carotid dissection and in serial follow-up vascular imaging without invasiveness or contrast agents. This may guide therapeutic decisions such as discontinuation of anticoagulation on healing of luminal stenosis; however, MR angiography may provide misleading images with thrombosis wrongly "visualized" as a patent lumen, whereas turbulence and sluggish flow may result in overestimation of the degree of luminal stenosis. MR angiography, in its present technical state, should be cautiously interpreted in vascular dissection in conjunction with other studies including conventional MR imaging in the axial plane (Figure 6).

Pathophysiology

The anatomic substrate of the luminal narrowing and aneurysm formation is more correctly referred to as a *dissecting intramural hematoma*. Pathologic material from surgical and autopsy specimens of the extracranial carotid artery reveal the abnormality occurring almost exclusively within the media. Associations with diseases known to affect the media include fibromuscular dysplasia, Marfan's disease, syphilis, atherosclerosis, and polyarteritis nodosa.[17,42] Fibromuscular dysplasia is present in approximately 20% of patients with dissections. The histologically verified cases of fibromuscular dysplasia affecting the carotid artery consist of the medial form rather than the intimal or periarterial forms.[64] Most specimens, however, are histologically normal or show only modest disorganization of the elastic fibers in the transition zone from the large elastic arteries to the medium-size muscular branches.

The role of an apparently minor trauma precipitating the dissection remains intriguing but elusive. Many patients retrospectively report a recent involvement in various sports activities, at times strenuous such as weightlifting, and other exertional events such as violent coughing, nose blowing, childbirth, or intraoperative hypertension.[27,73] There have also been reports of excessive or repetitive neck movements such as from chiropractic manipulation and riding a roller coaster. For dissections that occur at the C1-2 vertebral level, compression of the cervical carotid against the transverse process of the upper cervical vertebra with hyperextension rotation may be the source of injury; however, this would not explain dissections affecting other areas of the cervicocephalic vessels.[3,43]

Intracranial Carotid Artery Dissection

Dissections involving the intracranial carotid artery and its branches are sufficiently different both clinically and pathologically from dissections involving the extracranial carotid arteries to warrant separate consideration. Less than 50 cases have been reported in the literature affecting patients of all ages, with a mean reported age of 21 years. Fifty percent involve the middle cerebral artery and an additional 20% involve both the middle cerebral and the intracranial internal carotid artery. A rapidly progressive clinical course with sudden severe focal ischemia followed by fatal cerebral edema within 1 week has been the typical clinical presentation and course, but this may represent a bias since

the case reports are overrepresented by pathologic autopsy studies.[41] Isolated intrapetrous dissection has been described in two 42-year-old adults with a good clinical outcome.[63] Many intracranial arterial stenoses that have been reported to resolve spontaneously may actually have represented dissections.

The underlying vascular pathology characteristically involves the subintima with disruption of the internal elastica. The subintimal location of the hematoma has less resistance to luminal narrowing and occlusion than the thicker media and may explain the more rapidly progressive course and fatal outcome. Pathologic abnormalities include reduplication, absence, fraying, and splitting of the internal elastic lamina; absence of reticular fibers next to the internal elastic lamina has also been described.[28,49,54] Saccular aneurysms associated with the intracranial dissections are rare, but since they pathologically share many of the same abnormalities of the internal elastic lamina, a common congenital vascular abnormality has been suggested.

Intracranial arterial dissections are also encountered in the elderly and may be associated with atherosclerosis and more diffuse vascular ectasia.[20,75] They can result in ischemia from perforating branch occlusion or thromboembolism. Hemorrhage has also been reported in the setting of intracranial arterial dissection presumed secondary to atherosclerotic ectasia.[20]

Extracranial Vertebral Artery Dissection

Like extracranial carotid dissections, extracranial vertebral artery dissections tend to occur in young adults with a mean age of 40 years. In clinical series, the most common presentation is an ipsilateral, usually occipital, headache with or without cervical pain followed by delayed vertebrobasilar ischemic symptoms. Headache is present in approximately half of the patients initially, but it develops in 75% at some point along their clinical course. Up to 80% of reported cases develop vertebrobasilar ischemic symptoms usually manifested as a lateral medullary or cerebellar infarction, although the prevalence of less symptomatic cases is not known.[14,26] The acute and severe nature of the occipital headache associated with neck stiffness can sometimes mimic subarachnoid hemorrhage, but true documented subarachnoid hemorrhage has not been described with purely extracranial vertebral artery dissections.

Roughly half the patients have unilateral vertebral dissections that, if proximal, would not be expected to produce posterior circulation ischemia on a hemodynamic basis because of contralateral collateral supply; however, the site of dissection can serve as a source of thrombosis or thromboembolism (Figure 7), which has been the proposed mechanism of the delayed ischemic symptoms. This has prompted the clinical practice of anticoagulant or antiplatelet therapy until resolution of anatomic luminal anomalies. Short-term outcome in small series seems to be improved with anticoagulant rather than antiplatelet or no therapy, although the overall neurologic outcome is good in 70% to 80% of patients.[26]

Nearly 70% of vertebral artery dissections are extracranial in distribution. The most common level of vessel disruption is at the C1-2 level near its exit from the transverse foramen of the axis and extending horizontally as the artery travels over the posterior arch of the atlas.[39] Extradural aneurysms are often saccular with a broad neck parallel to the long axis of the artery (Figure 7).

Angiographic follow-up has documented improvement in 26% to 33% of cases, normalization in 61% to 63%, and progression to occlusion in 6% to 11%.[45,51] Marked angiographic improvement has been described as early as 7 days and normalization as early as 3 weeks with most vessels destined to do so improving by the third month. Of patients who undergo four-vessel angiographic studies, 23% to 33% manifest simultaneous bilateral carotid dissections.[45] This raises interesting questions about the true incidence of dissections when patients present with less obvious symptoms. This also is consistent with the concept of an underlying host-

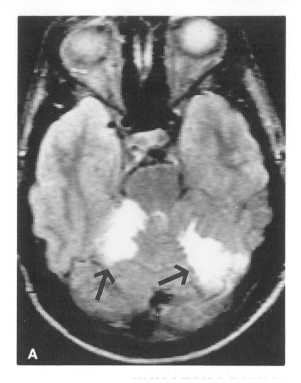

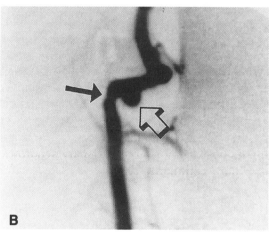

Figure 7. This young man had sudden onset of headache and violent nausea and vomiting several days after vigorous football training. *(A)* MR imaging revealed bilateral multifocal cerebellar infarctions (straight arrows) consistent with thromboembolism. *(B)* Vertebral angiography revealed slight luminal irregularity of the vessel at the level of C1 (closed arrow) with aneurysmal dilatation more distally (open arrow). This patient was treated with anticoagulation and is being followed with serial angiography. If there is progressive narrowing of the vascular lumen, or progressive expansion of the aneurysmal dilatation, balloon occlusion of the artery will be entertained.

related vasculopathy in spontaneous and traumatic dissections.

A distinctive Doppler ultrasound pattern in extracranial vertebral artery dissection consists of increased arterial diameter associated with decreased pulsativity, presence of intravascular echoes, and other hemodynamic signs of stenosis or occlusion.[67] Improvement in dissection can be followed noninvasively by this method. MR can also be effectively used to demonstrate the dissecting hematoma as well as any posterior fossa infarction.[60]

As with extracranial carotid dissections, pathologic involvement is typically medial.[54] Minor trauma, neck manipulation, or repetitive or sudden head rotation has also preceded symptoms similar to extracranial carotid dissections, suggesting a role of trauma.[8,14]

Intracranial Vertebral Artery Dissection

Primary intracranial dissection or intracranial extension of an extradural vertebral artery dissection occurs in up to a third of vertebral artery dissections.[31] Presenting symptoms are similar to those seen in extracranial vertebral artery dissections with the prominent exception that subarachnoid hemorrhage and more extensive brain stem infarctions than a lateral medullary syndrome are more commonly seen. Occasionally, dissecting aneurysms may achieve giant aneurysm proportion producing mass effect within the posterior fossa.[13]

Angiography typically demonstrates irregular luminal narrowing and aneurysm formation near or at the level of the posterior-inferior cerebellar artery. The dissecting hematoma compressing the intima proximal to the aneurysm may produce enough luminal narrowing to obscure aneurysm filling. In the presence of subarachnoid hemorrhage without aneurysm visualization, dissection between the media and adventitia should be suspected, and repeat angiography or MR scanning should be performed.[13]

In cases of subarachnoid hemorrhage from posterior circulation dissecting aneurysms, recurrent hemorrhage is likely to occur within 7 days of the initial ictus with an extremely poor outcome.[13,75] Although intracranial vertebral aneurysms have been reported to resolve spontaneously, the threat of devastating subarachnoid hemorrhage should prompt definitive obliteration of the aneurysm in most patients who are in suitable neurologic condition.[13,20,54,75] To prevent rupture of dissecting aneurysms, proximal clipping, trapping, and wrapping have all been recommended, but they should not be performed without careful evaluation of competence of the collateral circulation. Intravascular balloon techniques allow the safe testing of tolerance to occlusion with patients awake prior to permanent vascular occlusion.

The pathologic location within the vessel wall is less predictable with both medial and subintimal lesions reported.[54] Dissection between the elastica and media more typically presents with posterior circulation ischemia, whereas dissection between the media and adventitia is more likely to present with subarachnoid hemorrhage.[75] The extradural portion of the muscularis and adventitia thins by two-thirds, and the internal elastic lamina is lost at the intradural transition of the vertebral artery, which may account for adventitial rupture and subarachnoid hemorrhage with intracranial vertebral artery dissection.

Conclusions

The growing recognition of cervical and cerebral arterial dissections has led to a better understanding of their myriad neurologic manifestations and often relatively benign clinical course. Although the diagnosis can be suspected in patients presenting with cerebral or retinal ischemia associated with abrupt neck or face pain, a high index of suspicion is required in individuals who present with pain alone or with less obvious constellations of pulsatile tinnitus, oculosympathetic paresis, cranial nerve palsies, or subarachnoid hemorrhage. In the setting of overt trauma, a high index of suspicion is essential to prompt diagnosis and timely therapy.

Although many patients do well in association with a resolution of their dissecting arterial wall hematoma and concomitant angiographic abnormalities, the risk of delayed thrombosis or thromboembolism is one of the most serious and potentially preventable complications. The nonuniform manner of management in many of the case reports precludes definitive management recommendations. In the absence of an anticoagulation contraindication (e.g. intracranial hemorrhage, intracranial extension of a vertebral dissection, large completed cerebral infarction), we opt for short-term anticoagulation with heparin followed by warfarin until an angiographically documented resolution of the dissection occurs. The time interval for angiographic follow-up is usually between 3-6 months, but more data need to be collected from serial noninvasive modalities that would more accurately guide the length of therapy. MR angiography appears to allow safe and reliable follow-up as a guide to discontinuation of anticoagulants.

Surgical options, including direct repair of a dissection or excision of the disrupted arterial segment, are reserved for cases where anticoagulation is contraindicated and the whole extent of vascular disruption is accessible (exceptional cases). Interventional techniques currently allow the exclusion from the circulation of many dissecting aneurysms acting as a source of embolism or potential hemorrhage.

More information regarding the fate of dissecting aneurysms is needed. Intracranial aneurysms have been reported to rupture with sometimes devastating results, but the risk of this in the early and late phases of dissection is poorly understood. Extracranial dissecting aneurysms have not been described to rupture but may remain as a persistent embolic source requiring obliterative therapy. Little is currently known about factors favoring or interfering with healing of dissecting stenoses and aneurysmal disruptions. Anticoagulation, unless contraindicated, appears to provide the best available protection against thromboembolism and propagating thrombosis pending vascular healing.

References

1. Aarabi B, McQueen JD. Traumatic internal carotid occlusion at the base of the skull. *Surg Neurol.* 1978;10:233-236.
2. Ajir F, Tibbetts JC. Post-traumatic occlusion of the supraclinoid internal carotid artery. *Neurosurgery.* 1981;9:173-176.
3. Anson J, Crowell RM. Cervicocranial arterial dissection. *Neurosurgery.* 1991;29:89-96.
4. Anyanwu CH, Ude AC, Swarup AS. Traumatic left carotid aneurysm with hemiplegia. *J R Coll Surg Edinb.* 1982;27:181-182.
5. Arseni C, Maretsis M, Dumitrescu L. Comments on the aetiology of indirect traumatic thrombosis of the internal carotid: a case study of 22 cases. *Neurochirurgia (Stutts).* 1980;23:25-34.
6. Batnitzky S, Price HI, Holden RW, et al. Cervical internal carotid artery injuries due to blunt trauma. *AJNR.* 1983;4:292-295.
7. Batzdorf U, Bentson JR, Machleder HI. Blunt trauma to the high cervical carotid artery. *Neurosurgery.* 1979;5:195-201.
8. Biller J, Hingtgen WL, Adams HP, et al. Cervicocephalic arterial dissections: a ten-year experience. *Arch Neurol.* 1986;43:1234-1238.
9. Bogousslavsky J, Despland PS-A, Regli F. Spontaneous carotid dissection with acute stroke. *Arch Neurol.* 1987;44(2):137-140.
10. Bok APL, Kieck CF, DeVilliers JC. Head injury associated with carotid occlusion due to blunt cervical trauma. *S Afr J Surg.* 1984;22:43-50.
11. Bradac GB, Kaernbach A, Bolk-Weischedel D, et al. Spontaneous dissecting aneurysm of cervical cerebral arteries: report of six cases and review of the literature. *Neuroradiology.* 1981;21:149-154.
12. Capanna AH. Traumatic intracranial aneurysm and Gradenigo's syndrome secondary to gunshot wound. *Surg Neurol.* 1984;22:263-266.
13. Caplan LR, Baquis GD, Pessin MS, et al. Dissection of the intracranial vertebral artery. *Neurology.* 1988;38:868-877.
14. Caplan LR, Zarins CK, Hemmati M. Spontaneous dissection of the extracranial vertebral arteries. *Stroke.* 1985;16:1030-1038.
15. Cusick JF, Daniels D. Spontaneous reversal of internal carotid artery occlusion: case report. *J Neurosurg.* 1981;54:811-813.
16. Davies L. A case of vagal palsy due to dissecting aneurysm of the carotid artery. *Med J Austr.* 1987;147:352-353.
17. De Baets P, Delanote G, Jackers G, et al. Atherosclerosic dissection of the cervical internal carotid artery—a case report. *Angiology.* 1990;41:161-163.
18. Fisher CM, Ojemann RG, Roberson GH. Spontaneous dissection of cervico-cerebral arteries. *Can J Neurol Sci.* 1978;5:9-19.
19. Francis KR, Williams DP, Troost BT. Facial numb-

ness and dysesthesia: new features of carotid artery dissection. *Arch Neurol.* 1987;44:345-346.

20. Friedman AH, Drake CG. Subarachnoid hemorrhage from intracranial dissecting aneurysm. *J Neurosurg.* 1984;60:325-334.

21. Gee W, Kaupp HA, McDonald KM, et al. Spontaneous dissection of internal carotid arteries: spontaneous resolution documented by serial ocular pneumoplethysmography and angiography. *Arch Surg.* 1980;115:944-949.

22. Goldberg HI, Grossman RI, Gomori JM, et al. Cervical internal carotid artery dissecting hemorrhage: diagnosis using MR. *Radiology.* 1986;158:157-161.

23. Goldwasser MS, Lorson EL, Tucker DF, et al. Internal carotid artery thrombosis associated with a fracture. *J Oral Surg.* 1978;36:543-545.

24. Graham JM, Miller T, Stinnett DM. Spontaneous dissection of the common carotid artery: case report and review of the literature. *J Vasc Surg.* 1988;7:811-813.

25. Hanigan WC, Wright RM, Berkman WA, et al. MR imaging of a false carotid aneurysm. *Stroke.* 1986;17:1317-1319.

26. Hart RG. Vertebral artery dissection. *Neurology.* 1988;38:987-989.

27. Hart RG, Easton JD. Dissections of cervical and cerebral arteries. *Neurol Clin.* 1983;1:155-182.

28. Hegedüs K. Reticular fiber deficiency in the intracranial arteries of patients with dissecting aneurysm and review of the possible pathogenesis of previously reported cases. *Eur Arch Psychiatry & Neurol Sci.* 1985;235:102-106.

29. Hennerici M, Steinke W, Rautenberg W. High-resistance Doppler flow pattern in extracranial carotid dissection. *Arch Neurol.* 1989;46:670-672.

30. Hilton-Jones D, Warlow CP. Non-penetrating arterial trauma and cerebral infarction in the young. *Lancet.* 1985;1:1435-1438.

31. Hoang The Dan P, Pourriat JL, Lapandry C, et al. Dissection de la carotide interne. *Ann Fr. Anesth Reanim.* 1984;3:388-391.

32. Hoffmann TH, Richardson JD, Flint LM. Intimal disruption of major cerebral vasculature following blunt trauma. *Surgery.* 1980;87:441-444.

33. Jentzer A. Dissecting aneurysm of the left internal carotid artery. *Angiology.* 1954;5:232-234.

34. Källerö KS, Björck C-G, Bergqvist D. Carotid artery injury caused by blunt cervical trauma. *Acta Chir Scand.* 1987;153:155-160.

35. Kaps M, Dorndorf W, Damian MS, et al. Intracranial haemodynamics in patients with spontaneous carotid dissection: transcranial Doppler ultrasound follow-up studies. *Eur Arch Psychiatry Neurol Sci.* 1990;239:246-256.

36. Karlin RM, Marks C. Extracranial carotid artery injury. *Am J Surg.* 1983;146:225-227.

37. Krajewski LP, Hertzer NR. Blunt carotid artery trauma: report of two cases and review of the literature. *Ann Surg.* 1980;191:341-346.

38. LeBlanc KA, Benzel EC. Trauma to the high cervical carotid artery. *J Trauma.* 1984;24:992-996.

39. Leys D, Lesoin F, Pruvo JP, et al. Bilateral spontaneous dissection of extracranial vertebral arteries. *J Neurol.* 1987;234:237-240.

40. Lieschke GJ, Davis S, Tress BM, et al. Spontaneous internal carotid artery dissection presenting as hypoglossal nerve palsy. *Stroke.* 1988;19:1151-1155.

41. Linden MD, Chou SM, Furlan AJ, et al. Cerebral arterial dissection: a case report with histopathologic and ultrastructural findings. *Cleve Clin J Med.* 1987;54:105-114.

42. Lomeo RM, Silver RM, Brothers M. Spontaneous dissection of the internal carotid artery in a patient with polyarteritis nodosa. *Arthritis Rheum.* 1989;32:1625-1626.

43. Luken MG III, Ascherl GF Jr, Correll JW, et al. Spontaneous dissecting aneurysms of the extracranial internal carotid artery. *Clin Neurosurg.* 1979;26:353-375.

44. Maitland CG, Black JL, Smith WA. Abducens nerve palsy due to spontaneous dissection of the internal carotid artery. *Arch Neurol.* 1983;40:448-449.

45. Mas J-L, Bousser M-G, Hasboun D, et al. Extracranial vertebral artery dissections: a review of 13 cases. *Stroke.* 1987;18:1037-1047.

46. Maurer PK, Plassche W, Green RM. Blunt trauma to the carotid artery with transient deficit and early repair. *Surg Neurol.* 1984;21:110-112.

47. McNeill DH Jr, Dreisbach J, Marsden RJ. Spontaneous dissection of the internal carotid artery: its conservative management with heparin sodium. *Arch Neurol.* 1980;37:54-55.

48. Milandre L, Pérot S, Salamon G, et al. Spontaneous dissection of both extracranial internal carotid arteries. *Neuroradiology.* 1989;31:435-439.

49. Mizutani T, Goldberg HI, Parr J, et al. Cerebral dissecting aneurysm and intimal fibroelastic thickening of cerebral arteries: case report. *J Neurosurg.* 1982;56: 571-576.

50. Moar JJ. Traumatic rupture of the cervical carotid arteries: an autopsy and histopathological study of 200 cases. *Forensic Sci Int.* 1987;34:227-244.

51. Mokri B, Houser OW, Sandok BA, et al. Spontaneous dissections of the vertebral arteries. *Neurology.* 1988;38:880-885.

52. Mokri B, Sundt TM Jr, Houser OW, et al. Spontaneous dissection of the cervical internal carotid artery. *Ann Neurol.* 1986;19:126-138.

53. Morgan MK, Besser M, Johnston I, et al. Intracranial carotid artery injury in closed head trauma. *J Neurosurg.* 1987;66:192-197.

54. O'Connell BK, Towfighi J, Brennan RW, et al. Dissecting aneurysms of head and neck. *Neurology.* 1985;35:993-997.

55. Panisset M, Eidelman BH. Multiple cranial neuropathy as a feature of internal carotid artery dissection. *Stroke.* 1990;21:141-147.

56. Pellegrini RV, Manzetti GW, DiMarco RF, et al. The direct surgical management of lesions of the high internal carotid artery. *J Cardiovasc Surg (Torino).* 1984;25:29-35.

57. Perry MO, Snyder WH, Thal ER. Carotid artery injuries caused by blunt trauma. *Ann Surg.* 1980;192:74-77.

58. Petro GR, Witwer GA, Cacayorin ED, et al. Spontaneous dissection of the cervical internal carotid artery: correlation of arteriography, CT, and pathology. *AJR.* 1987;148:393-398.

59. Popowich L. Blunt carotid artery trauma associated with maxillofacial injuries: report of three cases. *J Oral Maxillofac Surg.* 1984;42:462-465.

60. Quint DJ, Spickler EM. Magnetic resonance demonstration of vertebral artery dissection: report of two cases. *J Neurosurg.* 1990;72:964-967.

61. Reyna TM, Cabellon S Jr., Fallon WF Jr. Delayed recognition of carotid artery injury due to blunt trauma. *Military Medicine*. 1986;151:450-451.

62. Rothrock JF, Lim V, Press G, et al. Serial magnetic resonance and carotid duplex examinations in the management of carotid dissection. *Neurology*. 1989;39:686-692.

63. Saeed SR, Hinton AE, Ramsden RT, et al. Spontaneous dissection of the intrapetrous internal carotid artery. *J Laryngol Otol*. 1990;104:491-493.

64. Sato S, Hata J. Fibromuscular dysplasia: its occurrence with a dissecting aneurysm of the internal carotid artery. *Arch Pathol Lab Med*. 1982;106: 332-335.

65. Sila CA, Furlan AJ, Little JR. Pulsatile tinnitus. *Stroke*. 1987;18:252-256.

66. Sweeney PJ, Assaf M, Kosmorsky G, et al. Subadventitial extracranial carotid artery dissection with normal angiography. *Ann Neurol*. 1991;30:247.

67. Touboul P-J, Mas J-L, Bousser M-G, et al. Duplex scanning in extracranial vertebral artery dissection. *Stroke*. 1988;19:116-121.

68. Tucci JM, Maitland CG, Pesolyar DW, et al. Carotid-cavernous fistula due to traumatic dissection of the extracranial internal carotid artery. *AJNR*. 1984; 5:828-829.

69. Vanezis P. Techniques used in the evaluation of vertebral artery trauma at post-mortem. *Forensic Sci Int*. 1979;13:159-165.

70. Vijayan N, Watson C. Spontaneous internal carotid artery dissection and abnormal facial sweating. *Arch Neurol*. 1980;37:468.

71. Waespe W, Niesper J, Imhof H-G, et al. Lower cranial nerve palsies due to internal carotid dissection. *Stroke*. 1988;19:1561-1564.

72. Welling RE, Kakkasseril JS, Peschiera J. Pseudoaneurysm of the cervical internal carotid artery secondary to blunt trauma. *J Trauma*. 1985; 25:1108-1110.

73. Wiebers DO, Mokri B. Internal carotid artery dissection after childbirth. *Stroke*. 1985;16:956-959.

74. Williams F, Awad IA, Spetzler RF, et al. Neurological complications after non-penetrating trauma to the cervical carotid artery. Presented to the Annual Meeting of the American Association of Neurological Surgeons; April 13-17, 1986; Denver, Colo.

75. Yonas H, Agamanolis D, Takaoka Y, et al. Dissecting intracranial aneurysms. *Surg Neurol*. 1977;8: 407-415.

76. Young PH, Smith KR Jr, Crafts DC, et al. Traumatic occlusion of the carotid artery. *Surg Neurol*. 1981;16:432-437.

77. Zelenock GB, Kazmers A, Whitehouse WM Jr, et al. Extracranial internal carotid artery dissections. *Arch Surg*. 1982;117:425-432.

CHAPTER 11

Vertebrobasilar Occlusive Disease

Fernando G. Diaz, MD, PhD

Treatment of patients with vertebrobasilar insufficiency has been controversial since Kubick and Adams[24] first described thrombosis of the basilar artery and its presumed symptoms in 1946. No specific form of treatment was recommended until Millikan and coworkers[25,26] proposed anticoagulation in 1955. Since most patients were not evaluated angiographically, it has not been possible to determine whether the condition treated by Millikan et al was the result of vertebrobasilar occlusive disease or from other causes. Diagnostic procedures were avoided in these patients because of fear of possible complications from vertebral arteriography.[25,26,31]

However, since many pathologic disorders can cause vertebrobasilar insufficiency, proper diagnosis must be made to institute correct treatment.[31]

The vertebrobasilar system is formed by two arteries, one on either side of the neck, each originating from the subclavian artery. The vertebral arteries each have four portions: the first extending from their origin to their entry into the foramen transversarium of C6; the second running between the foramen transversarium of C6 and C1; the third exiting from the foramen of C1 and extending to their entrance into the dura through the atlanto-occipital membrane; and the fourth, subarachnoid portion, extending from their entrance into the dura to their point of convergence. The extracranial vertebral arteries are surrounded by an extensive venous plexus from their point of origin to their point of entry through the dura at the atlanto-occipital membrane.

The two vertebral arteries join at the level of the mid-pons to constitute the basilar artery, which extends from the mid-pons to the upper midbrain where it bifurcates, giving rise to the two posterior cerebral arteries. The entire brain stem, cerebellum, occipital lobes, and part of the temporal lobes are irrigated by the vertebrobasilar circulation. The main arteries arising from the vertebrobasilar system are the long circumferential arteries: i.e. the posterior inferior cerebellar artery (from the vertebral arteries); the anterior-inferior cerebellar artery (from the mid-portion of the basilar artery); and the superior cerebellar arteries (from the distal basilar arery prior to its termination). Besides these three pairs of main arteries, numerous short circumferential and intermediate circumferential arteries, as well as perforators originate from the basilar and vertebral arteries.[11,24]

Normal anatomic communication exists between the internal carotid arteries and the posterior cerebral arteries through the posterior communicating arteries. The posterior cerebral arteries develop embryologically from the internal carotid arteries at the level of what eventually become the posterior com-

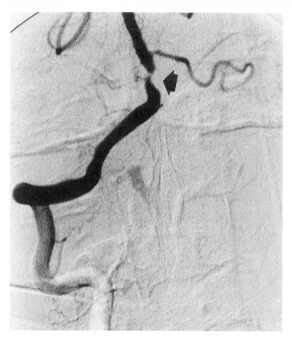

Figure 1. Angiogram of 48-year-old male with hyperlipidemia and multiple vascular risk factors, who presented with recurrent spells of diplopia, vertigo, and drop attacks despite antiplatelet therapy. The angiogram reveals severe stenosis at the proximal basilar artery (arrow). The patient was treated with anticoagulant therapy which resulted in total cessation of symptoms. He died of massive myocardiac infarction 8 months later. Such lesions represent a strong index for severe diffuse vascular disease, and a severe risk factor for subsequent myocardiac infarction and stroke (in any vascular territory). (Figure supplied courtesy of I.A. Awad, The Cleveland Clinic Foundation.)

municating arteries. These primitive posterior cerebral arteries join with the basilar artery at the level of its terminal bifurcation, and eventually the initial portion of the posterior cerebral arteries. After embryonic development, the posterior communicating arteries regress, becoming smaller than the initial portions of the posterior cerebral arteries arising from the basilar artery. Communication with the anterior circulation is functional in only 60% of individuals.[11,21] Four normal embryologic arterial connections may persist in some individuals after birth. These include the trigeminal artery, which connects the intracavernous carotid artery to the tip of the basilar artery; the otic artery, which connects the intrapetrous carotid to the midportion of the basilar artery; the hypoglossal artery, which connects the extracranial internal carotid artery to the intracranial vertebral artery; and the pro-atlantal artery, which connects the extracranial internal carotid artery to the extracranial vertebral artery at the C2 level.[12]

Clinico-Pathologic Correlation

Numerous pathologic processes can occur in the vertebrobasilar circulation. By far the most important are atherosclerotic plaques, which can develop at any level of the vertebrobasilar tree[12,31,32] most commonly occurring at the vertebral artery origin. Schwartz and Mitchell[32] described severe abnormalities of vertebrobasilar artery origin in a majority of unselected autopsies from a large group. Sites of less frequent involvement of the vertebrobasilar tree include the second portion of the vertebral arteries, generally as they pass through the foramen transversarium; the level at which the vertebral arteries enter the dura; and just prior to their confluence.[4,32] Any portion of the basilar artery can also be affected by atherosclerosis (Figure 1).[21,24,25] The frequency of atherosclerosis is variable, although most agree that the arteriosclerotic changes observed in the vertebrobasilar system are less frequent than those seen in the carotid artery territory.[12] Atherosclerosis and chronic arterial hypertension may result in dolichoectatic changes in the vertebrobasilar system, which predispose to dissecting aneurysms with secondary ischemic (Figure 2) or hemmorhagic complications.

Other pathologic conditions of the vertebrobasilar system include spontaneous dissection of the vertebral arteries with the formation of pseudoaneurysms (Figure 3) or varying degrees of occlusion. Spontaneous dissection is frequently observed in association with fibromuscular hyperplasia of the vertebral arteries or the carotid arteries.[25,31] Direct trauma to the vertebral artery by penetrating

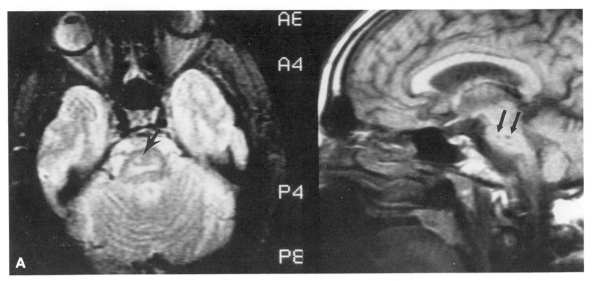

Figure 2. A 42-year-old severely obese, hypertensive male with advanced coronary artery disease presented with acute onset of left hemiplegia, horizontal gaze palsy, and right nuclear facial nerve palsy. **(A)** MRI reveals multiple lacunar infarctions within the pons (arrows). **(B)** MRA reveals distal stenosis of one vertebral artery (single arrow) and dolichoectasia of the basilar trunk with a dissecting aneurysm (triple arrows). Brain stem ischemia was presumed secondary to occlusion of pontine perforators by atherosclerotic dissection and/or thrombosis. (Figure supplied courtesy of I.A. Awad, MD, The Cleveland Clinic Foundation.)

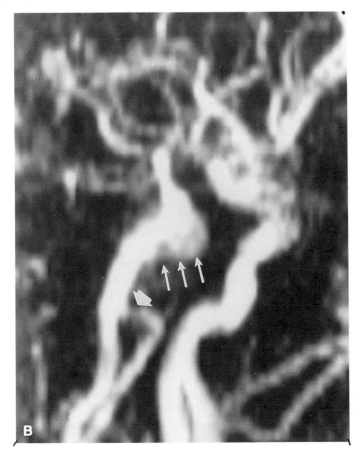

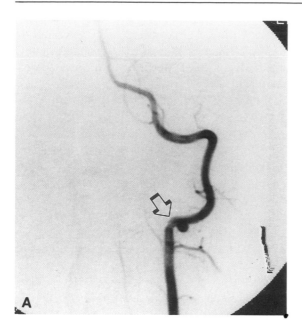

Figure 3. This 22-year-old college football quarterback suffered sudden onset of vertigo and gait and limb ataxia 3 weeks following a severe "neck sprain" sustained in training. *(A)* Right vertebral angiogram reveals luminal irregularity and a broad-based aneurysmal dilation of the vertebral artery at the level of the second cervical vertebrae (arrow), consistent with traumatic dissection. *(B)* MRI reveals multiple wedge-shaped cerebellar infarctions, likely representing artery-to-artery embolism from the site of arterial dissection (arrows). *(Figure supplied courtesy of I.A. Awad, The Cleveland Clinic Foundation.)*

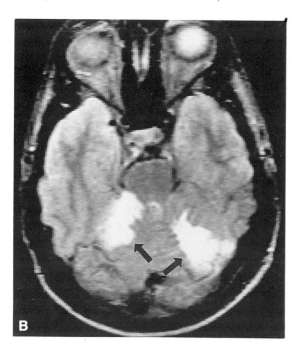

wounds or severe cervical spine fracture dislocations can result in occlusion, dissecting pseudoaneurysms, or ateriovenous fistula of the vertebral artery.[29] Traumatic occlusion or dissection of the vertebral arteries, which may extend into the basilar artery, has been reported after aggressive chiropractic manipulation of the neck.[29] The effect of trauma to the vertebral arteries induced by chiropractic manipulation is not necessarily age dependent or related to pre-existing pathology. External encroachment on the vertebral artery from osteophytic spurs arising from the cervical vertebrae may compress the second portion of the vertebral artery.[20,33] "Subclavian steal"[9,10,27] and ligamentous bands from the anterior scalene muscle compressing the vertebral artery at C6,[33] can also cause vertebrobasilar insufficiency. Many emboli in the vertebrobasilar territory originate from sources other than the vertebral arteries, including the heart valves or diseased myocardium; atrial thrombi; atrial myxomas; arteriosclerotic plaques of the aorta, subclavian, or innominate arteries; and pathologic emboli of systemic origin.[31]

In general, vertebrobasilar insufficiency syndrome is characterized by intermittent neurologic dysfunction episodes that usually include multiple symptoms. These usually repetitive symptoms can be progressive, or can occur as singular, sudden, severe events with complete and permanent neurologic dysfunction. Whisnant et al[32] describes vertebrobasilar insufficiency as occurring in patients who have at least two of the following symptoms: (1) motor or sensory symptoms, or both, occuring bilaterally and simultaneously in an attack; (2) ataxia of gait or dysmetria; (3) diplopia; (4) dysarthria; (5) bilateral homonymous hemianopsia. Additional symptoms compatible with this syndrome are vertigo, tinnitus, multiple cranial nerve involvement (usually contralateral to the major sensory deficit), or motor involvement of the extremities. Dizziness alone, syncope, drop attacks, and transient global amnesia are not given much weight in establishing the diagnosis of vertebrobasilar insufficiency. If any of these symptoms occurs singly, other causes besides vertebrobasilar insufficiency should be considered.[31,37] A systematic correlation between the symptoms of vertebrobasilar insufficiency and corresponding angiographic lesions has not yet been established.

The differential diagnosis of vertebrobasilar disease should exclude cardiac problems, such as dysrhythmias, myocardial insufficiency, and emboli (from an old infarction, from valvalar origin, or secondary to subacute bacterial endocarditis). Blood-related problems such as thrombocytosis, sickle cell disease, macroglobulinemias, or any disorder which may cause hypercoagulability should be ruled out. Women on contraceptives with associated events of basilar migraine, may develop symptoms that mimic vertebrobasilar ischemia. Bleeding disorders with intraparenchymal hemorrhages could result in the development of sudden neurologic dysfunction in the vertebrobasilar distribution, but the abrupt onset and marked severity would be comparable only to thrombosis of the basilar artery with complete loss of function of the brain stem. Other processes which may resemble vertebrobasilar insufficiency syndrome include demyelinating disease, usually occuring in younger individuals; and intracranial neoplasms, such as cerebellopontine angle region tumors or intra-axial tumors of the cerebellum. In some cases Ménière's syndrome could mimic vertebrobasilar insufficiency and therefore must be excluded.

Since the differential diagnosis can be difficult, complete ancillary tests are necessary to rule out other problems. Required routine laboratory examinations include a complete differential blood count with a blood smear and complete coagulation profile, a metabolic battery, a 12-lead electrocardiogram, and Holter monitoring for 24 or 36 hours. A computerized tomographic (CT) scan will likely exclude intracranial sources of nonvascular structural pathology.[31] With the recent introduction of positron emission tomography (PET) scanning, the metabolic function of the brain can be determined, although its application to the study of vertebrobasilar ischemic disease has been limited. A more useful current diagnostic modality for patients with ischemic disease of the vertebrobasilar circulation is magnetic resonance imaging (MRI). MRI permits a more detailed anatomic delineation of ischemic damage of the brain stem and cerebellar structures than CT scanning (Figures 2A and 3B), and may also permit metabolic study of these structures with magnetic resonance spectroscopy.

Selective cerebral angiography is the definitive diagnostic tool to establish the nature of the vascular involvement in the patient with vertebrobasilar insufficiency (See Figures 1-5).[11] Conventional cerebral angiography has been used for over 40 years;[15,21] the currently acceptable overall mortality rate is 0.6% with major complications under 1%.[11] The recent introduction of intra-arterial digital cerebral angiography has further reduced the concern because it requires lower doses of contrast infusion to obtain excellent diagnostic images, and because it reduces the contrast required in patients with serious renal or cardiac problems who may be at risk with large volumes of contrast material. An even more exciting diagnostic tool of vascular imaging is now in process of development—magnetic resonance angiography (Figure 2B). This noninvasive procedure does not require the administration of contrast material. As the diagnostic accuracy and precision of MR angiography increases, it will become the ideal diagnostic tool for evaluation of the cerebral circulation.

Medical Treatment

No medical treatment was effective in the management of patients with vertebrobasilar insufficiency until the mid-1950s when Millikan et al.[26] introduced systemic anticoagulation. In a group of patients assumed to have vertebrobasilar insufficiency, there was a decline in the mortality rate (from 43% in an untreated group of patients to 14% in the treated group). Angiography was not performed on any of these patients, other major causes of symptoms were not ruled out, and patients were nonrandomly assigned to the treatment group. All patients were assumed to have impending basilar occlusion prior to treatment. In a 15-year follow-up study of patients with vertebrobasilar ischemic symptoms who did not systematically receive angiograms, Whisnant et al.[37] reported a drop in stroke incidence (from 35% to 15% within 4 years) when these patients received oral anticoagulants. A treatment group and a control group were chosen, but most of these patients had not received angiograms, and were nonrandomly assigned to the two treatment groups.

Other forms of treatment, such as antiplatelet therapy, are used to treat patients with vertebrobasilar disease, but their effectiveness in averting strokes cannot be reliably predicted. Systemic or locally infused streptokinase and urokinase has been used by some patients with angiographically confirmed impending basilar artery occlusion, caused by a local thrombus or from a systemic embolus. Hemorrhagic complications and questionable efficacy have generally discouraged their use, however. The local application of streptokinase met with some success and lead to the introduction of tissue plasminogen activator (TPA) administered in a simlar manner, but the high cost of TPA has been a major limiting factor in its use. Comparative studies evaluating the differences between TPA and streptokinase in cardiac patients, have not shown a significant benefit of one over the other for intravascular clot lysis.

Strict blood pressure control should be discouraged in patients who have angiographically demonstrated, hemodynamically significant lesions of the vertebrobasilar tree. With severe lesions, a drop in blood pressure could acutely alter the perfusion to the ischemic brain and create a watershed area of ischemia.[18,31] Hypertension in these patients could reflect ischemia of the brain stem and may be necessary to maintain brainstem perfusion.

Surgical Treatment

The surgical management of patients with vertebrobasilar insufficiency has been a matter of great controversy since Crawford et al[15] reported the surgical approach to lesions of the extracranial vertebral artery in 1958. The initial surgical procedures,[18,19,22] including vertebral endarterectomy through the vertebral artery wall or through the subclavian artery,[22] were poorly received because they were associated with many complications including occlusion of the vertebral artery, postoperative hematomas, phrenic nerve paresis, lymphoceles, chyle fistulae, and others. It was not until the early 1970s that Edwards and Wright[19] reported a successful series of extracranial vertebral artery reconstructions for the treatment of patients with vertebrobasilar insufficiency.

Several procecures are currently in use to treat extracranial vertebral artery lesions. The most common is the transposition of the vertebral artery from its origin to a new location, generally the ipsilateral common carotid artery (Figure 4).[9,10,18,19] The vertebral artery is exposed through a supraclavicular incision placed 2 centimeters above the clavicle and just across the midline. The vertebral artery can be found easily by dissecting medial to the sternocleidomastoid muscle, first exposing the common carotid artery. The vertebral artery can be found as it travels from its origin to the foramen transversarium of C6, lateral to the longus coli muscle, medial to the anterior scalene muscle, and deep to the vertebral vein and sympathetic chain. Sufficient length of vertebral artery may be gained for an anastomosis by dissecting the entire vertebral artery from its origin to the foramen transversarium. The vertebral artery is transected after it has been ligated at its origin and temporarily clipped at the foramen transversarium. A fish-mouth stoma is prepared on the free end of the vertebral artery, and the common carotid artery is then clamped proximally and distally. A fenestration is made on the lateral wall of the carotid artery and an end-to-side anastomosis is completed under magnification between the vertebral and the common carotid arteries.

In cases of subclavian steal syndrome secondary to a subclavian artery occlusion, transposition of the subclavian artery to the common carotid artery has been performed.[19]

This procedure is preferable to the vertebral-to-carotid transposition, only in those patients who have intermittent claudication of the upper extermity. Other angioplastic procedures include patch graft of the vertebral artery origin with removal of the atherosclerotic plaque or angioplastic reconstruction, which widens and shortens the vertebral

Figure 4. (A) Technique of vertebral artery-to-common carotid artery transposition for proximal vertebral artery stenosis. (B) Typical case of symptomatic right vertebral artery stenosis amenable to such procedure. (C) Postoperative angiogram showing antegrade filling of the transposed vertebral artery on right common carotid injection. The metal clip marks the proximal stump of the vertebral artery. (Figure supplied courtesy of R.F. Spetzler, Barrow Neurological Institute.)

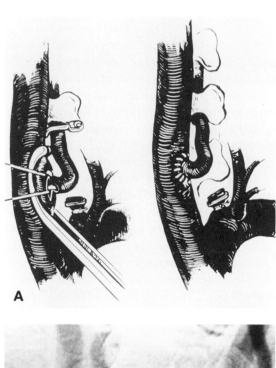

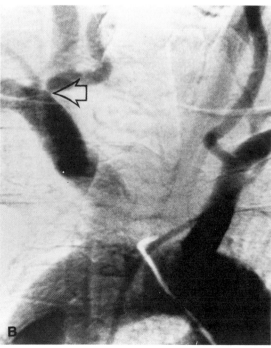

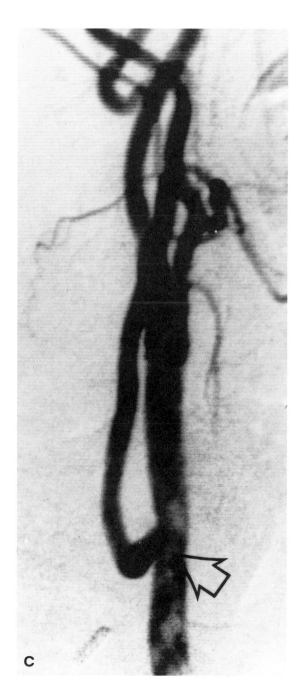

artery in cases of poststenotic ectasia of the first portion of the artery.[22] Saphenous vein grafts and prosthetic grafts have also been made from the subclavian artery to the vertebral artery or from the common carotid to the vertebral artery distal to the area of stenosis.[8,17] Balloon angioplasties have been performed successfully, but nearly 35% of cases have recurrence within the first 6 months postangioplasty.

Decompressive procedures have been used to treat lesions in the second portion of the vertebral artery. Fibrous bands originating from the anterior scalene muscle can easily be released at the level of entry of the vertebral artery into the C6 foramen.[14,18,22] Decompressive osteotomies of the foramina transversaria can be performed at single or multiple levels throughout the course of the vertebral artery from C6-C1 foramina via an anterior or lateral route.[20,33] When the foramina are removed for decompression, it is necessary to remove the periosteum surrounding the vertebral artery, since areas of constriction could persist if it is not removed.

Vascular reconstruction using a long saphenous vein graft or prosthetic graft from the subclavian or from the common carotid artery to the vertebral artery distal to the point of stenosis has also been reported.[13,14] Anastomosis of a branch or of the trunk of the external carotid artery to the second portion of the vertebral artery is an alternative bypass procedure for supply of blood distal to a stenotic area in the vertebral artery.[14,28] To accomplish this procedure, the anterior surfaces of one or two of the foramina above the level of stenosis are exposed through an anterior incision placed along the sternocleidomastoid muscle. The common carotid and the bifurcation are dissected in the usual manner and retracted laterally to expose the deep cervical fascia. The transverse processes are identified and the longus coli muscle is dissected off the anterior surface of the transverse process. The anterior and lateral walls of the transverse processes are removed and the periosteum adjacent to the vertebral artery canal is resected. The venous plexus surrounding the vertebral artery is carefully separated, cauterized, and transected to expose the vertebral artery. It is generally necessary to remove two or three foramina to expose enough of the vertebral artery. When the vertebral artery is free, a clamp may be placed at either end, and a longitudinal arteriotomy may be performed. The external carotid branch or the graft can then be anastomosed end-to-side to the dissected vertebral artery.

For arteriosclerotic lesions in the first or second foraminal level of the vertebral artery, it is sometimes possible to perform an anastomosis of the occipital artery or a saphenous vein graft to the third portion of the vertebral artery. The vertebral artery is exposed through an anterolateral incision that extends from the anterior border of the sternocleidomastoid muscle below the angle of the jaw, to the highest point of the mastoid bone, along the path of the external occipital artery. The vertebral artery is exposed through an anterolateral incision that extends from the anterior border of the sternocleidomatoid muscle below the angle of the jaw, to the highest point of the mastoid bone, along the path of the external occipital artery. The mastoid attachment of the muscle is transected and the posterior portion of the digastric is disinserted, to expose the external occipital artery. The superior and inferior oblique muscles are transected at the level of the lateral mass of C1 as the vertebral artery exits from the foramen. The vertebral artery is freed of the surrounding vertebral venous plexus and dissected from the foramen transversarium of C1 to its entrance into the skull at the atlanto-occipital membrane. If the segment of vertebral artery dissected is not enough for the anastomosis, the atlanto-occipital membrane and dura mater may be opened to expose the fourth position of the vertebral artery. Temporary clips are applied at the most proximal and distal ends of the vertebral artery, a longitudinal arteriotomy is performed, and an end-to-side anastomosis or a saphenous vein graft is completed with the occipital artery.

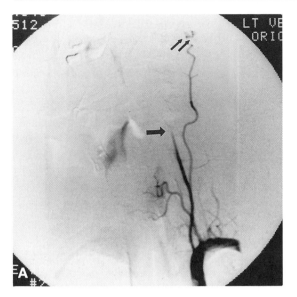
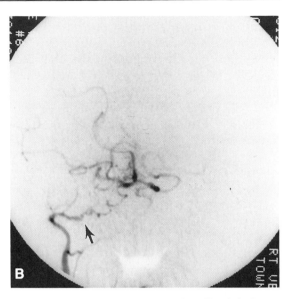

Figure 5. A 65-year-old diabetic hypertensive male who presented with recurrent stereotyped spells of diplopia, dysarthria, and drop attacks precipitated by upright posture. (A) Left subclavian angiogram shows occlusion of the left vertebral artery at its midportion (single arrow); ascending cervical muscular collaterals appear to fill the cerebellar circulation faintly via transdural collateralization (double arrows). (B) Right vertebral angiogram shows occlusion of that vessel as well, just distal to the posterior inferior cerebellar artery (arrow); the latter artery fills the more rostral vertebrobasilar circulation via leptomeningeal collaterals. The patient has remained asymptomatic for 25 months on anticoagulant therapy and liberalization of hypertension control (to 160-180 mmHg). Should he fail medical therapy, this patient would be an excellent candidate for occipital artery-to-posterior inferior cerebellar artery bypass. (Figure supplied courtesy of I.A. Awad, MD, The Cleveland Clinic Foundation.)

Vertebral artery endarterectomies have been performed to treat stenotic lesions of the third and fourth portions of the vertebral artery by Allen et al[1] and Ausman et al.[4] Sundt[35] also attempted balloon dilatation of the distal vertebral artery under direct observation. The results of endarterectomy were initially promising, but on subsequent evaluation many complications arose, like those experienced by Sundt during balloon angioplasties. Neither endarterectomy nor angioplasty of the distal vertebral artery are recommended now.

For bilateral occlusion or high-grade stenosis of the distal vertebral artery (Figure 5), various forms of extracranial-to-intracranial anastomosis have been described. The occipital artery (OA) may be anastomosed to the postmedullary portion of the posterior-inferior cerebellar artery (PICA).[6,7,23,30] The occipital artery is dissected with the patient in the lateral position, from the level of the mastoid process to the inion. A lateral suboccipital craniectomy is then performed and the postmedullary portion of PICA is dissected to free it from the area of the lateral medulla. This portion of PICA is generally free of any branches to the brain stem and can be temporarily clamped for an anastomosis. The OA is clamped proximally, the distal end is cleaned of periadventitial tissue, and a fish-mouth end is fashioned on its most distal portion. A longitudinal arteriotomy is performed on the segment of PICA that has been dissected and clamped, and an end-to-side anastomosis is completed from the occipital artery to the PICA. For occlusive lesions of the vertebrobasilar junction, an anastomosis of the occipital artery to the second portion of the anterior inferior cerebellar artery (AICA) may be performed.[2] The procedure is essentially the same as the one described for OA-PICA anastomosis regarding the position, dissection of the OA, and suboccipital craniectomy, but the dissection of the AICA is performed on the anterior surface of the cerebellum just lateral to the foramen of Luschka. The rostral and caudal branches of AICA may be found at that level, and there are usually no branches to the brain stem or the cerebellum at that point. The largest of the two branches is dissected and isolated, and an anastomosis of this occipital artery to AICA may then be completed in the same manner described for the OA-PICA anastomosis.

Other bypass procedures for the vertebrobasilar circulation, which have been used predominantly for mid- and distal basilar artery stenosis, but which have also been applied more proximal lesions, include superficial temporal artery (STA) and superior cerebellar artery (SCA) anastomosis. With the patient in the supine position and with the ipsilateral shoulder elevated, the head is placed flat on the table and rotated to the opposite side. The largest branch of the STA is dissected and a craniotomy is placed centered on the ear, with its inferior margin level with the floor of the middle fossa. The temporal lobe is elevated, preserving the posterior temporal lobe veins draining into the transverse sinus. The tentorial edge is identified and the tentorium is incised from the tentorial incisura, behind the point of penetration of the fourth cranial nerve, towards the lateral cranial wall. The two tentorial flaps are elevated and fixed to the dural base, exposing the circum-mesencephalic cistern, the cerebral peduncles and the superior cerebellar arteries. The larger of the two SCA branches is dissected as it nears the anterior border of the cerebellum, where there are no branches to the brain stem. The distal end of the STA is then prepared in the same manner described for the OA anastomosis, taking care to leave enough so that the STA reaches the level of the cerebral peduncles. Twelve to fifteen centimeters of STA are usually required to complete the anastomosis without tension. Temporary clips are then applied to the SCA, a longitudinal arteriotomy is completed, and an end-to-side anastomosis is performed from the STA to the SCA.

The superficial temporal artery may also be anastomosed to the posterior cerebral artery (PCA).[3,34,36] The procedure is essentially the same as the one described for the STA-SCA anastomosis, but it requires more retraction of the temporal lobe because the PCA is somewhat higher than the superior cerebellar artery, and enters the posterior interhemispheric fissure soon after it passes the posterolateral margin of the cerebral peduncle. The STA-PCA anastomosis is more risky because it requires temporary occlusion of the arterial supply to the visual cortex. An interposition reversed saphenous vein segment may be grafted from the extracranial carotid artery (or its branches) to the PCA[36] or to the SCA.[34,36] The vein graft is obtained from the leg. It must be handled carefully so that the graft is oriented properly when the anastomoses are completed, since these grafts have a greater tendency to become occluded than artery-to-artery grafts.

All these surgical approaches have been designed to treat patients with symptoms suggestive of vertebrobasilar insufficiency, for whom the best available medical therapy has failed, and who have a specific arterial lesion demonstrated by selective cerebral angiography compatable with their clinical picture. However, no attempt has been made to assign patients to a randomized controlled study.

The surgical results have been encouraging for those patients who have had an extracranial reconstructive procedure of the vertebral artery, with a neurologic morbidity of 2% and mortality of 1%, as reported by Diaz and Ausman.[16] The intracranial reconstructive procedures, including angioplasties of the fourth portion of the vertebral artery, and all types of extracranial-to-intracranial anastomoses have had a greater number of complications. Ausman and Diaz[5] reported that the safest procedure overall is the STA-SCA anastomosis, followed by the OA-PICA anastomosis. The highest number of complications were observed in patients who had unstable neurologic syndromes with signs of progressing ischemia or stroke in evolution.

Summary

Since symptoms suggestive of vertebrobasilar insufficiency may reflect a variety of pathoetiologic mechanisms, it is necessary to establish an accurate diagnosis before a treatment modality is chosen. Differential diagnostic possibilities include vascular and nonvascular pathologies that should be considered before treatment is begun. The natural histories of patients with symptomatic vertebrobasilar insufficiency and arteriosclerotic lesions of the vertebrobasilar tree have not been well delineated. Available information indicates that the stroke risk for untreated patients with symptomatic vertebral basilar ischemia is 35% within 4 years of the onset of symptoms.[37] Risk of stroke decreased to 15% in symptomatic patients treated with anticoagulants,[37] although there was no angiographic proof that these patients had significant arterial lesions compatible with their symptomatology. The surgical morbidity for patients with angiographically proven, significant vertebral or basilar artery lesions is reported to be 5% and surgical mortality is 3%.[53,17] However, there has been no randomized controlled study of medically treated versus surgically treated patients. Further study of the natural histories of these patients, along with well-controlled randomized comparisons of medical and surgical treatment, should solve the current problem of choosing a specific therapy for patients with vertebrobasilar ischemia.

References

1. Allen GS, Cohen RJ, Preziosi TJ. Microsurgical endarterectomy of the intracranial vertebral artery for vertebrobasilar transient ischemic attacks. *Neurosurgery*. 1981;8:56-59.
2. Ausman JI, Diaz FG, de los Reyes RA, et al. Anastomosis of occipital artery to anterior inferior cerebellar artery for vertebrobasilar junction stenosis. *Surg Neurol*. 1981;16:99-102.
3. Ausman JI, Diaz FG, de los Reyes RA, et al. Microsurgical techniques in cerebral revascularization. *Henry Ford Hosp Med J*. 1983;31:125-132.
4. Ausman JI, Diaz FG, Pearce JE, et al. Endarterectomy of the vertebral artery from C2 to posterior inferior cerebellar artery intracranially. *Surg Neurol*. 1982;18:400-404.
5. Ausman JI, Diaz FG, Vacca DF, et al. Superficial temporal and occipital artery bypass pedicles to superior, anterior inferior, and posterior inferior cerebellar arteries for vertebrobasilar insufficiency. *J Neurosurg*. 1990;72:554-558.
6. Ausman JI, Lee MC, Klassen AC, et al. Stroke: What's new? Cerebral revascularization. *Minn Med*. 1976;59:223-227.
7. Ausman JI, Nicoloff DM, Chou SN. Posterior fossa revascularization: anastomosis of vertebral artery to PICA with interposed radial artery graft. *Surg Neurol*. 1978;9:238-286.
8. Berguer R, Bauer RB. Vertebral artery reconstruction: a successful technique in selecting patients. *Ann Surg*. 1981;193:441-447.
9. Bohmfalk GL, Storey JL, Brown WE, et al. Subclavian steal syndrome, I: Proximal vertebral to common carotid artery transposition in three patients, and historical view. *J Neurosurg*. 1979;51:628-640.
10. Bohmfalk GL, Storey JL, Brown WE, et al. Subclavian steal syndrome, II: Intraoperative vertebral artery blood flow measurement. *J Neurosurg*. 1979;51:641-643.
11. Caplan LR, Rosenbaum AE. Role of cerebral angiography in vertebrobasilar occlusive disease. *J Neurol Neurosurg Psychiatry*. 1975;38:601-612.
12. Cerebral Angiograph. In: Traveras JM, Wood EH, eds. *Diagnostic Neuroradiology*, 2nd ed. Baltimore, MD: The Williams & Wilkins Company; 1976:543-986.
13. Clark K, Perry MO. Carotid vertebral anastomosis: an alternate technic for repair of the subclavian steal syndrome. *Ann Surg*. 1966;163:414-416.
14. Corkill G, French BN, Michas C, et al. External carotid-vertebral artery anastomosis for a vertebrobasilar insufficiency. *Surg. Neurol*. 1977;7:109-115.
15. Crawford ES, DeBakey, ME, Fields WS. Roentgenographic diagnosis and surgical treatment of basilar artery insufficiency. *JAMA*. 1958;168:509-514.
16. Diaz FG, Ausman JI. Surgical therapy in vascular brainstem diseases. In: Hofferberth B, Brune GG, Sitzer G et al, eds. *Workshop on Vascular Brainstem Diseases*, Gütersloh Basel, New York, NY: Karger; 1990:270-281.
17. Diaz FG, Ausman JI, de los Reyes RA. et al. Surgical correction of lesions affecting the vertebral artery. *Surg Forum*. 1982;33:495-497.
18. Diaz FG, Ausman JI, de los Reyes, et al. Combined reconstruction of the vertebral and carotid artery in one single procedure. *Neurosurgery*. 1983;12:629-635.
19. Edwards WH, Wright R. A new surgical technique for relief for subclavian stenosis. *Hosp Pract*. March 1972;7:78-87.
20. Hardin C. Vertebral artery insufficiency produced by cervical osteoarthritic spurs. *Arch Surg*. 1965;90:629-633.
21. Hass WK, Fields WS, North RR, et al. Joint study of extracranial arterial occlusion, II: Arteriography, techniques, sites, and complications. *JAMA*. 1968;203:961-968.
22. Imparato AM. Surgery for extracranial cerebrovascular insufficiency. In Ransohoff, ed. *Neurosurgery*. Kisco, NY: Futura; 1979;14:1-38.
23. Khodadad G. Occipital artery-posterior inferior cerebellar artery anastomosis. *Surg Neurol*. 1976; 5:225-227.

24. Kubick CS, Adams RD. Occlusion of the basilar artery—a clinical and pathological study. *Brain.* 1946;69:73-121.

25. Millikan CH, Siekert RG. Studies in cerebrovascular disease, I: The syndrome of intermittent insufficiency of the basilar arterial system. *Mayo Clin Proc.* 1955;30:61-68.

26. Millikan CH, Siekert RG, Shick RM. Studies in cerebrovascular disease, III: the use of anticoagulant drugs in the treatment of insufficiency or thrombosis within the basilar arterial system. *Mayo Clin Proc.* 1955;30:116-126.

27. A new vascular syndrome—"The subclavian steal." *N Engl J Med.* 1961;265:912-913. Editorial.

28. Pritz MB, Chandler WF, Kindt GW. Vertebral artery disease: radiological evaluation, medical management, and microsurgical treatment. *Neurosurgery.* 1981;9:524-530.

29. Rosenwasser R, Delgado, T, Buckheit W. Cerebrovascular complications of closed neck and head trauma: injuries to the carotid artery. *Surg Rounds.* June 1983;6:56-65.

30. Roski RA, Spetzler RF, Hopkins LN. Occipital artery to posterior inferior cerebellar artery bypass for vertebrobasilar ischemia. *Neurosurgery.* 1982; 10:44-49.

31. Sahs AL, Hartman EC. *Fundamentals of Stroke Care.* Washington, DC: US Department of Health, Education and Welfare, Public Health Service, Health Resources Administration, Bureau of Health Planning and Development; 1976.

32. Schwartz CJ, Mitchell JRA. Atheroma of the carotid and vertebral arterial systems. *Br Med J.* 1961;2: 1057-1063.

33. Sheehan S, Bauer RB, Meyer JS. Vertebral artery compression in cervical spondylosis. *Neurology.* 1960;70:968-986.

34. Sundt TM Jr, Piepgras DG, Houser OW, et al. Interposition saphenous vein grafts for advanced occlusive disease and large aneurysms in the posterior circulation. *J Neurosurg.* 1982;56:205-215.

35. Sundt TM Jr, Smith HC, Campbell JK, et al. Transluminal angioplasty for basilar artery stenosis. *Mayo Clin Proc.* 1980;55:673-680.

36. Sundt TM Jr, Whisnant JP, Piepgras DG, et al. Intercranial bypass grafts for vertebrobasilar ischemia. *May Clin Proc.* 1978;53:12-18.

37. Whisnant JP, Cartlidge NEF, Elvebach LR. Carotid and vertebral-basilar transient ischemic attacks: effect of anticoagulants, hypertension, and cardiac disorders on survival and stroke occurrence—a population study. *Ann Neurol.* 1978;3:107-115.

CHAPTER 12

Extracranial-Intracranial Bypass Surgery: Current Indications and Techniques

Issam A. Awad, MD, MS, FACS

No subject in the field of cerebrovascular surgery has evoked more debate and controversy in the past decade than extracranial-intracranial (EC-IC) bypass surgery. Potential revascularization of the ischemic brain has been a subject of great appeal to neurosurgeons for many years. Technical difficulties preventing such a procedure were surmounted in the late 1960s with the successful application of microsurgical techniques to microvascular anastomosis.

In subsequent years, the procedure of superficial temporal artery to middle cerebral artery (STA-MCA) bypass gained increasing acceptance among neurosurgeons for a variety of indications associated with brain ischemia. In 1986, results of a major international cooperative trial failed to demonstrate any benefit of the procedure over medical therapy alone in commonly accepted indications.[25] Since then, there has been significant controversy about any indications and therapeutic merit of revascularization procedures in any clinical setting.

In this chapter, we review the background and rationale of EC-IC bypass surgery. We summarize the methodology, results, and clinical impact of the international EC-IC Bypass Study, including pathophysiologic implications, limitations, and methodologic lessons learned from that cooperative trial. Possible current indications for the procedure in light of available alternative therapies are explored along with the spectrum of surgical techniques for EC-IC bypass. We conclude with an overview of ethical considerations and future outlook regarding the procedure.

Background and Rationale

Focal brain ischemia results when regional cerebral blood flow (rCBF) in an area of the brain is insufficient to meet the regional metabolic demands of that area. Experimental studies have demonstrated consistent rCBF thresholds for functional impairment and structural integrity of neural tissue. Sustained rCBFs below these thresholds invariably result in neuronal dysfunction and tissue damage, respectively.[29] A variety of mechanisms contribute to brain ischemia from occlusive cerebrovascular disease. These include artery to artery embolism, progressive hemodynamic compromise, and small-vessel occlusive disease.[8,17,48,49,52] Up to 15% of patients with previous carotid transient ischemic attacks or minor stroke have vascular lesions that are inaccessible to conventional carotid endarterectomy and that might play a role in subsequent brain ischemia.[7,10,48,49] Although antiplatelet therapy has decreased incidence of subsequent stroke in these patients, progressive ischemic insults can still occur despite this therapy.[19,20] Direct measurements within MCA branches reveal markedly decreased perfusion pressures in many symptomatic patients with intracranial occlusive lesions.[20,46] The microsurgical creation of an EC-IC bypass in these patients is conceptually attractive as an alternative collateral channel and a conduit for additional blood flow.[5,21,27,31,35]

Since the introduction of EC-IC bypass surgery almost three decades ago, several large published series have confirmed low perioperative morbidity and mortality and high bypass patency rates.[1,4,15,33,45,47,51] Augmentation of rCBF has been documented in several studies[5,21,27,31,35] and seems more pronounced in regions with more profound ischemia[21,31]; however, the ability of EC-IC bypass surgery to favorably alter the natural history of ischemic cerebrovascular disease remained in question.[11]

A prospective randomized multicenter cooperative study, initiated in 1977, randomized 1,377 patients through 1982.[13,25,26] The findings of this study were published in 1985 and failed to confirm the hypothesis that the procedure prevents further symptomatic cerebral ischemia in patients with atherosclerotic internal carotid artery (ICA) occlusion, intracranial stenosis, or MCA disease.[25]

EC-IC Bypass Study

Surgical Indications Prior to EC-IC Bypass Study

The concept of "inaccessible vascular lesion" prevailed heavily in clinical practice in the years leading up to the EC-IC Bypass Study.[2,11,26,51] It referred to a vascular occlusive lesion that is not amenable to direct endarterectomy, either because of complete occlusion of the vessel or because of inaccessibility of the stenosis (intracranial arterial stenosis). Symptomatic brain ischemia in the setting of such lesions could not be relieved by surgical endarterectomy and direct restoration of vessel patency. It was felt that such patients would alternatively benefit from surgical revascularization of the territory of inaccessible occlusive lesions via bypass.

With the perfecting of techniques of the STA-MCA bypass, a consensus of indications

for such a procedure emerged.[2,11,13] Suitable candidates were thought to be patients with minor stroke or transient ischemia in the territory of an occluded cerebral artery, or in the setting of intracranial arterial stenosis. Asymptomatic patients with such lesions were thought to be unsuitable candidates because of the perceived benign natural history, whereas patients with more debilitating stroke were thought to present forbidding operative risks while not likely to benefit from further protection. The most common vascular lesions in the anterior circulation thought to be amenable to STA-MCA bypass included the ICA occlusion, the intracranial ICA stenosis, and the MCA stenosis or occlusion.

Surgical indications in the era prior to the results of the EC-IC bypass study rarely differentiated between symptoms at the time of an arterial occlusion from symptoms beyond a documented occlusion.[13,26] This would later prove to be a critical differentiation, since most symptomatic patients at the time of an arterial occlusion can go on to have no further symptoms beyond the documented occlusion. Furthermore, the majority of ischemic symptoms accompanying arterial occlusion are now understood to be thromboembolic in nature and seldom recur beyond the phase of unstable thrombosis within the acutely occluded vessel. Also, indications in that era rarely distinguished patients with documented hemodynamic compromise from other symptomatic patients with well-developed collateral channels. This resulted in bypass surgery in numerous patients with stroke from nonhemodynamic mechanisms ipsilateral to an arterial stenosis or occlusion, regardless of the relationship of brain ischemia to the large-vessel lesion. Indications for EC-IC bypass surgery rarely distinguished patients who may or may not have failed a previous trial of medical therapy including antiplatelet agents or anticoagulation.[13,26]

Methodology and Results

The study examined the role of STA-MCA bypass surgery in patients with ante-

All Fatal and Nonfatal Strokes

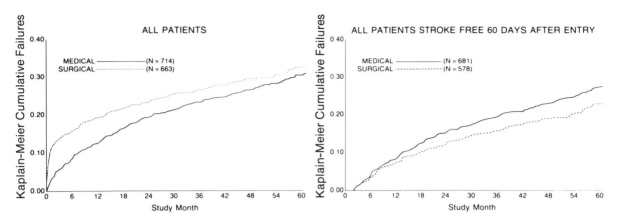

Figure 1. *Kaplan-Meier cumulative failure curves for all strokes (fatal and nonfatal) in the EC-IC Bypass Study. Left. All patients entered in the study. Note the higher rate of early morbidity and mortality in the surgical group who were stroke-free two months after entry. Note the lower rate of new events in the surgical group beyond the period of perioperative morbidity and mortality. (Data courtesy of the Statistical Center of the EC-IC Bypass Study Group furnished on request, March 1986. Reproduced from Awad and Spetzler.[6])*

rior circulation transient ischemia or minor infarction, and vascular lesions inaccessible to endarterectomy.[25,26] It accepted 1,377 patients between 1977 and 1982. Patients were assigned through stratified prospective randomization into two groups matched for age, sex, and clinical and angiographic parameters. One group (714 patients) received the best available medical therapy, essentially consisting of hypertension control and antiplatelet therapy with aspirin. The second group (663 patients) received similar medical therapy plus the EC-IC bypass operation. Crossover between the groups was minimal and bypass patency rates averaged 96%. The operative morbidity rate from ischemic events was 12.2%, the major stroke rate (fatal and nonfatal) was 3.1%, and the mortality rate was 0.6% in operated patients within 30 days of surgery. There was no difference in cumulative stroke rates or death rates between the two groups after an average follow-up of 5 years.[25]

No clinical or angiographic category showed a trend for surgical benefit in secondary analyses of the various subgroups, and the results were no different when ipsilateral or major ischemic events were examined separately.[12,25] Other attempts at further sub-

division of patients into groups with and without ophthalmic artery collaterals and groups with and without "prominent arterial filling via the bypass" also failed to reveal any significant benefit.[12,14] Among patients who were stroke-free 2 months after entry into the study (eliminating perioperative risks in the surgical group and time-matched morbidity in the medical group), there was a trend toward less fatal and nonfatal strokes in operated patients (Figure 1), although this trend did not reach statistical significance.[6,23] Patients operated on in Asian centers also showed a trend toward benefit with surgical intervention, although this trend was again not statistically significant.[12] Since patency rates were similar in Asian and non-Asian centers, such a trend toward better outcome in Asian centers was attributed by some investigators to a difference in the pathology of occlusive disease in Asian patients, whereas other investigators claimed that this was a spurious statistical finding not achieving any objective degree of significance.

It is important to emphasize that the EC-IC Bypass Study was not designed to assess, with statistical reliability, benefit or lack of benefit from the procedure in specific subgroups of patients.[1,6,23] The absence of benefit in secondary analyses of multiple clinical and angiographic categories is not statistically valid, given the study design and the numbers of patients in each category.

The study failed to reliably examine the benefit of the procedure in two particular groups of patients, which in retrospect would have been most likely to benefit from the procedure.[1,6,23] One group of patients not adequately addressed in the trial were those with clearly documented hemodynamic compromise.[7,49,53] Over one-third of the patients in the study had ICA occlusion without subsequent symptoms, whereas many others had hemodynamically insignificant lesions probably unrelated to ischemic symptoms. By including all patients with brain ischemia without regard to the pathophysiology of each subgroup, the study may have been diluted with a large number of patients who, by current understanding of the disease, would not have been suitable candidates for a revascularization procedure.[7] Another group of patients that should have been examined separately with statistical reliability consists of patients failing the best available medical therapy. Over 50% of the patients admitted to the study did not have a trial on medical therapy, even aspirin, prior to consideration for surgery. Patients who have no further symptoms on medical therapy may be less likely to require or benefit from additional revascularization than patients who have further brain ischemia despite antiplatelet therapy or anticoagulation.[6]

Given these observations, it is conceivable that a limited number of patients with clear hemodynamic compromise or failure of medical therapy, or both, may have benefitted from the procedure. The study was not designed to uncover benefit in such patients.[1,6,7,23]

Pathophysiologic Implications

The EC-IC Bypass Study clearly demonstrated that the indiscriminate use of EC-IC bypass surgery in brain ischemia was not justified.[6,12,14,25] Furthermore, it indicated that the prevailing indications for the procedures, i.e. transient ischemia or minor infarction associated with a so-called inaccessible lesion, were not appropriate. The failure of EC-IC bypass surgery in such patients has profound pathophysiologic implications.

Over the past few years, a more comprehensive view of the pathology of brain ischemia has emerged. Thromboembolism is now recognized as the major mechanism in most transient ischemic spells and minor strokes, whereas hemodynamic factors seem to be operating in a minority of cases.[7,10] Hemodynamic ischemic events can result from occlusive disease of large vessels in the absence of competent collateral pathways or from progressive small-vessel disease of perforating end vessels.[7,48,49,52] Often, multiple factors are operating simultaneously.[7] Also, the role of the ECA and the ICA stump as potential sources of ocular and cerebral emboli in patients with ICA occlusion is now better appreciated.[10] Patients with neurologic symptoms accompanying ICA occlusion (38% of the patients in the EC-IC Bypass Study) are now known to have a benign prognosis, with only a few patients suffering subsequent symptomatology. Ischemic symptoms accompanying ICA occlusion are often thromboembolic and are related to the unstable thrombus within the lumen of the occluded vessel.[8] The EC-IC Bypass Study confirmed that revascularization is of no benefit in such patients.

Patients with neurologic events after a known (previously documented) ICA occlusion (20% of patients in the study) are also a heterogenous group.[3,10,17] Many such patients have significant ECA disease or a prominent ICA stump, and excellent collateralization into the territory of the occluded ICA. In many such patients, there does not appear to be any hemodynamic compromise whatsoever, and further symptoms may be due to incidental small-vessel disease, disease in other vascular territories, or embolic sources in the collateral pathways. A minority of patients do appear to have significant hemodynamic compromise and inadequate collaterals.[6,7,49,53]

The benefit or lack of benefit of EC-IC bypass in such cases specifically has not been adequately studied.

The lack of benefit of EC-IC bypass surgery in patients with intracranial arterial stenoses may now be clearly explained pathophysiologically.[4] These lesions are often sources of microemboli to the eye or brain and are infrequently associated with decreased rCBF or cortical artery pressures.[21,45] Intracranial stenoses are dynamic lesions subject to spontaneous resolution, progression, or occlusion.[4] Furthermore, bypass surgery has been shown to promote symptomatic occlusion of such stenoses, whereas in other cases stenoses may resolve, making the need for bypass surgery obsolete.[4] In later years of the EC-IC Bypass Study but prior to publication of its final results, many investigators warned about the pitfalls of revascularization surgery in the setting of arterial stenoses.[4] Such investigators reserved surgery for cases with documented lesion progression on repeat angiography or persistence of symptoms despite anticoagulant therapy.

Several years after the publication of the results of the EC-IC bypass, there appears to be convincing pathophysiologic evidence why such revascularization surgery is not beneficial in the majority of symptomatic patients with so-called inaccessible occlusive lesions.[6,7]

Impact

The results of the EC-IC Bypass Study had an immediate and profound impact on the clinical management of cerebrovascular occlusive disease.[12] The practice of the procedure came to an immediate halt in community hospitals where it was estimated that hundreds of such procedures were heretofore performed yearly. In large academic cerebrovascular centers, the practice of the procedure fell off abruptly immediately following publication of the results of the EC-IC Bypass Study and diminished more gradually in subsequent years. It is estimated that no more than a handful of bypass procedures are currently performed each year by any one of a few large cerebrovascular centers in North America.

There are scientific and nonscientific reasons for such a profound impact of a single scientific study on clinical practice. The cooperative EC-IC Bypass Study was well planned, methodologically sound, and well executed.[38] Its scientific findings were clear, blunt, and indisputable: The EC-IC bypass procedure provides no benefit in the setting of prevailing indications.[25] The findings led many scientists and investigators to a thoughtful reexamination of pathophysiologic factors operating in brain ischemia and to a scientific rationale for the lack of surgical benefit (see preceding section). Clearly, the procedure had been overused, and the majority of patients thought to be surgical candidates would derive no benefit from it. This has led referring physicians, neurologists, and surgeons to spare numerous patients obviously needless operations.

Other nonscientific factors played a prominent role in magnifying the impact of the EC-IC Bypass Study. The 1980s were a decade of reexamination of the benefits of surgical procedures in a wide variety of settings.[38] Potential benefits of carotid endarterectomy were seriously questioned, and there were serious calls against any surgical intervention in cerebrovascular disease. Results of the EC-IC Bypass Study provided significant momentum for such arguments. Scientific debate of the findings of the EC-IC Bypass Study was discouraged, and surgeons who appeared to be struggling to defend the use of the procedure in a rare selected subgroup of patients were accused of "hanging on" to an obsolete and ineffective therapeutic modality.[12,14] Some hailed the bypass study as the end of an era of surgical intervention for cerebrovascular disease in general. Government and third-party payers rapidly capitalized on this antisurgical atmosphere and would refuse coverage for any revascularization surgery thereafter—even in the setting of indications not addressed by the EC-IC Bypass Study (recent decision by HCFA)!

Such powerful backlash effectively tended to polarize the issue and discourage rational scientific arguments. Cooperative prospective studies are often performed when major advances in the understanding of the disease, patient selection, and surgical techniques are taking place.[36,42] The impact of these advances is often not appreciated until sometime later. The first cooperative study on subarachnoid hemorrhage in the 1960s gave incorrect impressions about rebleeding times and rates and failed to detect a clear benefit from aneurysm surgery as practiced at that time.[43] Similarly, early studies on myocardial revascularization for stable angina failed to detect a benefit in the majority of patients.[37,50] Subsequent studies have placed these initial results in better perspective. Prospective collection of data in large registries allows the survey of a greater spectrum of patients. Although nonrandomized, this observational data base approach examines changes in medical and surgical therapy over time and has certain advantages over randomized trials.[30,36,42,50] No single study, no matter how well planned, methodologically perfect, and well executed, should be allowed to discard altogether a potentially beneficial treatment modality.[28,36] Similarly, the findings of an apparent benefit in a clinical trial should not be allowed to cause a backlash in the opposite direction, where the procedure would subsequently be recommended in an indiscriminate fashion.[28] Regardless of the methodologies, acceptance or rejection of a treatment modality, except in rare instances, should always be confirmed by multiple studies.[6,23,42,50] This is especially true in ischemic cerebrovascular disease, where the effectiveness of one agent such as aspirin in stroke prevention continues to be hotly debated despite several large collaborative trials using sound statistical methodology.[19,20]

A closer examination of the wide and complex spectrum of ischemic cerebrovascular disease and of the methodology of the trial would caution us against "discarding the baby with the bath water."[6,7,23,44] The EC-IC Bypass Study did not address hemodynamic cases or cases failing medical therapy in a statistically reliable fashion. The findings of

the study should not be extrapolated to these patients or to other secondary subgroups. There may be other indications for the procedure that have not been examined at all by this study. Despite the appropriate caution imposed on us by the findings of the study, outright rejection of the procedure for all indications is not scientifically justifiable.

Limitations and Methodologic Lessons

The EC-IC Bypass Study was truly a "remarkable piece of clinical investigation" with exemplary planning and nearly perfect execution.[38] The stratified randomization process effectively eliminated assignment bias and balanced the treatment groups for most patient characteristics.[13,26] Even though much effort was expended to attain objectivity in data collection and processing, several methodologic weaknesses persisted. It is recognized that most of these were not avoidable in a trial of this nature; however, these should be acknowledged and discussed because they may have affected the results of the study in unpredictable ways.[1,6,23] Some of these questions address the limitations of clinical trials in the evaluation of surgical procedures. The discipline of neurologic surgery had not faced these questions previously.

Lesson I: *A trial should be limited to patients thought likely to benefit from the procedure.*[1,6,7,23] Patients with ICA occlusion and no further symptoms represented 38% of cases entered into the trial. Several clinical studies have subsequently demonstrated an extremely low risk of stroke in this subgroup of patients. Similarly, patients without further symptoms on antiplatelet therapy accounted for over 50% of cases entered into the trial. This raised questions as to whether the trial should have included a large number of patients symptom-free on this very low-risk medication or should have instead been limited to cases failing medical therapy. At the very least, clinical trials should be stratified to allow the examination of such important factors in a statistically reliable fashion. This was not performed in the EC-IC Bypass Study. Overall, the trial was criticized for having been diluted with low-risk patients not likely to benefit from an operation so as to achieve a given sample size.[1,6,23]

Lesson II: *There should be a uniform consensus regarding what represents the "correct procedure."* Debate continues among neurologic surgeons regarding the use of a low-flow versus a high-flow bypass.[5,24,33] Also, there is continued disagreement about the advisability of using a direct anastomosis versus an interpositional vein graft, and whether the recipient artery should represent a small cortical artery or a larger, more proximal vessel. Other specific technical considerations regarding preoperative, intraoperative, and postoperative care might also have an impact on surgical outcome.[45] In summary, clinical trials should be stratified to allow for examination of therapeutic heterogeneity.

Lesson III: *The design of a trial should allow examination of benefit in patients who tolerate the procedure without immediate complications* (Figure 1). A number of patients suffered strokes prior to surgery and in the immediate postoperative period.[6,9] Other patients tolerated the procedure well. The risk of subsequent stroke in surgical patients who were stroke-free 60 days after randomization was lower than the risk of subsequent stroke in medical patients who were stroke-free after the same period (Figure 1).[6] This suggests some therapeutic benefit of the bypass procedure in patients who tolerated surgery without complications. Therapeutic benefit in some patients may be masked by perioperative morbidity in other patients.

Lesson IV: *A "surgery versus medicine" trial can minimize but can never eliminate "observational" bias and "randomization to treatment" bias.*[28,32] In such a trial, patient and therapists are never blinded. The identification, grading, and reporting of events are the responsibility of a party that should be clearly and objectively unbiased. In addition, there is the problem of patients randomized

to the surgical group who suffer complications prior to surgery. No statistically valid way exists dealing with these cases. There may be an argument to include these among the "medical complications." Study design should minimize the impact of such potential bias on eventual outcome to make it insignificant.

Lesson V: *Patients eventually entered into a trial may not be representative of the whole population of eligible cases.*[1,6,14,23] Many eligible patients do not undergo necessary diagnostic evaluation or referral because of physician bias, patient bias, therapeutic attitudes, misdiagnosis, or referral patterns. Some are treated medically because they are considered "not to be surgical candidates," whereas others are treated surgically outside the trial because they are felt to "need surgery." Other patients refuse randomization. The ongoing trial may affect referral and treatment patterns in a complex and unpredictable fashion. Patients randomized into the trial may represent a highly biased sample of eligible cases. The compliance of participating investigators is not the most important factor in this preselection bias. Studies should allow outcome monitoring of eligible cases not entered into a trial for any reason. Scientific methodology must be designed to verify that the sample studied is representative of the patient population eligible for the procedure.

Lesson VI: *Secondary analysis of multiple subgroups has no statistical merit when there is no significant difference in the sample at large.*[12,22,28,50] Stratified randomization does not guarantee equal distribution of all risk factors (especially unknown factors) in the medical and surgical subgroups. The significance level for any subgroup analysis should be more stringent (Bonferoni's principle). In most cases, there would not be a sufficient number of patients in each subgroup to reach a significant negative or positive conclusion. The suggestion that some subgroups may have fared significantly better or worse with surgery is invalid and misleading, since such significance was not demonstrated at the more stringent p-level. In summary, a clinical trial is designed to answer a single broad question. Subsequently, postquestions can seldom be accurately answered by the same trial.

Lesson VII: *A trial should have built-in plasticity to accommodate technical innovations and improved understanding of the disease.*[6] Several major clinical and technical advances occur during the execution of a clinical trial.[4,10,17] These advances could not be incorporated in an ongoing randomized trial; however, they altered attitudes toward patient selection and management during the study. An observational data base approach is more flexible in this regard.[36,42]

Lesson VIII: *A single therapeutic modality cannot be expected to be effective against widely different pathophysiologic mechanisms.*[7] It has become clear that ischemic cerebrovascular diseases are associated with a wide range of pathophysiologic heterogeneity in different patients. Bypass surgery is not expected to help patients with nonhemodynamic phenomena (e.g. thromboembolism, small end-vessel disease). Pathophysiologic heterogeneity dictates individualization of therapeutic options, and clinical trials should attempt to stratify the randomization process in accordance with this heterogeneity.[6,7] Unfortunately, many advances in the understanding of pathophysiology and in the identification of different pathophysiologic mechanisms may occur after the design or during execution of clinical trials.

These methodologic lessons are not mentioned to discredit in any way the findings of the EC-IC Bypass Study; however, clinical trials addressing surgical procedures on heterogenous disease processes do have significant methodologic limitations. These limitations should be understood and addressed in the design and interpretation of future clinical trials in neurologic surgery.[6,18,28] The surgical community should be educated about these limitations and should evaluate the results of trials accordingly.[18,32] Some of these limitations are inherent to the nature of clinical trials, surgical procedures, and management of surgical disease and cannot be avoided

altogether.[18,32] It is therefore imperative that a surgical procedure not be accredited or discredited totally based on a single clinical trial.

The design and execution of recently completed and ongoing carotid endarterectomy trials have taken in consideration most of these methodologic lessons. Stratification has been more stringent, and sample size has been estimated to allow meaningful statistical analysis of different subgroups. Also, a variety of trials were designed to be carried out more or less simultaneously, to provide confirmatory information. Last, more stringent criteria have been adopted for the monitoring of eligible nonrandomized patients and for the consideration of such patients in the final analysis and interpretation of data.

Current Indications
Atherosclerotic Occlusive Disease

In light of the EC-IC Bypass Study, symptomatic brain ischemia in the setting of so-called inaccessible occlusive lesions is clearly not sufficient indication for revascularization surgery.[25] In the setting of arterial occlusion, persistent symptoms should follow documentation of arterial occlusion. There should be clear evidence of hemodynamic compromise,[1,3,5,6,7,15,27,31,35,40,53] including the following:

1. Parenchymal infarction or ischemia in the border zone territory on imaging studies (computed tomography or magnetic resonance imaging).
2. Impaired physiologic collaterals (atretic or incompetent ophthalmic, anterior circle of Willis, or posterior circle of Willis collaterals).
3. Visualization of certain pathologic collaterals suggestive of severe chronic ischemia (e.g. moyamoya collaterals, retrograde leptomeningeal collaterals, transdural collaterals).
4. Demonstrated functional hypoperfusion by rCBF or metabolic measurements between spells.

In addition to the aforementioned evi-

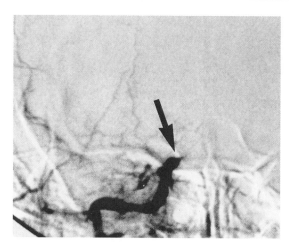

Figure 2. Twenty-three-year-old diabetic woman with progressive symptomatic basal occlusive disease. Right common carotid angiogram reveals occlusion of the distal internal carotid artery. The contralateral internal carotid artery was also occluded. (Reproduced from Awad and Spetzler.[6])

dence of hemodynamic compromise, patients should reasonably be given a *trial of all available medical therapy* prior to consideration for EC-IC bypass surgery.[6,7] This should include at the very least antiplatelet therapy and modification of risk factors. A trial of anticoagulant therapy should also be instituted unless contraindicated.

At the Cleveland Clinic Foundation, patients fulfilling the above criteria of *hemodynamic compromise* and *failure of medical therapy* are still offered the option of revascularization surgery. Such patients are presented with this option on the grounds that no clear scientific evidence supports a lack of benefit in this specific setting, and no other alternative therapies may be reasonably expected to offer benefit at the present time. Patients fulfilling all of these criteria are not commonly encountered. No more than a handful of such patients present to our center each year despite a very large volume of clinical practice in ischemic cerebrovascular disease.

In the setting of posterior circulation ischemia from atherosclerotic disease, we adopt similar criteria. It is important to recognize that there has been no controlled scientific

trial whatsoever of any therapeutic intervention for vertebrobasilar occlusive disease.

The strict criteria for revascularization surgery suggested above do not guarantee surgical benefit.[12,39] Patients with advanced ischemic symptoms of hemodynamic nature despite anticoagulant therapy may pose grave perioperative risks. The natural history in these patients may be such that surgical intervention may be of no benefit whatsoever[39]; however, in the absence of any alternative therapy that may be remotely effective, the option of revascularization surgery in this select subgroup is reasonable based on pathophysiologic rationale and published noncontrolled evidence of possible benefit.[6,15,21,23,31,35,47]

Nonatherosclerotic Occlusive Disease

Some nonatherosclerotic obstructive vasculopathies result in hemodynamic ischemic compromise to the cerebral circulation with progressive parenchymal infarction despite all available medical therapy. The most prevalent entity in this category is the so-called idiopathic basal occlusive disease or moyamoya disease.[41,45] The disease appears idiopathic in Japan and in other Asian countries but may be associated with known vascular risk factors including diabetes and hyperlipidemia in North American patients.[41,45] The disease involves occlusion of moderate-sized cerebral arteries at or near the circle of Willis (Figure 2). Such occlusive disease also compromises physiologic collateral pathways of the ophthalmic artery and the circle of Willis. Such occlusive basal vasculopathies are chronic and are accompanied by a pathologic attempt at collateralization, involving proliferation of arterioles and small penetrating arteries near the perforating substance. Such proliferation of deep collaterals provides the typical angiographic appearance of a "puff of smoke," hence the Japanese term *moyamoya*. There also may be other attempts at collateralization via transdural collateral channels, thereby providing a "natural" EC-IC bypass. Such pathologic collateralization is

seldom sufficient to prevent progressive parenchymal infarction.

Anticoagulation therapy has been shown
to be ineffective in moyamoya disease and
may predispose to hemorrhagic complications
from basal pathologic proliferative vessels.
These vessels are highly friable and are associated with subarachnoid and intracerebral
hemorrhage.[45]

Chronic ischemia has been shown to favor
the development of natural EC-IC collaterals
from muscle or omentum juxtaposed on the
surface of the brain. This has provided the
rationale for such procedures as encephalomyo-synangiosis or encephalo-omental-
synangiosis. These procedures have been
shown to encourage the development of natural EC-IC collaterals and may favorably alter
the course of progressive hemodynamic brain
ischemia; however, such synangiosis procedures would not be expected to provide
immediate revascularization in unstable patients with progressive symptoms of hemodynamic compromise. More conventional EC-
IC bypass surgery should be considered as an
adjunct to synangiosis procedures in such
cases.

The role of EC-IC bypass surgery for nonatherosclerotic occlusive disease has not been
addressed in any scientific study.

Planned Large-Vessel Occlusion

Planned large-vessel occlusion may be entertained as an adjunct to the treatment of base
of skull neoplasms or certain giant aneurysms.[34] Brain ischemia may complicate such
planned large-vessel occlusions and may result
from a variety of mechanisms. Propagating
thrombosis and thromboembolism may compromise vascular territories downstream by
obstructing previously competent physiologic
collateral pathways. Insufficient collaterals may
lead to hemodynamic compromise.

Gradual vessel occlusion in the awake
patient had been advocated on the grounds
that it may encourage the development of
collateral circulation and may be reversed at
the first sign of brain ischemia.[34] More re-

cently, we and others have advocated the
practice of endovascular trial occlusions in
the awake patient under full anticoagulation.
Monitoring of intracranial collateral circulation using transcranial Doppler or rCBF, or
both, may further enhance the safety of such
planned arterial occlusions.[34]

A subgroup of patients remains with insufficient hemodynamic collateral reserve who
do not tolerate planned arterial occlusion.
Prophylactic elective EC-IC bypass surgery
may allow safe arterial occlusion in such
patients.

It is our belief that prophylactic EC-IC
bypass surgery is not necessary in all planned
arterial occlusions.[34] At the Cleveland Clinic,
we perform trials of arterial occlusion using
an endovascular balloon under full anticoagulant therapy and under transcranial Doppler
monitoring of intracranial collaterals. In the
absence of clinical symptoms after arterial
occlusion for more than 15 minutes, and in
the presence of documented angiographic and
transcranial Doppler collaterals, permanent
occlusion of the vessel is performed without
revascularization surgery. Anticoagulation is
continued for at least 24 hours and is tapered
gradually to minimize the risk of thromboembolic complications from the acutely
occluded artery. Prophylactic EC-IC bypass
surgery is reserved for patients who do not
clinically tolerate arterial occlusion under
anticoagulation or who have demonstrably
impaired collateral circulation.

Chronic Cerebral Vasospasm

There have been anecdotal reports of EC-
IC bypass surgery reversing symptomatic brain
ischemia in the setting of chronic cerebral
vasospasm (following subarachnoid hemorrhage) that has been refractory to all other
medical measures.[16] The role of such heroic
intervention in this setting has not been
clearly defined. Furthermore, the timing of
revascularization surgery has not been clarified in relation to the development of parenchymal infarction on neuroimaging studies.
Also, there is no consensus opinion regarding

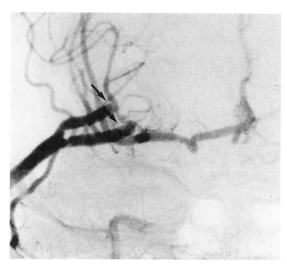

Figure 3. High-flow interpositional EC-IC saphenous vein graft with "double barrel" y-shaped anastomosis into MCA branches within the sylvian fissure. Note the high-flow revascularization of the whole right carotid territory via the graft. (Reproduced from Awad and Spetzler.[6])

the role of EC-IC bypass surgery versus balloon angioplasty or other investigational interventional approaches. In the absence of clear scientific evidence, much clinical judgment is needed in the management of individual clinical scenarios with progressive refractory clinical symptomatology.

Surgical Technique

Spectrum of Procedures

Cerebral revascularization surgery does not consist of a single uniform surgical procedure.[5,24,33,45] The spectrum of operations includes a variety of donor arteries in the extracranial circulation, a variety of anastomosis techniques, and a number of potential recipient vessels.

Donor vessels most commonly consist of the STA or its branches. These may be anastomosed directly to a cortical recipient vessel (see below) or via an interposed vein graft. Interpositional bypass procedures offer the advantage of higher-flow conduits and may be used even when the distal STA is occluded or diseased (Figure 3).[5,33] Other donor ves-

sels may be used in the setting of an occluded STA and include the internal or external carotid arteries in the neck, or even the subclavian artery (via long vein interpositional grafts). The occipital artery is conveniently useable for anastomosis to the posterior-inferior cerebellar artery (PICA) or anterior-inferior cerebellar artery (AICA) for posterior circulation ischemia.[45]

In anterior circulation ischemia, recipient vessels consist of a cortical branch of the MCA, most commonly an angular branch or a frontal branch. These typically have a diameter of 1-2 mm and can easily accommodate an end to side anastomosis of a STA branch of similar size (Figure 4). Higher-flow conduits for anterior circulation revascularization typically consist of an interpositional vein graft between the STA at the level of the zygoma and an M2 or M3 branch of the MCA within the sylvian fissure.[24]

In posterior circulation ischemia, the occipital artery or the STA (via a vein graft) is anastomosed to the PICA (for distal vertebral artery occlusions), to the AICA (for vertebrobasilar occlusive lesions distal to PICA), or to the posterior cerebral artery or superior cerebellar artery in the ambient cistern (for basilar occlusive lesions distal to the AICA).[45]

Figure 4. Diagram illustrating commonly used recipient cortical arteries for direct STA-MCA anastomosis. (Drawing courtesy of Robert F. Spetzler, MD.)

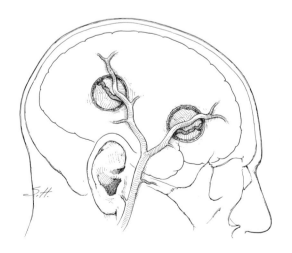

Superficial Temporal Artery to Middle Cerebral Artery Bypass Technique

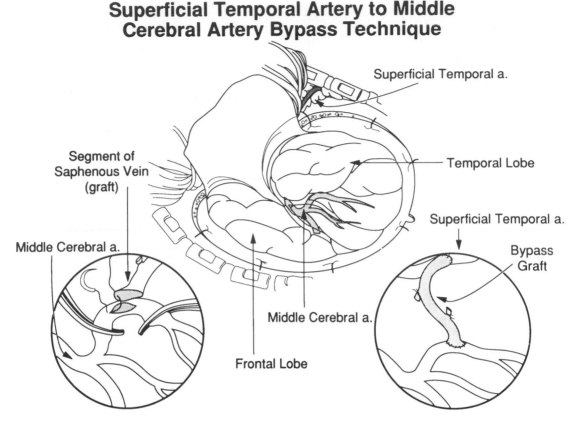

Figure 5. *Surgical technique of anterior circulation EC-IC bypass via short-vein graft from the STA at the zygoma to a main MCA branch within the sylvian fissure. This procedure is currently the most widely used by the Cerebrovascular Surgery Service at the Cleveland Clinic.*

Spectrum of Techniques

The precise choice of patient positioning, skin flap, craniectomy, and so forth is dictated by the particular bypass procedure to be performed (see previous discussion). For direct artery-to-artery anastomosis, the donor artery is mapped and marked using a transcutaneous ultrasound probe, and an incision is made along the course of the artery isolating as long a segment as is needed for anastomosis. A craniectomy is then performed over the proposed recipient artery, with a cruciate dural opening and direct arachnoidal opening over the proposed recipient artery (Figure 3). End-to-side arterial anastomosis is then performed between the donor and recipient arteries.

For interpositional vein graft EC-IC bypass procedures, a shorter segment of donor artery is exposed, preferably in line with the same incision to be used for exposure of the recipient artery. End to side artery to vein anastomosis is performed starting at the recipient vessel. A clip is then placed across the reversed vein graft segment that had been prefilled with heparinized saline, and flow is reestablished in the donor artery. A second artery to vein end to side anastomosis is performed at the donor artery, with subsequent reestablishment of flow in the donor artery and through the graft (Figure 4). Patency of the graft is easy to visualize by direct inspection and is confirmed by palpation. Tactile manipulation of a new bypass graft should be minimal to minimize endothelial injury and resulting thrombosis.

The end to side anastomosis remains the

cardinal technical procedure for all EC-IC bypass operations (Figure 5). It is performed by isolating the segment of artery between two atraumatic (temporary) vessel clips. Systemic heparinization is usually not necessary, but the lumen of the temporarily occluded vessel should be vigorously irrigated with heparinized saline. A longitudinal arteriotomy is performed, typically 2-3 mm in length. The end vessel (artery or vein) to be anastomosed is prepared by trimming its adventitia and fish mouthing it obliquely to create a stoma of comparable size to the arteriotomy in the side of the recipient artery. The actual end to side anastomosis may be performed using a continuous or interrupted microvascular suturing technique. Special 9-0 or 10-0 monofilament sutures are used with corresponding microvascular needles and needle holders and jeweler's forceps of varying lengths. An end to side anastomosis is typically completed in less than 30 minutes in experienced hands.

Hemostasis at the suture line is seldom a problem on reinstitution of flow, as long as precise suturing was performed at regular intervals. Mild oozing at the suture line can be stopped by the gentle application of a Gelfoam patty soaked in thrombin solution. Mechanical pressure on a fresh suture line should be avoided. Any vigorous bleeding at the suture line or any bleeding not arrested easily with the aforementioned technique should be stopped by the precise application of a single 10-0 suture at the bleeding point. Reclamping is rarely necessary unless bleeding is profuse.

Wound closure should ensure that no layer is causing any compromise whatsoever on the bypass graft. Dural leaflets are loosely approximated, or left open altogether. If a craniotomy flap was elevated (as opposed to a craniectomy), a window of bone should be created by rongeur in the flap to prevent any kinking or compression of the EC-IC bypass graft. Similarly, muscle and galeal closure should be done in such a way to ensure total freedom of the underlying graft. Extreme care should be undertaken during skin closure

to avoid injury to the underlying graft. Skin closure should be watertight in view of the wide opening in the underlying dura.

In cases where an encephalo-myo-synangiosis is performed in conjunction with an EC-IC bypass procedure, a flap of vascularized temporalis muscle is allowed to come in direct contact with the pial brain surface. This may be tacked to the edges of the dural leaflets. The underlying arachnoid membrane may be fenestrated to encourage more rapid synangiosis.

Recommended Technique of STA-MCA Bypass

The preferred procedure currently performed for anterior circulation EC-IC bypass at our institution interposes a reversed short segment of saphenous vein between the STA at the level of the zygoma (in an end to side fashion) to an M2 or M3 segment of the MCA within the sylvian fissure (also in an end to side fashion) (Figure 4).[24,33] This allows the creation of a high-flow conduit (see Figure 2B) with high short-term and long-term patency rates and an immediate measurable increase in rCBF in the ischemic vascular territory.[5] This procedure is associated with low operative morbidity in well-selected patients. It must be emphasized that this is one of many possible technical approaches to provide a bypass between the extracranial and intracranial circulations.

The STA is exposed at the level of the zygomatic arch after marking the skin by palpation of the STA pulse or by transcutaneous ultrasound localization. Microsurgical technique is used to isolate a segment of STA approximately 1.5 cm long. The overlying skin incision is then extended in a question mark fashion anteriorly. The skin and underlying temporalis muscle are turned as a unit anteriorly and inferiorly, making sure not to injure the isolated STA segment. A small pterional free bone craniotomy flap is then elevated and centered on the pterion, thereby exposing the sylvian region. The sylvian dura is opened in a Y-shaped fashion and the dural leaflets are flapped so as to expose the underlying sylvian fissure. The sylvian fissure is opened using microsurgical techniques, and a frontal opercular M4 branch is followed proximally into the sylvian fissure until the MCA bifurcation is visualized. A segment of M2 or M3 vessel is then identified as a recipient artery. The precise choice of recipient artery in this region depends on the region of the brain most in need of revascularization (e.g. frontal versus temporal, anterior versus posterior). The precise techniques of anastomosis have been discussed before. This recommended procedure is illustrated in Figure 4.

Ethical Considerations and Future Outlook

Conflicting ethical considerations surround the use of EC-IC bypass surgery in the era following the bypass study. On the one hand, each patient must be informed that the procedure has never been shown to be effective in a scientific study. Patients with atherosclerotic occlusive disease must be informed in lay terms about the general findings of the EC-IC Bypass Study. The patient must be presented with a clear rationale why he or she may still be considered a candidate for the procedure despite these findings.

A consensus among many cerebrovascular surgeons and neurologists is that a small group of patients with arterial occlusive disease, impaired collaterals, and clearly demonstrated progressive symptomatic ischemia despite anticoagulant therapy may benefit from revascularization surgery despite the findings of the EC-IC Bypass Study.[1,6,23] Two strict criteria must be met to justify a bypass procedure in such cases: (1) demonstrated hemodynamic compromise (severely impaired collaterals and preferably a confirmatory study demonstrating rCBF compromise), and (2) failure of optimal medical therapy.

From an ethical perspective, it is also important to inform patients falling in this category that the EC-IC Bypass Study was not designed to examine effectiveness of the procedure in their specific clinical situation; however, we should not be inclined to imply that bypass surgery has been shown to be effective in this setting. The question of possible effectiveness of EC-IC bypass surgery in the setting of clear intractable hemodynamic compromise despite medical therapy has not been settled scientifically.[30]

In the absence of an alternative effective medical therapy or clear evidence that EC-IC bypass surgery is not helpful, we have felt it ethically unjustified in our center to arbitrarily deny such patients bypass surgery altogether. In individualized clinical situations, which are effectively quite rare, we obtain convergent multidisciplinary opinions including those of a neurology consultant and a neurosurgeon. In addition, the patient and referring primary physician are clearly informed about the controversies and available options. They are informed that third-party payers may or may not agree with our joint decision to proceed with the procedure. We believe that these conditions constitute a truly informed consent, which takes into consideration all information available at the present time.

A similar cautious and exhaustive preparation is undertaken prior to considering EC-IC bypass surgery for any other indication, including nonatherosclerotic disease, planned artery occlusion (with failure of temporary occlusion tests), and chronic vasospasm.

It is obvious in any of the aforementioned situations that the operating surgeon is responsible for demonstrating that (1) the patient is likely to deteriorate further without EC-IC bypass surgery, and (2) all alternative treatment measures have been exhausted and have failed.

Cases fulfilling the strict criteria listed here will likely continue to be rare. Such cases will also likely reflect the end stage in the spectrum of the disease of hemodynamic ischemia and carry an inherently worse prognosis. In view of limited numbers of patients in these special clinical scenarios, it is unlikely that benefit of EC-IC bypass surgery will be demonstrated scientifically in a controlled setting. The procedure will probably remain, for the foreseeable future, at large, experienced cerebrovascular centers a last-resort attempt to improve hemodynamic ischemia in a handful of patients failing all other therapeutic measures.

References

1. Ausman JI, Diaz FG. Critique of the extracranial-intracranial bypass study. *Surg Neurol.* 1986;26:218-221.
2. Austin G, Laffin D, Hayward W. Physiologic factors in the superficial temporal artery-to-middle cerebral artery selection of patients for anastomosis. *Surgery.* 1974;75:861-868.
3. Awad I, Little JR, Modic MT, et al. Intravenous digital subtraction angiography: an index of collateral cerebral blood flow in internal carotid artery occlusion. *Stroke.* 1982;13:469-472.
4. Awad IA, Furlan AJ, Little JR. Changes in intracranial stenotic lesions after extracranial-intracranial bypass surgery. *J Neurosurg.* 1984;60:771-776.
5. Awad IA, Little JR, Bryerton B, et al. Regional cerebral blood flow in extracranial-intracranial bypass surgery. *J Cereb Blood Flow Metab.* 1983;3:S596-597.
6. Awad IA, Spetzler RF. Extracranial-intracranial bypass surgery: a critical analysis in light of the international cooperative study. *Neurosurgery.* 1986;19:655-664.
7. Awad IA, Spetzler RF, Liu SS. Pathophysiology of ischemic symptoms in patients with lesions amenable to EC-IC bypass surgery. In: Gagliardi G, Benvenuti L, eds. *Controversies in EIAB for Cerebral Ischemia.* Monduzzi Editore; 1988:73-78.
8. Balow J, Alter M, Resch JA. Cerebral thromboembolism: a clinical appraisal of 100 cases. *Neurology.* 1966;16:559-564.
9. Barba D, Peerless SJ. The international cooperative study of extracranial to intracranial anastomosis (EC-IC bypass study): surgical complications. *Stroke.* 1986;17:142. Abstract.
10. Barnett HJM. Delayed cerebral ischemic episodes distal to occlusion of major cerebral arteries. *Neurology.* 1978;28:769-774.
11. Barnett HJM. Is there a place for cerebral revascularization? *Clin Neurosurg.* 1979;26:314-329.
12. Barnett HJM, Fox A, Hachinski V, et al. Further conclusions from the extracranial-intracranial bypass trial. *Surg Neurol.* 1986;26:227-235.
13. Barnett HJM, McCormick CW. The collaborative study on STA-MCA anastomosis: a progress report. *Surg Neurol.* 1980;13:409-412.
14. Barnett HJM, Sackett D, Taylor DW, et al. Are the results of the extracranial-intracranial bypass trial generalizable? *N Engl J Med.* 1987;316:820-824.
15. Baron JC, Bousser MG, Rey A, et al. Reversal of focal "misery-perfusion syndrome" by extracranial-intracranial arterial bypass in hemodynamic cerebral ischemia. A case study with ^{15}o-positron emission tomography. *Stroke.* 1981;12:454-459.
16. Batjer H, Samson D. Use of extracranial-intracranial bypass in the management of symptomatic vasospasm. *Neurosurgery.* 1986;19:235-246.
17. Bogousslavsky J, Regli F, Hungerbühler J-P, et al. Transient ischemic attacks and external carotid artery. *Stroke.* 1981;12:627-630.
18. Bonchek LI. Are randomized trials appropriate for evaluating new operations? *N Engl J Med.* 1979;301:44-45.
19. Britton M, Helmers C, Samuelson K. High dose acetylsalicylic acid after cerebral infarction: a Swedish cooperative study. *Stroke.* 1986;17:132. Abstract.
20. The Canadian Cooperative Study Group. A randomized trial of aspirin and sulfinpyraxone in threatened stroke. *N Engl J Med.* 1978;299:53-59.
21. Carter LP, Hadley MN, Spetzler RF. Regional cortical blood flow during extracranial-intracranial bypass. In: Spetzler RF, Carter LP, Selman WR, et al. eds. *Cerebral Revascularization for Stroke.* New York, NY: Thieme-Stratton Inc; 1985:136-142.
22. David HA. *Order Statistics.* New York, NY: John Wiley & Sons;1970.
23. Day AL, Rhoton AL Jr, Little JR. The extracranial-intracranial bypass study. *Surg Neurol.* 1986;26:222-226.
24. Diaz FG, Umansky F, Mehta B, et al. Cerebral revascularization to a main limb of the middle cerebral artery in the sylvian fissure. *J Neurosurg.* 1985;63:21-29.
25. The EC/IC Bypass Study Group. Failure of extracranial-intracranial arterial bypass to reduce the risk of ischemic stroke: results of an international randomized trial. *N Engl J Med.* 1985;313:1191-1200.
26. The EC/IC Bypass Study Group. The international cooperative study of extracranial/intracranial arterial anastomosis (EC/IC bypass study): methodology and entry characteristics. *Stroke.* 1985;16:397-406.
27. Gibbs JM, Wise RJS, Thomas DJ, et al. Cerebral hemodynamic changes after extracranial-intracranial bypass surgery. *J Neurol Neurosurg Psychiatry.* 1987;50:140-150.
28. Haines SJ. Randomized clinical trials in the evaluation of surgical innovation. *J Neurosurg.* 1979;51:5-11.
29. Jones TH, Morawetz RB, Crowell RM, et al. Thresholds of focal cerebral ischemia in awake monkeys. *J Neurosurg.* 1981;54:773-782.
30. Kassell NF, Torner JC. The international cooperative study on timing of aneurysm surgery—an update. *Stroke.* 1984;15:566-570.
31. Leblanc R, Tyler JL, Mohr G, et al. Hemodynamic and metabolic effects of cerebral revascularization. *J Neurosurg.* 1987;66:529-535.
32. Lee KL, McNeer JF, Starmer CF, et al. Clinical judgment and statistics: lessons from a simulated randomized trial in coronary artery disease. *Circulation.* 1980;61:508-515.
33. Little JR, Furlan AJ, Bryerton B. Short vein grafts for cerebral revascularization. *J Neurosurg.* 1983;59:384-388.
34. Little JR, Rosenfeld JV, Awad IA. Internal carotid artery occlusion for cavernous segment aneurysm. *Neurosurgery.* 1989;25:398-404.
35. Little JR, Yamamoto YL, Feindel W, et al. Cerebral blood flow in superficial temporal artery to middle cerebral artery anastomosis. In: Peerless SJ, McCormick CW, eds. *Microsurgery for Cerebral Ischemia.* New York, NY: Springer-Verlag;1980:59-66.

36. Mohr JP. Stroke data banks. *Stroke.* 1986;17:171-172.
37. Murphy ML, Hultgren HN, Detre K, et al. Treatment of chronic stable angina. A preliminary report of survival data of the randomized Veterans Administration cooperative study. *N Engl J Med.* 1977; 297:621-627.
38. Plum F. Extracranial-intracranial arterial bypass and cerebral vascular disease. *N Engl J Med.* 1977;297: 621-627. Editorial.
39. Powers WJ, Grubb RL Jr, Raichle ME. Clinical results of extracranial-intracranial bypass surgery in patients with hemodynamic cerebrovascular disease. *J Neurosurg.* 1989;70:61-67.
40. Powers WJ, Press GA, Grubb RL Jr, et al. The effect of hemodynamically significant carotid artery disease on the hemodynamic status of the cerebral circulation. *Ann Intern Med.* 1987;106:27-35.
41. Quest DO, Correll JW. Basal arterial occlusive disease. *Neurosurgery.* 1985;17:937-941.
42. Rosati RA, Lee KL, Califf RM, et al. Problems and advantages of an observational data base approach to evaluating the effect of therapy on outcome. *Circulation.* 1982;65 (Suppl 2):II-27-I-32.
43. Sahs AL, Perret GE, Locksley HB, et al. eds. *Intracranial Aneurysms and Subarachnoid Hemorrhage: A Cooperative Study.* Philadelphia, PA: J.B. Lippincott Company; 1969.
44. Spetzler RF. *BNI Quarterly.* 1985;1:1-2. Editorial.
45. Spetzler RF, Carter LP, Selman WR, et al. *Cerebral Revascularization for Stroke.* New York, NY: Thieme-Stratton, Inc; 1985.
46. Spetzler RF, Roski RA, Zabramski J. Middle cerebral artery perfusion pressure in cerebrovascular occlusive disease. *Stroke.* 1983;14:552-555.
47. Sundt TM Jr, Whisnant JP, Fode NC, et al. Results, complications, and follow-up of 415 bypass operations for occlusive disease of the carotid system. *Mayo Clin Proc.* 1985;60:230-240.
48. Transient ischemic attacks. In: Toole JF, ed. *Cerebrovascular Disorders.* New York, NY: Raven Press; 1984:101-116.
49. Vorstrup S, Paulson OB, Lassen NA. How to identify hemodynamic cases. In: Spetzler RF, Carter LP, Selman WR, et al, eds. *Cerebral Revascularization for Stroke.* New York, NY: Thieme-Stratton, Inc; 1985:120-126.
50. Ware JH. Comparison of medical and surgical management of coronary artery disease: methodologic issues. *Circulation.* 1982;65: (suppl 2):II-32-II-36.
51. Weinstein PR, Rodriguez y Baena R, Chater NL. Results of extracranial-intracranial arterial bypass for intracranial internal carotid artery stenosis: review of 105 cases. *Neurosurgery.* 1984;15:787-794.
52. Wodarz R. Watershed infarctions and computed tomography: a topographical study in cases with stenosis or occlusion of the carotid artery. *Neuroradiology.* 1980;19:245-248.
53. Yonas H, Gur BC, Good BC, et al. Stable xenon CT blood flow mapping for evaluation of patients with extracranial-intracranial bypass surgery. *J Neurosurg.* 1985;62:324-339.

CHAPTER 13

Endovascular Thrombolysis and Angioplasty

Bruce Mackay, MD

The success of thrombolytic agents in the treatment of myocardial infarction, pulmonary embolus and deep venous thrombosis motivated stroke investigators to evaluate this form of treatment in acute stroke patients. In uncontrolled studies the initial impressions on their efficacy and safety has been quite favorable. The next step, now in progress, is to subject this treatment to randomized, controlled trials of sufficient size and rigor to establish whether the initial impressions are valid. Several excellent recent reviews offer further background details.[6,29,97,98]

Mechanisms of Clot Formation and Lysis

The regulation of clot formation, although highly complex, can be conceptualized as involving three interacting arms: (1) fibrin formation and crosslinking, (2) platelet aggregation, and (3) fibrin breakdown. Several mechanisms exist for initiation or inhibition of each of these processes, with the goal of maintaining vessel patency and protecting blood vessel integrity. Because there are many excellent recent reviews on hemostasis, this discussion addresses only the most important aspects as they relate to therapeutic thrombolysis.[16,92]

The initial step in sealing a rent in the vessel wall is activation and deposition of platelets with formation of a hemostatic plug. Platelet activation occurs in three steps: platelet adhesion, the release reaction, and platelet aggregation. Damage to the endothelium with exposure of collagen, fibronectin, laminin, and microfibrils in the subendothelium stimulates platelet adhesion by means of von Willebrand factor. This factor binds to these subendothelial substances, changes its conformation and then binds to the platelet via the platelet membrane glycoprotein Ib (GPIb).

Next, the release reaction occurs with release of the alpha granules and dense bodies. Alpha granules release beta-thromboglobulin, platelet factor 4, platelet-derived growth factor (PDGF), von Willebrand factor (vWF), factor V, fibrinogen, and thrombospondin; dense bodies release adenosine diphosphate (ADP), adenosine triphosphate (ATP), calcium, and serotonin. Platelet aggregation then occurs, increasing the size of the platelet plug. A wide variety of agents, including ADP, epinephrine, collagen, thrombin, immune complexes, and platelet-activating factor, can cause platelet aggregation. Platelets are linked by means of fibrinogen which attaches to them by means of the glycoprotein IIb/IIIa receptor (GPIIb/ IIIa). This GPIIb/IIIa-fibrinogen association is the final common pathway for all platelet aggregation.

TABLE 1
Comparison of Thrombolytic Agents

Variable	Streptokinase	APSAC	Urokinase	tPA	scuPA
Antigenic	Yes	Yes	No	No	No
Dose	1.5 mil units IV x 60 min	30 units IV x 2-3 min	3 mil units IV x 30-90 min	100 mg IV x 1-3 hrs	70 mg IV x 1-3 hrs
Half-life (min)	23	90	16	5	7
Fibrin Enhancement	1+	1+	2+	3+	2+
Plasma Proteolytic State	4+	4+	2+	1+	2+
Frequency of Reocclusion (estimated %)	15	10	10	20	NA
Bleeding Complications	4+	4+	4+	4+	4+
Cost per Treatment	$200	$1,700	$2,800	$2,200	NA

APSAC = acylated plasminogen-streptokinase activated complex
tPA   = tissue plasminogen activator
scuPA   = single chain urokinase plasminogen activator
NA   = not available

Formation of the platelet plug is followed by fibrin deposition by means of the coagulation cascade. There are extrinsic and intrinsic pathways to fibrin formation. The first pathway is called "extrinsic" because of the requirement for a factor outside of the plasma (tissue thromboplastin) to initiate it. The intrinsic pathway can be initiated by plasma constituents (factor XII or Hageman factor). They both lead to generation of thrombin by means of the prothrombin activation complex consisting of factors Xa and Va, Ca++, and phospholipids. The relative importance of the two sytems in vivo is not known.

Thrombin then converts fibrinogen to fibrin and factor XIII to XIIIa which stabilizes fibrin polymer by covalent crosslinking, forming an insoluble fibrin clot. Thrombin also activates other coagulation proteins such as prothrombin and factors V and VIII, as well as the anticoagulant protein C. It also can stimulate vascular endothelial cells to increase their production and secretion of PGI2 (prostacyclin), vWf, and tissue plasminogen activator inhibitor (tPA-I). In addition, platelets contribute substantially to the coagulation process by providing a surface which speeds the cascade.

Many mechanisms control coagulation. One of the most important is the fibrinolytic system which breaks down fibrin. This occurs primarily by the conversion of plasminogen to plasmin, a serine protease which hydrolyzes susceptible lysine and arginine bonds in many proteins, including, fibrin, fibrinogen, factor V, and factor VIII. The breakdown of fibrin and fibrinogen creates fibrin degradation products which inhibit platelet aggregation and thrombin function. Plasminogen can be activated to plasmin by several activators, including tissue plasminogen activator and urokinase. The relative significance of these different activators in vivo is not known.

Thrombolytic Agents

All thrombolytic agents have in common the ability to cause conversion of plasminogen to plasmin, thus initiating thrombolysis.[17,68,69,91] They differ in relation to their antigenicity, cost, fibrin selectivity, mechanism of action, half-life, ease of administration, speed of recanalization, and incidence of recanalization (Table 1). Four clinical agents are available: streptokinase (SK), urokinase (UK), acylated plasminogen-streptokinase activated complex (APSAC) and tissue plasminogen activator (tPA). Other agents have been developed which offer different have been developed which offer different advantages such as single-chain urokinase plasminogen activator (scuPA) and a modified tPA with a longer half-life (Fb-Fb-CF). Others are being developed. Ancrod, a protein from Russell viper venom, causes fibrinogenolysis, and indirectly initiates fibrinolysis.

Streptococcal bacteria produce SK (Streptase—Hoechst-Roussel, Kabikinase—Smith-Kline-Beecham) which functions by binding to plasminogen, changing this zymogen's conformation to a form which can convert other plasminogen molecules to plasmin. SK has no enzymatic activity of its own. The SK-plasminogen complex has similar specificity for both circulating fibrinogen and fibrin in clot. This breakdown of circulating fibrinogen creates the "lytic state," a condition in which circulating fibrinogen levels are decreased and circulating fibrin/fibrinogen degradation products are increased, creating an anticoagulated state.

This lytic state has both positive and negative theoretical consequences—theoretical in that none of these considerations have been proven to be of importance in the clinical situation. On the positive side, it decreases serum viscosity by decreasing the amount of circulating fibrinogen and its secondary antithrombotic effect provides further protection against thrombosis for a period of time after discontinuation of the drug. There has been concern that the lytic state may increase bleeding complications, but the evidence for this is mixed.[68]

Certainly in the context of myocardial infarction this concern has been laid to rest by the Third International Study of Infarct Survival (ISIS-3) where it was shown that tPA and APSAC actually have a slightly higher intracerebral hemorrhage incidence than SK (0.6, 0.7, and 0.3%, respectively). Another concern about SK is its antigenicity: allergic reactions and an unpredictable active drug level due to blocking antibodies. Allergic reactions have been shown to occur in about 5.0% of patients and vary from fever, hypotension or serum sickness to, rarely, anaphylaxis. These complications

have not been of great significance except that patients should not be treated twice with this medication within a period of 6 months.

Attempts to determine the circulating levels of antibody against SK in order to calculate the necessary dose have not been practical for clinical use. The present suggested dose is based on these calculations, though, and represents the dose which will be effective in 90% of patients, based on previous measurements of blocking antibodies.[116] SK remains the most widely used and well accepted thrombolytic drug worldwide, primarily because it is much less expensive than the alternatives and seems to have equivalent clinical efficacy in most situations.

Urokinase (Abbokinase — Abbott) is the second oldest thrombolytic agent. It cleaves plasminogen directly, without modification or binding. It is found naturally in the body and is thus not antigenic. It has a serum half-life similar to SK (about 15 minutes). Like SK, it cleaves both circulating plasminogen and plasminogen on clot, thus creating a systemic lytic state. It costs around $235.00 for 250,000 units, about $2,800.00 for a 3-million unit dose as opposed to SK which is about $150 to $200 for a 1.5-million unit dose. Some believe that it is more effective than SK and has been used widely for intra-arterial treatments of peripheral vascular occlusions.[17]

More recently developed thrombolytic agents have taken advantage of clot selectivity. The two agents with this characteristic are tissue plasminogen activator (tPA-Activase—Genentech) and single chain urokinase plasminogen activator (scuPA, pro-urokinase), both naturally occurring substances that work by different mechanisms.

Of these two, tPA has by far been used the most. It consists of a heavy chain and a light chain, the former containing the kringle domains and the latter the active site for plasminogen activation. The kringle domains are the sites that bind to fibrin. When fibrin binding occurs, the conformation of tPA changes so that it has much more affinity for plasminogen. This increase in affinity is what gives this structure its fibrin selectivity. Very little fibrinogen is broken down in the serum because of tPA's low affinity for circulating plasminogen when it is not bound to fibrin. It is nonantigenic and has been shown to provide more rapid and more frequent recanalizations than SK in acute MI.[12] As a therapeutic agent, its primary weakness is its cost, which is about $1,100/50 mg or $2,200 per 100 mg dose. Endogenous tPA is synthesized in endothelial cells and circulates bound to PAI-1 (plasminogen activator inhibitor -1).

The other fibrin selective plasminogen activator, scuPA, is not as well understood. It circulates in an inert form but can be converted to the active form by plasmin. This, though, does not occur except in the presence of fibrin. The mechanism of this selectivity for fibrin is not understood.

Other thrombolytic agents have been developed by various means, including genetic engineering. These agents were designed either to prolong the half-life or increase fibrin selectivity. APSAC (acylated plasminogen/streptokinase activated complex [Eminase—Beecham]) has a half-life of 90 minutes and has some clot selectivity because the active site is acylated and does not become active until it binds to fibrin, which makes it susceptible to deacylation. Because of its long half-life, it can be given as a single bolus injection. It remains antigenic and costs about $1,700 per 30-unit dose.

No other thrombolytic agents are presently available, but many are being developed.

Ultra-Early Evaluation of the Stroke Patient

Animal studies have repeatedly shown that reperfusion must occur within the first few hours following stroke onset in order to salvage ischemic tissue at risk for infarc-

tion.[1,21,49,53,54,59,101] Animal experiments using cats, dogs, and baboons suggest that reperfusion of ischemic tissue within several hours of the initial occlusion may decrease infarct size.[21,59,101] Thrombolytic studies in acute myocardial infarction (MI) show a very time-dependent clinical response, with a much better response when treatment begins within 1 hour of symptom onset.[43] Previous studies and current clinical practice have allowed a leisurely approach to acute stroke care, considering this short therapeutic window.

The reasons for these delays in diagnostic evaluation and treatment are manifold, including: the patient's and family's recognition of the symptoms, the sense of urgency by medical care providers, and the availability and speed of performance of pretreatment tests. Many think that a pervasive sense of futility has had a powerful impact on these treatment delays. This sense of futility will clearly be perpetuated if treatments continue to be given at times in which there is very little potential for clinical benefit.

On the other hand, despite the fact that the public has been informed extensively on the symptoms of MI, recent studies have shown that patients already present for medical attention nearly as fast for stroke as for MI.[2] The development of effective treatment strategies for acute stroke should shorten these treatment intervals further by increasing the sense of urgency and decreasing the pervasive nihilistic attitudes.

The first hurdle will be to have patients with acute stroke present soon after the onset of their stroke. This will presumably take extensive public education. It has been shown that efforts toward education of the public and other health professionals can significantly increase the proportion of patients presenting to the hospital within 24 hours. Furthermore, the Phase I portion of the tPA in acute stroke trial demonstrated that treatment within 90 minutes of onset is feasible.[7,109]

Many diagnostic issues may assume importance if thrombolytic therapy is shown to be beneficial in a subset of patients. These issues are likely to require use of diagnostic technologies which can measure cerebrospinal fluid (CBF), document occlusion of vessels, show regions of fixed vessel stenosis, and determine the viability and integrity of vascular endothelium and brain tissue in order to determine the risk of hemorrhage and the potential for tissue salvage.

In this context, the speed with which the test may be performed and interpreted may well be as important as the nature of the information obtained. Work has begun in this area using several different technologies—computed tomography (CT), cerebral angiography, single photon emission computed tomography (SPECT), and transcranial doppler (TCD). Each of these offers distinct advantages and limitations. The history and clinical examination remains the most rewarding source for diagnostic, prognostic and mechanistic information, although its accuracy has not been thoroughly evaluated in this early time frame.

Because stroke may have many different causes, it may also require different therapies. The determination of the mechanism underlying an acute stroke can be challenging even when ample time is available, but when time is short, the challenge increases. The use of potentially dangerous treatments requires that the selection of patients be directed only toward those that are the most likely to benefit. Therefore, the challenge of identifying the mechanism of a patient's stroke will probably increase with the development of more aggressive treatments. Efforts toward this end have begun.

Computed tomography has dramatically improved early diagnosis by reliably excluding hemorrhage. In addition, it can sometimes demonstrate intracranial arterial thrombi, in which case it indicates a poor prognosis.[111,112] Infarction, though, is not well characterized soon after onset by CT alone. Some means of evaluating the cerebral vasculature and cerebral blood flow is needed.

This has been provided traditionally by angiography, which remains the most definitive method of demonstrating vascular anatomy. Intra-arterial digital subtraction angiography has recently been used in animal studies to demonstrate relative side-to-side perfusion by taking pictures of the capillary and venous phases.[62]

Fieschi and others evaluated 80 patients with acute stroke by several different means, including: clinical examination, angiography, CT, SPECT, and TCD.[36] These patients were all studied within 6 hours of onset and many within 4 hours. These investigators documented that 66% of the patients will demonstrate an intracranial occlusion which appears to be embolic. Furthermore, as many as 80% are potentially embolic in that they had potential embolic sources.

Besides demonstrating intracranial arterial occlusions, they also showed that the presence of collateral flow through leptomeningeal vessels correlates with a better clinical outcome. Although angiography remains the most definitive means of evaluating the cerebral vasculature, it also has risks and time constraints. In this study, 2 of the 80 patients appeared to decline in a manner suggesting that angiography was responsible. Other safer, more rapid, means of studying the cerebral vasculature are needed.

To this end, TCD and SPECT were also evaluated. The simplest, least expensive, quickest, and most mobile technique is the transcranial Doppler. This technique has limitations, however, in that it can only access the proximal portions of the middle cerebral artery (MCA) and anterior cerebral artery (ACA), and signals cannot be obtained in some patients.

Certain findings, though, are very reliable and therefore may obviate the need for angiography and provide real-time monitoring capabilities for documenting reperfusion. In this study, demonstration of an MCA trunk occlusion was completely reliable. A completely normal study provided reliable evidence against the presence of a proximal trunk occlusion.

Kushner et al also compared TCD and angiography findings in patients within 6 hours of onset of acute stroke.[64] The TCD results were highly predictive of the angiographic findings and the eventual infarct pattern on CT. Of the 42 patients studied, 15 showed no flow in the proximal MCA by TCD. Of these 15, 9 developed large, multilobar infarcts, 2 died, and 3 developed large single lobe infarcts. Only 1 developed a small, superficial infarct. All but 1 of these demonstrated an MCA or distal internal carotid artery (ICA) occlusion on angiography performed soon after the TCD exam. No patient who developed a multilobar infarction had a normal TCD.

Based on this study, a severely abnormal TCD performed soon after the onset of symptoms is highly predictive of the development of a large infarct, and, conversely, a normal study predicts that the infarct will not be multilobar. This could be important information in determining the risk/benefit ratio of a reperfusion treatment.

Another easily performed study, which could be useful in the acute setting, is SPECT. With technetium-99m hexamethylpropyleneamine oxime (^{99m}Tc HM-PAO) the tracer is easily obtained, quickly prepared, and can be used with conventional gamma cameras.[32,95] It reaches maximal brain uptake within 1 to 2 minutes and has little redistribution over the subsequent hours, so that its distribution represents relative blood flow during the period of uptake. These characteristics make it an excellent means of determining relative regional, tomographic CBF soon after the moment of presentation.

The primary limitations of the technique are its inability to give actual CBF values and the time that it takes for data acquisition, which is about 30 to 40 minutes using a single-headed gamma camera. Because of the lack of redistribution of the tracer, this data acquisition phase can be delayed several hours, allowing time for other treatments or diagnostic procedures.

Giubilei et al evaluated the predictive value of this technique in patients with acute stroke within 6 hours of onset.[40] Compared to the clinical examination as represented by the score on the Canadian Stroke Scale, SPECT predicted a poor outcome at 1 month more reliably (92% predictive value using SPECT criteria versus 78% using the clinical examination). The combination of the two was 100% predictive.

Stable xenon CT is another technique which can measure CBF quickly and noninvasively.[41,58,102] The studies can be performed in several minutes and the equipment is commercially available. Calculations provide actual CBF values and the study can be performed immediately after a routine CT with the precise anatomical correlation that the CT gives. Its value in the evaluation of the acute stroke patient has not been investigated, but it would appear to have some important advantages.

Magnetic resonance (MR) imaging could conceivably eliminate all other imaging modalities in the evaluation of the acute stroke patient. In the near future it may be able to rule out hemorrhage with gradient echo techniques, demonstrate blood vessel anatomy and the presence of clot by MR angiography,[31,82] show CBF by dynamic techniques,[89] document the metabolic status of the brain by MR spectroscopy,[42,56] show early infarction using diffusion techniques,[63,76] and show evidence of previous infarction with routine spin echo studies.

Some significant barriers must be overcome before all of these capabilities become possible or practical, and much validation remains to be done. The most important problem is the time which it takes to perform these studies, but the sequences continue to get shorter and shorter. At this time, no work has been done to evaluate the value of these techniques in the hyperacute clinical setting, primarily because of the difficult logistic issues involved with this kind of study. The versatility of this technique, though, holds much promise for the future.

Much more work needs to be done on the evaluation of the acute stroke patient in the first few hours after onset.

TABLE 2
Summary of Major Cardiac Thrombolytic Trials

Study	Onset to Treatment	Number of Pts	Treatment	Results (%) Mortality
Yusuf (pooled results of earlier studies)[121]		6,000 IV 900 UC	SK vs P SK vs P	19% decrease in Mortality 15% decrease in Mortality
Western Washington IC SK Trial[60,61]	< 6 hrs	250	IC SK vs P	3.7% vs 11.2%
GISSI-1[43]	< 6 hrs	11,806	IV SK vs Conventional	8.2% vs 17.7% @ 1 yr
ISAM[57]	< 3 hrs	1,741	IV SK vs P	20% decreased in Mortality
Dutch Interuniversity Trial[96]	< 4 hrs	533	IC SK ± IV SK vs Conventional	9% vs 16%
Western Washington[70]	< 4 hrs	368	IV SK vs Conventional	6.3 vs 9.7 p > .05
New Zealand tPA SK[117]	< 6 hrs	219	IV SK vs	2.5% vs 12.9%
TIMI-1[110]	< 6 hrs	313	IV tPA vs SK	5 vs 8 Mortality reperfusion rate 60% vs 35%
European Cooperative Study Group[115]	< 6 hrs	129	IV tPA vs SK	patency 70% vs 55%
German Activator Urokinase[78]		245	IV tPA vs UK	patency 64% vs 68%
ISIS-3	< 6 hrs	46,000	IV tPA vs APSAC vs SK	10.3% vs 10.67% vs 10.5%

Relevant Results from Cardiac Studies

The results of many randomized, blinded studies involving many thousands of patients have now been reported (Table 2) on the use of thrombolytic agents in the treatment of acute MI.[113] Since there are important similarities between cerebral infarction and myocardial infarction, much can be learned from these studies which may help investigators anticipate the future of stroke trials. Both myocardial and cerebral infarction are caused by occlusion of an artery by thrombus. Animal studies suggest that the therapeutic window for tissue reperfusion may be very similar.

On the other hand, it must also be recognized that important differences also exist. Most importantly, the complications of reperfusion hemorrhage are considerably more serious in the brain because of the rigid, closed space of the skull. It has also been shown that the majority of large vessel ischemic strokes are due to embolism of clot into a normal artery rather than thrombotic occlusion at a site of fixed stenosis.[36]

Following is a highly abbreviated list of some of the most important results from acute MI studies:

1. Clinical response (mortality, ventricular function) is related to elapsed time from onset of symptoms to treatment.[90]
2. Clinical response occurs only in the context of reperfusion. Stated alternatively, patients treated with thrombolytic agents fare no differently than placebo-treated controls if their infarct-related artery is not recanalized.[60,61]
3. The documented differences in mortality between treated and untreated patients persist out to at least 1 year.[90]
4. The incidence of reocclusion is directly related to the severity of residual stenosis.[46]

5. No significant safety differences have been found between SK, tPA, and APSAC, and there is no relationship between the systemic "lytic state" and complications.[68,69] Recently, the ISIS-3 study showed a statistically significant lower intracranial hemorrhage (ICH) incidence in patients treated with SK (0.3%) compared to tPA (0.7%) and APSAC (0.6%).

6. Bleeding complications occur primarily at sites of invasive procedures.[68,69]

7. Intracranial hemorrhage occurs at a rate of around 0.5-1.0%.[68,69]

8. tPA has the best recanalization rate compared to SK (approximately 75%)[15] but highest reocclusion rate (approximately 25%)[110,115] although the reocclusion rate can be diminished by the use of heparin[55] and coumadin.[100]

9. Delayed angioplasty has been shown to have equivalent efficacy to immediate post-treatment angioplasty.[80]

10. Preclinical work suggests that accelerated tPA protocols may cause earlier reperfusion and fewer bleeding complications. Accelerated protocols give a relatively greater proportion of the medicine early, in the first few minutes, rather than evenly over the subsequent 60-90 minutes.

Thrombolysis in Animal Models of Focal Cerebral Ischemia

A growing amount of literature exists on the effects of thrombolytic agents in animal models of focal cerebral ischemia. These studies have addressed issues regarding recanalization, clinical recovery, differences in infarct size, incidence and severity of hemorrhagic conversion, the effect of adjuvant therapies, and the differences between the available fibrinolytic agents.

The angiographically demonstrated recanalization rates of different thrombolytic agents including tPA,[10,11,37,62,81,84] SK,[9] and UK[29,51] have been compared to placebo in embolic stroke models. These have repeatedly shown a more rapid rate or a higher incidence of recanalization with the use of a thrombolytic agent. This has been shown most frequently with tPA, but it has also been shown with urokinase and Fb-Fb-CF, a tPA compound modified to have a longer serum half-life.

The relative efficacy of the different agents has also been compared. Streptokinase in a dose of 25,000U/kg was ineffective in recanalizing an embolic occlusion at 3 hours (1 of 7) after embolization, whereas the tPA analog, Fb-Fb-CF, was successful in recanalizing 6 of 10 with a dose of 0.8 mg/kg.[85] In another study, SK was just as effective as tPA in recanalizing vessels, but created more hemorrhagic infarction.[66] The mean time to reperfusion for the tPA analog was 70 minutes. Urokinase fared better against tPA than SK. Again in rabbits, UK showed equivalent efficacy to tPA in reducing the number of emboli found at postmortem microscopic examination of the cerebral vessels.[4] The area of infarction was not significantly different between the two agents, although the incidence of infarction was less with tPA.

Of some interest is the finding of decreased thrombolytic efficacy of tPA in extranial carotid arteries compared to intracranial arteries, particularly since this finding has also been suggested in human trials. The reasons for this could be multiple: increased size of embolus, decreased delivery of lytic agent, or undefined physiological differences in the two arteries. The efficacy in recanalizing the extracranial ICA improved by delivering the medication via local intra-arterial infusion.[11]

The timing of drug administration has been evaluated in order to find the outer limits of time in which the treatment can be efficacious. In the rabbit model, tPA has been shown to be effective in reducing neurologic damage as late as 45 minutes after embolization but not at 60 minutes.[122,123,124] tPA can recanalize vessels as late as 3 hours after embolization.[83] In a baboon model in which the MCA is occluded by an external silastic balloon, benefit has been obtained from intraarterial urokinase when given after 3 hours of reversible occlusion.[29]

Massive hemorrhagic conversion remains the biggest concern as to whether thrombolytic agents will be effective treatments for cerebral infarction in humans. In animal focal ischemia studies, despite the fact that petechial hemorrhagic conversion is common in untreated animals, it has been repeatedly and consistently shown that thrombolytic agents do not increase the frequency or severity of hemorrhagic conversion when given in the first few hours of embolic occlusion.[13,22,25,28,67,85,97] It has even been shown that hemorrhagic conversion is not increased when given as late as 8 or 24 hours after embolization in rabbits.[66] In a different rabbit model using common carotid artery (CCA) and MCA ligations combined with 2 hours of hypotension, SK was given 1 hour after occlusion and either SK, tPA, high-dose heparin, or placebo 24 hours after occlusion. Only excessive anticoagulation or thrombolytic therapy given 24 hours after occlusion caused gross hemorrhage, whereas rabbits given SK at 1 hour and untreated rabbits showed no significant hemorrhage.[97] In one study, SK caused more hemorrhagic conversion than tPA or saline.[83]

Overall, it is clear from animal studies that thrombolytic agents are capable of recanalizing intracranial occlusions due to autologous emboli or due to mechanical occlusion with in situ thrombosis. Whether this recanalization can be clinically beneficial in humans is not completely clear in that the therapeutic window of 45 minutes obtained from rabbit models seems too short to be clinically applicable to the care of patients, whereas the time window of 3 hours determined from baboon studies indicates that there may be a clinically meaningful therapeutic window. Presumably, the results from the primate model can be considered to be more applicable to the situation in humans.

Intra-Arterial Thrombolytic Trials

Seven recent reports of intra-arterial thrombolytic therapy have been published.[19,27,44,71,72,86,106] They are summarized along with the intra-venous studies in Tables 3 and 4. Intra-arterial therapy has several advantages over intravenous (IV) treatment: (1) occlusion and recanalization can be documented angiographically; (2) the lytic agent can be delivered in a more concentrated fashion with less systemic lytic effects and be discontinued when the desired effect is obtained; and, (3) in the future it may allow mechanical dilatations of fixed stenoses or possibly injection of lytic agents directly into the clot as has been done in some systemic vessels.

Disadvantages include the added time which is required to begin treatment, the unavailability of the needed technology and expertise at many sites, and the inherent risk. For instance, it has been shown in cardiac studies that hemorrhagic complications are increased dramatically by the use of invasive procedures. These studies, though, add critical information on the relationship between reperfusion and clinical improvement, the relative risk of treating different locations and types of occlusion, and preliminary information on the types of patients most likely to recanalize.

Therapy was initiated at a mean of 4.5,[71] 7.6,[28] and 7.2[106] hours after onset in the studies of anterior circulation emboli. Recanalization was repeatedly shown to be associated with improved outcome.

In the Mori et al series 10 of 22 patients recanalized; of these 10, 5 had an excellent outcome and 3 had a good outcome. In patients who did not recanalize, 1 of 12 had an excellent outcome and 3 of 12 a good outcome.[71] In the Del Zoppo et al series, 15 of 20 recanalized completely, 3 of 20 partially, and 2 of 20 none at all. Of who that recanalized completely, 6 had complete or near complete recovery, 4 partial, 4 none, and 1 died. Among those with partial recanalization, 2 had partial recovery and 1 died. Of the 2 who remained completely occluded, 1 remained unchanged, and 1 died.[28]

Among the 8 Theron et al patients with embolic occlusions, all showed some recanalization and there was only 1 death, and the remainder showed either partial or excellent recovery.[106] Compared to previous series of patients with proximal MCA occlusions,[93,119]

TABLE 3
Thrombolytic Therapy In Acute Stroke

Agent	Time	Treated (%) Improved/ Total	Controls (%) Improved/ Total	Early Recanilization # (%)	Stroke Type
IA UK or SK[44]	< 2 Weeks (29 ≤ 24 hr)	10/43 (23%)	3/22 (14%)	19 (44%)	Vertebrobasilar
IA UK or SK[26,28]	1 Hr-24 Hrs (7.6 Hr Mean)	6/20 (30%)	—	15 (75%)	Carotid
IA UK	45 Min-12 Hrs	NA/43	—	15/43 (35%)	Carotid/Basilar
IA SK (1 IA UK)	30 Hrs-3 Wks	6/12 (50%)	—	12/12 (100%)	Carotid
IA SK[19]	24 Hrs-7 Days	7/15 (46%)	—	7 (47%)	Carotid (9) Vertebrobasilar (6)
IA UK	24 Hrs-7 Days	22/81 (27%)	See Below	NA	Carotid Only
IV UK plus[39] (Dextran Sulfate)	24 Hrs-7 Days	32/62 (52%)	See Above	NA	Carotid Only
IV UK or SK[77]	5 Hrs-4 Days	2/4 (50%)	—	NA	Vertebrobasilar
IV UK[94]	1-2 Days	4/9 (44%)	6/12 (50%)	NA	Embolic
IV tPA[7]	≤ 90 min	29/74 (39%)	—	NA	Carotid
IV tPA[45]	> 90, ≤ 180	5/21 (24%)	—	NA	Vertebrobasilar
IV tPA[104]	≤ 8 Hrs	NA/104	—	33 (32%)	Vertebrobasilar
IV tPA[73]	≤ 6 Hrs	NA/19	NA/12	9/19 (47% Treated) 3/12 (25% Controls)	Carotid Carotid

A = Intra-arterial   UK = Urokinase
K = Streptokinase   IV = Intravenous
CA = Middle Cerebral Artery   NS = Not Specified
CA = Internal Carotid Artery NA = Not Evaluated
CME = Interval between stroke onset & thrombolytic therapy

this seems to represent an improvement in outcome, but without a simultaneous, randomized control group, no definitive statements can be made regarding the therapy's effect on outcome.

Of the 50 patients mentioned above, 11 showed hemorrhagic conversion on post-treatment CT scans. Eight of these 11 demonstrated recanalization. Six were symptomatic and 3 died. All hemorrhages occurred in the region of the lenticulostriate arteries. The mean time to treatment for those who had CT demonstrable hemorrhage was 381 minutes and 367 minutes for those who demonstrated no hemorrhage.[28,71,106]

Overall, the studies suggest that early recanalization confers a better outcome in patients with anterior circulation occlusions. It is likely that thrombolytic therapy is shortening the interval to reperfusion, but not certain, for recanalization frequently occurs spontaneously. Hemorrhage remains a concern. Its overall impact on outcome remains to be worked out with randomized studies comparing thrombolysis to placebo.

Only one sizeable series of vertebrobasilar occlusive disease has been reported in a formal paper.[44] This series compared 22 historical control patients with basilar artery thrombosis to 43 patients with the same dis-

TABLE 4
Intracerebral Hemorrhage Following Thrombolytic Therapy

Thrombolytic Agent	Anticoagulant	# ICH / # Treated	# Symptomatic	# Fatal
IA UK or SK[44]	Yes	4 / 43	3	4
IA UK or SK[26,28]	Yes	4 / 20	0	0
IA UK[73]	6 / 22	8 / 43	4 (?)	2
IV tPA[104]	No	3 / 74	2	1
IV tPA[24]	No	33 / 104	12	6
IA SK or UK[106]	No	3 / 12	2	1
IV UK[39]	No	1 / 143	1	0
IV UK[94]	No	5 / 9	NS	NS
IV tPA[45]	No	2 / 21	2	2
IV tPA[73]	No	10 / 19	0 (?)	0 (?)
Treated Placebo	No	5 / 12	0 (?)	0 (?)

IA = Intra-arterial   IV = Intravenous   SK = Streptokinase
UK = Urokinase   NS = Not Specified   ? = Not Clearly Stated

order who were treated with intra-arterial thrombolytic agents. Nineteen of the untreated controls died and the remaining 3 were severely disabled. Nineteen of the treated patients recanalized. Ten of these had a favorable outcome and 9 an unfavorable outcome (3 deaths). All 24 patients who did not recanalize died. Overall, 10 of 43 (23%) treated patients did well compared to 3 of 22 (13%) of the historical controls.

Again, recanalization appears to be required in order to obtain a clinical response. Hemorrhagic conversion developed in none of the historical controls, 2 of the recanalized treated patients and 2 of the nonrecanalized treated patients. Two appeared to succumb to the intracranial hemorrhage.

Conclusions regarding the type of patients most likely to recanalize must be considered very preliminary. The patterns of vertebrobasilar occlusion were divided into top of the basilar (TOP), middle basilar (MID), caudal vertebrobasilar (CVB), and mixed. TOP showed the best recanalization rate with 6 of 9 recanalizing, MID had the worst with only 5 of 15 recanalizing, and mixed almost as bad with 3 of 8 recanalizing. This may suggest that embolic occlusions, which are more common at the basilar bifurcation (TOP), may be more easily recanalized than throm-

botic ones, which are more common in the mid-basilar. Previous studies suggest that combined ICA and MCA occlusions, as well as combined MCA, anterior cerebral artery (ACA), and/or posterior cerebral artery (PCA) occlusions in the anterior circulation, recanalize less commonly than isolated MCA occlusions. This may imply that larger clots are more difficult to lyse than smaller ones, as one might expect.

These studies seem to offer a rationale for continuing to refine this means of treatment in the context of controlled trials.

Recent Studies of Intravenous tPA in Acute Stroke

Two open-label studies were executed recently using tPA in acute stroke patients, but have not yet been reported in complete form. Only abstracts are available for review.[7,45,104] The results of these studies as well as a recent randomized study and three other studies of IV treatment are summarized in Tables 3 and 4.

One study sponsored by Burroughs-Wellcome required the angiographic demonstration of an intracranial arterial occlusion.[104] Efficacy was defined by angiographically demonstrated recanalization of the occluded artery, and safety by lack of hemorrhagic conversion on CT accompanied by clinical deterioration. Treatment was required within 8 hours of onset and a continuous infusion of tPA over 1 hour was given. Repeat CT scans were performed at 24 hours and 14 days. A total of 139 were examined by angiography and 104 were treated. Only 94 were included for analysis. The dose was escalated gradually through 8 dose groups. Positive end points included only recanalization and negative end points hemorrhagic conversion and clinical deterioration.

Complete recanalization was achieved in only 4 patients and partial in 29, but some recanalization was achieved in all eight dose groups. The investigators did not believe that optimal recanalization had been achieved. Hemorrhagic conversion within 24 hours occurred in 22% of patients but only 6 showed clinical deterioration. This was not felt to be outside of the range to be expected in patients with acute stroke and no treatment. Hemorrhagic conversion did not appear to be dose dependent. Angiographic responders were said to have fared better than nonresponders, although a comparison of outcome results is not available. MCA occlusions were more likely to recanalize than mixed ICA and MCA occlusions.

A second trial is being conducted by the National Institutes of Health (NIH).[7,45] The phase I portion of this study did not require pre- or post-treatment angiography, but treatment within 90 minutes of onset was required. Recanalization could not be addressed because of the lack of pretreatment angiogaphy, and therefore thrombolytic efficacy could only be determined indirectly by the patient's clinical response. An "on-the-table" response was defined as improvement during the infusion of the drug.

Twenty-nine of the 74 patients reported demonstrated improvement during the drug infusion. Three patients developed intracerebral hemorrhage. No hemorrhages occurred in patients given doses of 0.9 mg/kg or less.

Two of these were symptomatic and 1 died. A major question of this study was whether such early treatment was feasible and the results confirm that it is.

An additional group of 22 patients was studied with treatment begun between 90 and 180 minutes of onset. Preliminary results suggest that this later time period will be associated with a somewhat higher incidence of hemorrhage and lower rate of clinical improvement. This study accrued 21 patients into 3 dose tiers. There were 3 dramatic responses at 2 hours and 5 at 24 hours. Two patients had fatal hemorrhages (9.5%), 1 at 32 mg/M2 and 1 at 37.5 mg/M2. The second phase of this study is randomized and blinded and an additional treatment group was added which will receive the medication between 90 and 180 minutes.

A recent double-blind, placebo-controlled trial of IV tPA in acute stroke patients was reported in abstract form.[73] The groups were treated as follows: 12 with placebo, 9 with 20 MIU tPA, and 10 with 30 MIU tPA. The tPA patients showed greater clinical improvement, but the actual results are not yet available. Angiography, performed immediately before and after a 1 hour infusion, showed recanalization in 3 of 12 given placebo, 4 of 9 given 20 MIU, and 5 of 10 given 30 MIU. Hemorrhagic complications were not significantly greater in the treated groups, although the numbers are too small to establish statistical significance.

Risks of Treatment

Intracerebral hemorrhage remains the most important safety concern in patients undergoing thrombolytic treatment (Table 4). It must be understood, though, that the presence of hemorrhagic conversion cannot be considered a negative outcome in itself. Hemorrhage into an infarct is common, particularly if sought prospectively by serial CT scans.[52,79] It is much more commonly asymptomatic than symptomatic, even occurring sometimes in the context of clinical improvement. Hemorrhagic conversion can occur in several forms: small, patchy, petechia without mass effect; patchy with worsening of mass effect; coalescent into a frank hematoma with mass effect. Futhermore, hemorrhage may occur outside the region of ischemia.

The incidence of hemorrhagic conversion has been evaluated by several different means, including autopsy, retrospective series, and prospectively using CT. The incidence has varied from 2.0% to 43%. Prospective CT studies suggest an incidence of around 40%. Hornig et al[52] found that 28 of 65 (43%) sequential stroke patients showed hemorrhagic conversion at some point after their stroke on serial CT scans performed on days 1, 3, 7, 14, 21, and 28. Frank hematomas with mass effect predominated early, whereas later transformation after about a week showed only cortical, gyral hemorrhage without mass effect. The development of hemorrhagic conversion correlated with the severity of the neurologic deficit, presence of mass effect, a cardiac source of embolus, early enhancement and involvement of the cortex. Three of these patients deteriorated due to the hemorrhage.

In another prospective study of 160 patients with a cardiac embolus, 65 (40.6%) developed hemorrhagic conversion.[79] In this study, the size of the infarct and the patient's age correlated with the incidence of conversion. Neither urokinase nor heparin appeared to influence the incidence of hemorrhagic conversion, although when hemorrhages occurred, they were more commonly massive with urokinase than with the other agents. Some other studies suggested that heparin also increases the severity, but to a lesser extent the incidence, of postinfarction hemorrhage.

So far, the evidence from thrombolytic trials suggests that when these agents are given within 6 hours of onset, they do not increase the incidence of hemorrhage dramatically.[7,24,43,45,71,72,73,104,105] Table 4 shows the incidence of ICH in the recent studies with post-treatment CT scans. One study showed an increased incidence of intracerebral hemorrhage when treatment began between 6 to 8 hours after onset.[104]

In a recently reported small, double-blind, placebocontrolled study of tPA in acute stroke,[73] a total of 31 patients were entered: 12 given placebo, 9 given 20 MIU of tPA, and 10 given 30 MIU of tPA. Hemorrhagic transformation of generally mild degree occurred in 5 of the placebo group, 6 of the 20 MIU group, and 4 of the 30 MIU group. This provides further support that thrombolytics can be given safely in this early period after stroke onset.

Angioplasty

Percutaneous transluminal angioplasty (PTA) has been used widely for coronary artery disease and has achieved acceptance as a therapeutic modality. Although it has been used almost as long in cerebrovascular patients (see Table 5 for a summary of previous reports), it has not become widely accepted as a therapeutic option.[48,114,121] The reasons for this are several:

1. Concern about the potential for distal embolization of atherosclerotic debris.[30]
2. For MCA and basilar artery stenosis, concern about inadvertent occlusion of perforators while crushing the plaque. As opposed to the heart and systemic arteries, occlusion of small, single perforators can be devastating in the brain.
3. The natural history of large-vessel occlusive disease outside of the ICA sinus has not been well defined. There is, therefore, reluctance to attempt potentially dangerous procedures when one does not know the likely consequences of the underlying disease.

Regarding the first concern, Theron et al[105] developed a triple coaxial catheter system designed to protect the cerebral circulation from distal embolization of thrombus and atherosclerotic debris. This protection is achieved by distal occlusion of the vessel by a second balloon with simultaneous irrigation and suction more proximally during balloon dilation. Fragments which are too large for suction presumably are diverted into the ECA.

These investigators feel that their method addresses the issue of distal embolization. Questions regarding the size and complexity of the equipment have been raised because of concerns that it may not be technically feasible in all or even most situations.[34] Whether or not this becomes an accepted technique, it has demonstrated exciting new potentials.

Certain types of stenotic lesions are fibrous, without atherosclerosis or other friable material. These include fibromuscular dysplasia, postendarterectomy fibrostenosis, and vasospasm. It also appears that certain sites of atherosclerosis, such as in the proximal vertebral arteries, are less frequently ulcerated or irregular and are usually smooth and fibrous.[121] These types of lesions may be more amenable to dilatation without concern for distal emboli.

Small, closely spaced vessels branch off the M1-MCA, A1-ACA and basilar arteries. These vessels do not have collateral supply. They supply highly critical regions of the brain, which if infarcted, create serious, even devastating neurological consequences. There is concern that fractured plaque could dissect through the wall of the parent vessel to occlude the ostium of perforating vessels.

In one of the two cases of basilar artery balloon dilation reported by Sundt,[103] a patient developed symptoms suggesting occlusion of a perforator, although recovery was good. Otherwise, there is very little in the neurological literature regarding the risk of perforator occlusion. Most dilation procedures have been performed in regions free of these vessels.

In coronary procedures, techniques have been developed which protect bisecting vessels from inadvertent occlusion. These may find some use in neurological applications, but it is unlikely that they will be useful in the 50-400 μm diameter perforating vessels

of the M1 and basilar perforators. The fact that plaque tends to develop on the ventral surface of the basilar artery[18] opposite to the perforators may imply that some plaque disruption may occur without jeopardizing the distal perforators. A similar case may be true also for the MCA, but it has not yet been addressed in the available literature.

The natural history of atherosclerotic occlusive disease has not been well defined, except perhaps in the case of proximal ICA stenosis. Other sites of stenosis such as in the MCA, ACA, PCA, basilar, and vertebral arteries have only preliminary information on their natural history and it appears to vary considerably with each site. Means of determining high-risk subgroups have not been developed.

Too frequently, "failure of medical therapy" refers to a devastating stroke which obviates the need for further preventive efforts. Hopefully, advancements in predicting an individual's risk of stroke will enable us to focus efforts on those most likely to benefit. The fear of inducing an iatrogenic stroke in a patient with an otherwise benign prognosis has limited the willingness of clinicians to submit their patients to unproven, potentially dangerous therapies. The most common site for athereosclerosis in arteries supplying the brain is the ICA sinus.

Recently, the North American Symptomatic Carotid Endarterectomy Trial (NASCET) demonstrated a powerful benefit for carotid endarterectomy (CEA) over medical therapy in patients with a stenosis of 70% to 99% and appropriate symptoms ipsilateral to the stenosis. Combined, morbidity/mortality was kept below 6% for the procedure. New approaches to treating carotid stenosis will need to demonstrate a complication rate at least this good in order to have any hope of acceptance, particularly now that the procedure is being performed routinely under local anesthesia with only a 2-3 day admission.

The rationale for avoiding surgery is nowhere nearly as convincing as it is in coronary bypass surgery where patients must have a thoracotomy and undergo cardiopul-

TABLE 5
Angioplasty for Fixed Stenosis of Cerebral Arteries

	Cervical ICA and Distal CCA	MCA	Vertebral	Basilar
# of Patients	52	1	32	3
# of Arteries	53	***	35	***
Indications for R$_x$				
Not Stated	18			
Stroke	4		2	
TIA	13	1	30	3
Asymptomatic Stenosis	6			
Symptomatic Restenosis	1			
Asymptomatic Restenosis	8			
Complications				
Stroke	0			2
TIA	2			1
Death	0			
None	50	1	32	
Technical Results				
Unsuccessful	8		11	
Good	45	1	24	3
Follow-Up				
No	20		1	1
Yes	29	1	31	1
Asymptomatic	32	1	30	
Stroke				
TIA	0		1	1

Results of angioplasty of fixed stenosis of the extracranial and intracranial arteries. The ICA angioplasties include lesions due to atherosclerosis, fibromuscular dysplasia, and post endarterectomy fibrotic stenosis. The other vessels are only involved by atherosclerosis.

Cervical ICA & Distal CCA[5,8,20,38,47,105,107,108,118]

MCA[87]

Vertebral[50,74,75]

Basilar[50,103]

monary bypass with all the attendant risks, discomforts, and costs which these procedures entail. CEA is comparatively a much less invasive procedure. Future applications of angioplasty should probably be directed toward more surgically inaccessible stenoses.

So far, angioplasty has been shown to be feasible at sites where alternative treaments are excellent (ICA sinus with CEA) or treatments are rarely necessary because of a benign natural history (proximal vertebral and subclavian steel). Application of this technique would have a much stronger rationale in distal vertebral, ICA siphon, or MCA stenosis where initial evidence suggests that

the prognosis may warrant a therapy with some potential risk. The technical difficulties at these sites will certainly be considerably greater, but the technology continues to improve dramatically and successful dilation of these sites will certainly be seen in the near future.

References

1. Astrup J, Siesjo BK, Symon L. Thresholds in cerebral ischemia—the ischemic penumbra. *Stroke.* 1981;12:723-725.
2. Barsan WG, Brott TG. Early treatment of acute ischemic stroke. *Stroke: Clinical Updates.* 1990;1:5-8.

3. Barsan WG, Brott T, Olinger CP, et al. Identification and entry of the patient with acute cerebral infarction. *Ann Emerg Med.* 1988;17:1192-1195.

4. Benes V, Zabramski JM, Boston M, et al. Effect of intra-arterial antifibrinolytic agents on autologous arterial emboli in the cerebral circulation of rabbits. *Stroke.* 1990;21:1594-1599.

5. Bockenheimer SAM, Mathias K. Percutaneous transluminal angioplasty in arteriosclerotic internal carotid artery stenosis. *AJNR.* 1983;4:791-792.

6. Brott T. Thrombolysis and stroke in clinical practice: past, present, and future. In: Sawaya R, ed. *Fibrinolysis and the Central Nervous System* Philadelphia, Pa: Hanley & Belfus, Inc.; 1990:189-197.

7. Brott TG, Haley EC Jr, Levy DE, et al. Tissue plasminogen activator (tPA) as very early therapy for cerebral infarction. *Circulation.* 1987;76(suppl 4): 142.

8. Brown M, Butler P, Gibbs J, et al. Feasibility of percutaneous transluminal angioplasty for carotid artery stenosis. *J Neurol Neurosurg Psychiatry.* 1990;53:238-243.

9. Centeno RS, Hackney DB, Rothrock JR. Streptokinase clot lysis in acute occlusions of the cranial circulation: study in rabbits. *AJNR.* 1985;6:589-594.

10. Chehrazi BB, Seibert AJ, Hein L, et al. Evaluation of tissue plasminogen activator (tPA) in embolic stroke. *Stroke.* 1988;19:133.

11. Chehrazi BB, Seibert JA, Hein L, et al. Differential effect of recombinant tissue plasminogen activator-induced thrombolysis in the central nervous system and systemic arteries. *Neurosurgery.* 1991;28: 364-369.

12. Chesebro JH, Knatterud G, Roberts R, et al. Thrombolysis in myocardial infarction (TIMI) trial, phase I: a comparison between intravenous tissue plasminogen activator and intravenous streptokinase. *Circulation.* 1987;76:142-154.

13. Clark WM, Madden KP, Zivin JA, et al. Intracerebral hemorrhage: tPA versus streptokinase thrombolytic therapy. *Neurology.* 1989;39(suppl 1):183.

14. Clarke RL, Cliffton EE. The treatment of cerebrovascular thrombosis and embolism with fibrinolytic agents. *Am J Cardiol.* 1960;6:546-551.

15. Colle D. Coronary thrombolysis: streptokinase or recombinant tissue-type plasminogen activator? *Ann Intern Med.* 1990;112:529-538.

16. Colman RW, Marder VJ, Salzman EW, et al. Overview of hemostasis. In: Colman RW, Hirsh J, Marder VJ, et al. eds. *Hemostasis and Thrombosis: Basic Principles and Clinical Practice.* Philadelphia, Pa: JB Lippincott Company, 1987:3-17.

17. Comerota AJ. ed. *Thrombolytic Therapy.* Orlando, Fl: Grune & Stratton, Inc. 1988.

18. Cornhill JF, Akins D, Hutson M, et al. Localization of atherosclerotic lesions in the human basilar artery. *Atherosclerosis.* 1980;35:77-86.

19. Courthéoux P, Théron J, Tournade A, et al. Percutaneous endoluminal angioplasty of post endarterectomy carotid stenoses. *Neuroradiology.* 1987;29: 186-189.

20. Courthéoux P, Théron J, Derlon M, et al. In situ fibrinolysis in supra-aortic main vessels. A preliminary study. *J Neuroradiology.* 1986;13:111-124.

21. Crowell RM, Marcoux FW, DeGirolami U. Variability and reversibility of focal cerebral ischemia in unanesthetized monkeys. *Neurology.* 1981;31: 1295-1302.

22. De Ley G, Weyne J, Demeester G, et al. Experimental thromboembolic stroke studied by positron emission tomography: immediate versus delayed reperfusion by fibrinolysis. *J Cereb Blood Flow Metab.* 1988;89:539-545.

23. De Ley G, Weyne J, Demeester G, et al. Streptokinase treatment versus calcium overload blockade in experimental thromboembolic stroke. *Stroke.* 1989;20:357-361.

24. Del Zoppo GJ, The RT-PA/Acute Stroke Study Group. An open, multicenter trial of recombinant tissue plasminogen activator in acute stroke. A progress report. *Stroke.* 1990;21(suppl 4):174-175.

25. Del Zoppo GJ, Copeland BR, Anderchek K, et al. Hemorrhagic transformation following tissue plasminogen activate or in experimental cerebral infarction. *Stroke.* 1990;21:596-601.

26. Del Zoppo GJ, Copeland BR, Hacke W, et al. Intracerebral hemorrhage following r-tPA infusion in a primate stroke model. *Stroke.* 1988;19:134.

27. Del Zoppo GJ, Copeland BR, Waltz TA, et al. The beneficial effect of intracarotid urokinase on acute stroke in a baboon model. *Stroke.* 1986;17:638-643.

28. Del Zoppo GJ, Ferbert A, Otis S, et al. Local intra-arterial fibrinolytic therapy in acute carotid territory stroke: a pilot study. *Stroke.* 1988;19:307-313.

29. Del Zoppo GJ, Zeumer H, Harker LA. Thrombolytic therapy in stroke: possibilities and hazards. *Stroke.* 1986;17:595-607.

30. DeMonte F, Peerless SJ, Rankin RN. Carotid transluminal angiopl asty with evidence of distal embolization. *Neurosurg.* 1989;70:138-141.

31. Edelman RR, Mattle HP, Atkinson DJ, et al. Cerebral blood flow: assessment with dynamic contrast-enhanced T2*-weighted MRI at 1.5 T. *Radiology.* 1990;176:211-220.

32. Ell PJ, Hocknell JM, Jarritt PH, et al. A ^{99m} Tc labelled radiotracer for the investigation of cerebral vascular disease. *Nucl Med Commun.* 1985;6: 437-441.

33. Fallon, JT. Pathology of arterial lesions amenable to percutaneous transluminal angioplasty. *AJR.* 1980;135:913-916.

34. Ferguson, R. Getting it right the first time. *AJNR.* 1990;11:875-877.

35. Fieschi C, Argentino C, Lenzi GL, et al. Therapeutic window for pharmacological treatment in acute focal cerebral ischemia. *Ann NY Acad Sci.* 1988;662-666.

36. Fieschi C, Argentino C, Lenzi GL, et al. Clinical and instrumental evaluation of patients with ischemic stroke within the first six hours. *J Neurol Sci.* 1989; 91:311-321.

37. Fisher M, Phillips DA, Smith TW, et al. Delayed treatment with a tPA analog in an embolic stroke model. *Stroke.* 1989;20:154.

38. Freitag G, Freitag J, Koch RD, et al. Percutaneous angioplasty of carotid artery stenoses. *Neuroradiology.* 1986;28:126-127.

39. Fujishima M, Omae T, Tanaka K, et al. Controlled trial of combined urokinase and dextran sulfate therapy in patients with acute cerebral infarction. *Angiology.* 1986;37:487-498.

40. Giubilei F, Lenzi GL, Di Piero V, et al. Predictive value of brain perfusion single-photon emission computed tomography in acute ischemic stroke. *Stroke.* 1990;21:895-900.

41. Good WF, Gur D. Xenon-enhanced CT of the brain: effect of flow activation on derived cerebral blood

flow measurements. *AJNR*. 1991;12:83-85.

42. Graham GD, Howseman AM, Rothman DL, et al. Proton magnetic resonance spectroscopy of metabolites after cerebral infarction in humans. *Stroke*. 1991;22:143.

43. Gruppo Italiano per lo Studio della Streptochinasi nell'Infarto Miocardico (GISSI). Effectiveness of intravenous thrombolytic treatment in acute myocardial infarction. *Lancet*. 1986;1:397-401.

44. Hacke W, Zeumer H, Ferbert A, et al. Intra-arterial thrombolytic therapy improves outcome in patients with acute vertebrobasilar occlusive disease. *Stroke*. 1988; 19:1216-1222.

45. Haley EC, Levy D, Sheppard G, et al A dose-escalation safety study of intravenous tissue plasminogen activator in patients treated from 90 to 180 minutes from onset of acute ischemic stroke. *Ann Neurol*. 1990;28:225.

46. Harrison DG, Ferguson DW, Collins SM, et al. Rethrombosis after reperfusion with streptokinase: importance of geometry of residual lesions. *Circulation*. 1984;69:991-999.

47. Hasso AN, Bird CR, Zinke DE, et al. Fibromuscular dysplasia of the internal carotid artery: percutaneous transluminal angioplasty. *AJNR*. 1981;2:175-180.

48. Health & Public Policy Committee, American College of Physicians. Percutaneous Transluminal Angioplasty. *Ann Intern Med*. 1983; 99:864-869.

49. Heiss W-D, Rosner G. Functional recovery of cortical neurons as related to degree and duration of ischemia. *Ann Neurol*. 1983;14:294-301.

50. Higashida RT, Hieshima GB, Tsai FY, et al. Transluminal angioplasty of the vertebral and basilar artery. *AJNR*. 1987;8:745-749.

51. Hirschberg M, Hofferberth B. Thrombolytic therapy with urokinase and pro-urokinase in a canine model of acute stroke. *Neurology*. 1987;37(suppl 1):132.

52. Hornig CR, Dorndorf W, Agnoli AL. Hemorrhagic cerebral infarction—a prospective study. *Stroke*. 1986;17:179-185.

53. Hossmann K-A, Kleihues P. Reversibility of ischemic brain damage. *Arch Neurol*. 1973;29:375-384.

54. Hossmann K-A, Olsson Y. Suppression and recovery of neuronal function in transient cerebral ischemia. *Brain Res*. 1970;22:313-325.

55. Hsia J, Hamilton WP, Kleiman N, et al. A comparison between heparin and low-dose aspirin as adjunctive therapy with tissue plasminogen activator for acute myocardial infarction. *N Engl J Med*. 1990; 323:1433-1437.

56. Hugg JW, Matson GB, Duyn JH, et al. MR spectroscopic imaging of stroke. *Stroke*. 1991;22:143.

57. ISAM Study Group. A prospective trial of intravenous streptokinase in acute myocardial infarction (I.S.A.M.): mortality, morbidity, and infarct size at 21 days. *N Engl J Med*. 1986;314:1465-1471.

58. Johnson DW, Stringer WA, Marks MP, et al. Stable xenon CT cerebral blood flow imaging: rationale for and role in clinical decision making. *AJNR*. 1991; 12:201-213.

59. Jones TH, Morawetz RB, Crowell RM, et al. Thresholds of focal cerebral ischemia in awake monkeys. *J Neurosurg*. 1981;54:773-782.

60. Kennedy JW, Ritchie JL, Davis KB, et al. Western Washington randomized trial of intracoronary streptokinase in acute myocardial infarction. *N Engl J Med*. 1983;309:1477-1482.

61. Kennedy JW, Ritchie JL, Davis KB, et al. The western Washington randomized trial of intracoronary streptokinase in acute myocardial infarction: a 12-month follow-up report. *N Engl J Med*. 1985;312: 1073-1078.

62. Kissel P, Chehrazi B, Seibert JA, et al. Digital angiographic quantification of blood flow dynamics in embolic stroke treated with tissue-type plasminogen activator. *J Neurosurg*. 1987;67:399-405.

63. Knight RA, Ordidge RJ, Helpern JA, et al. Investigation of brain ischemia imaging by MR diffusion. *Stroke*. 1991;22:138.

64. Kushner MJ, Zanette EM, Bastianello S, et al. Transcranial doppler in acute hemispheric brain infarction. *Neurology*. 1991;41:109-113.

65. Lyden P, Madden K, Clark W, et al. Effect of tPA thrombolysis on hemorrhage after stroke. *Stroke*. 1989;20:154.

66. Lyden PD, Madden KP, Clark WM, et al. Incidence of cerebral hemorrhage after antifibrinolytic treatment for embolic stroke in rabbits. *Stroke*. 1990; 21:1589-1593.

67. Lyden PD, Zivin JA, Alving LA, et al. The effect of thrombolysis and anticoagulation on post ischemic hemorrhage after experimental cerebral embolism. *Circulation*. 1987;76(suppl 4):141.

68. Marder VJ, Sherry S. Thrombolytic therapy: current status (first of two parts). *N Engl J Med*. 1988;318: 1512-1520.

69. Marder VJ, Sherry S. Thrombolytic therapy: current status (second of two parts). *N Engl J Med*. 1988; 318:1585-1595.

70. Martin GV, Stadius ML, Davis KB, et al. Western Washington intravenous streptokinase trial; effects of intravenous streptokinase on vessel patency and left ventricular function. *Circulation*. 1986;74(suppl 2):II-367.

71. Mori E, Tabuchi M, Shsumi Y, et al. Intra-arterial urokinase infusion therapy in acute thromboembolic stroke. *Stroke*. 1990;21(suppl 1):I-74.

72. Mori E, Tabuchi M, Yoshida T, et al. Intracarotid urokinase with thromboembolic occlusion of the middle cerebral artery. *Stroke*. 1988;19:802-812.

73. Mori E, Yoneda Y, Ohksawa S, et al. Double-blind, placebo-controlled trial of recombinant tissue plasminogen activator (rt-PA) in acute carotid stroke. *Neurology*. 1991;41(suppl 1):347.

74. Motarjeme A, Keifer JW, Zuska AJ. Percutaneous transluminal angioplasty of the vertebral arteries. *Radiology*. 1981;139:715-717.

75. Motarjeme A, Keifer JW, Zuska AJ. Percutaneous transluminal angioplasty of the brachiocephalic arteries. *AJR*. 1982;138:457-462.

76. Moseley ME, Kucharczyk J, Mintorovitch J, et al. Diffusion-weighted MR imaging of acute stroke: correlation with T2-weighted and magnetic susceptibility-enhanced MR imaging in cats. *AJNR*. 1990; 11:423-429.

77. Nenci GG, Gresele R, Taramelli M, et al. Thrombolytic therapy for thromboembolism of vertebrobasilar artery. *Angiology*. 1983;34:561-571.

78. Neuhaus KL for the G.A.U.S. Study Group. Thrombolysis in acute myocardial infarction: results of the German-Activator-Urokinase-Study (G.A.U.S.) *Eur Heart J*. 1987;8:49.

79. Okada Y, Yamaguchi T, Minematsu K, et al. Hemorrhagic transformation in cerebral embolism. *Stroke*. 1989;20:598-603.

80. O'Neill WO, Timmis GC, Bourdillon PD, et al. A prospective randomized clinical trial of intracoronary streptokinase versus coronary angioplasty for acute myocardial infarction. *N Engl J Med.* 1986; 314:812-818.

81. Papadopoulos SM, Chandler WF, Salamat MS, et al. Recombinant human tissue-type plasminogen activator therapy in acute thromboembolic stroke. *J Neurosurg.* 1987;67:394-398.

82. Pettigrew C, Lee C, Dean B, et al. Ultra-fast magnetic resonance perfusion mapping of brain infarction. *Stroke.* 1991;22:142.

83. Phillips DA, Fisher M, Davis MA, et al. Delayed treatment with a t-PA analogue and streptokinase in a rabbit embolic stroke model. *Stroke.* 1990;21: 602-605.

84. Phillips DA, Fisher M, Smith TW, et al. The safety and angiographic efficacy of tissue plasminogen activator in a cerebral embolization model. *Ann Neurol.* 1988;23:391-394.

85. Phillips DA, Fisher M, Smith TW, et al. The effects of a new tissue plasminogen activator analogue, Fb-Fp-CF, on cerebral reperfusion in a rabbit embolic stroke model. *Ann Neurol.* 1989;25:281-285.

86. Poeck K. Intraarterial thrombolytic therapy in acute stroke. *Acta Neurol Belg.* 1988;88:35-45.

87. Purdy PD, Devous MD Sr, Unwin DH, et al. Angioplasty of an atherosclerotic middle cerebral artery associated with improvement in regional cerebral blood flow. *AJNR.* 1990;11:878-880.

88. Ritchie JL, Davis KB, Williams DL, et al. Global and regional left ventricular function and tomographic radionuclide perfusion: The western Washington intracoronary streptokinase in acute myocardial infarction trial. *Circulation.* 1984;70:867-875.

89. Ross JS, Masaryk TJ, Modic MT, et al. Magnetic resonance angiography of the extracranial carotid arteries and intracranial vessels: a review. *Neurology.* 1989;39:1369-1376.

90. Rovelli F, De Vita C, Feruglio GA, et al. GISSI trial: early results and late follow-up. *J Am Coll Cardiol.* 1987;10(suppl B): 33B-39B.

91. Runge MS, Quertermous T, Haber E. Plasminogen activators: the old and the new. *Circulation.* 1989; 79:217-224.

92. Saito H. Normal hemostatic mechanisms. In: Ratnoff OD, Forbes CD, eds. *Disorders of Hemostasis.* Philadelphia, Pa: WB Saunders Company; 1991: 18-47.

93. Saito I, Segawa H, Shiokawa Y, Taniguchi M, Tsutsumi K. Middle cerebral artery occlusion: correlation of computed tomogra phy and angiography with clinical outcome. *Stroke.* 1987;18:863-868.

94. Sato Y, Mizoguchi K, Sato Y. Anticoagulant and thrombolytic therapy for cerebral embolism of cardiac origin. *Kurume Med J.* 1986;33:39-95.

95. Sharp PF, Smith FW, Gemmell HG, et al. Technetium-99m HM-PAO stereoisomers as potential agents for imaging regional cerebral blood flow: human volunteer studies. *J Nucl Med.* 1986;27: 171-177.

96. Simoons ML, Serruys PW, vanden Brand M, et al. Early thrombolysis in acute myocardial infarction: limitation of infarct size and improved survival. *J Am Coll Cardiol.* 1986;7:717-728.

97. Slivka A, Pulsinelli W. Hemorrhagic complications of thrombolytic therapy in experimental stroke. *Stroke.* 1987;18:1148-1156.

98. Sloan MA. Thrombolysis and stroke: past and future. *Arch Neurol.* 1987;44:748-768.

99. Sloan MA. Thrombolytic therapy in experimental focal cerebral ischemia. In: Sawaya R, ed. *Fibrinolysis and the Central Nervous System.* Philadelphia, Pa: Hanley & Belfus, Inc., 1990;177-188.

100. Smith P, Arnesen H, Holme I. The effect of warfarin on mortality and reinfarction after myocardial infarction. *N Engl J Med.* 1990;323:147-152.

101. Steen PA, Michenfelder JD, Milde JH. Incomplete versus complete cerebral ischemia: improved outcome with a minimal blood flow. *Ann Neurol.* 1979; 6:389-398.

102. Stringer WA. Accuracy of xenon CT measurement of cerebral blood flow. *AJNR.* 1991;12:86-87.

103. Sundt TM Jr, Smith HC, Campbell JK, et al. Transluminal angioplasty for basilar artery stenosis. *Mayo Clin Proc.* 1980;55:673-680.

104. The rt-PA/Acute Stroke Study Group. An open safety/efficacy trial of rt-PA in acute thromboembolic stroke: final report. *Stroke.* 1991;22:153.

105. Theron J, Courtheoux P, Alachkar F, et al. New triple coaxial catheter system for carotid angioplasty with cerebral protection. *AJNR.* 1990;11:869-874.

106. Theron J, Courtheoux P, Casasco A, et al. Local intraarterial fibrinolysis in the carotid territory. *AJNR.* 1989;10:753-765.

107. Theron J, Raymond J, Casasco A, et al. Percutaneous angioplasty of atherosclerotic and postsurgical stenosis of carotid arteries. *AJNR.* 1987;8:495-500.

108. Tievsky AL, Druy EM, Mardiat JG. Transluminal angioplasty in postsurgical stenosis of the extracranial carotid artery. *AJNR.* 1983;4:800-802.

109. Timerding BL, Barsan WG, Hedges JR, et al. Stroke patient evaluation in the emergency department before pharmacologic therapy. *Am J Emerg Med.* 1989;7:11-15.

110. TIMI Study Group: The thrombolysis in myocardial infarction (TIMI) trial. *N Engl J Med.* 1985;312: 932-936.

111. Tomsick TA, Brott TG, Chambers AA, et al. Hyperdense middle cerebral artery sign on CT: efficacy in detecting middle cerebral artery thrombosis. *AJNR.* 1990;11:473-477.

112. Tomsick TA, Brott TG, Olinger CP, et al. Hyperdense middle cerebral artery: incidence and quantitative significance. *Neuroradiology.* 1989;31: 312-315.

113. Topol EJ, ed. *Acute Coronary Intervention.* New York, NY: Alan R. Liss, Inc.; 1988.

114. Tsai FY, Higashida R. Balloon transluminal angioplasty of the carotid artery in the head and neck. In: Norris JW, Hachinski VC, eds. *Prevention of Stroke.* New York: Springer-Verlag, 1991;1:205-218.

115. Verstraete M, Bory M, Collen D, et al. Randomized trial of intravenous recombinant tissue-type plasminogen activator versus intravenous streptokinase in acute myocardial infarction. *Lancet.* 1985;1:842-847.

116. Verstraete M, Tytgat G, Amery A, et al. Thrombolytic therapy with streptokinase using a standard dosage. *Thromb Diath Haemorrh.* 1966;16(suppl 21):493.

117. White HD, Norris RM, Brown MA, et al. Effect of intravenous streptokinase on left ventricular function and early survival after acute myocardial infarction. *N Engl J Med.* 1987;317:850-855.

118. Wiggli U, Gratzi O. Transluminal angioplasty of stenotic carotid arteries: case reports and protocol. *AJNR.* 1983;4:793-795.

119. Yoshimoto T, Ogawa A, Seki H, et al. Clinical course of acute middle cerebral artery occlusion. *J Neurosurg.* 1986;65:326-330.

120. Yusuf S, Collins R, Peto R, et al. Intravenous and intracoronary fibrinolytic therapy in acute myocardial infarction: overview of results on mortality, reinfarction and side-effects from 33 randomized controlled trials. *Eur Heart J.* 1985;6:556-585.

121. Zeumer H. Survey of progress: vascular recanalizing techniques in interventional neuroradiology. *J Neurology.* 1985;231:287-294.

122. Zivin JA, Hemenway CC, DeGirolami U. Delayed therapy of embolic stroke with tissue plasminogen activator. *Ann Neurol.* 1986;20:154.

123. Zivin JA, Kochhar A, Lyden PD, et al. Delayed thrombolytic therapy with tPA reduces neurologic damage after experimental cerebral ischemia. *Circulation.* 1987;76(suppl 4):142.

124. Zivin JA, Lyden PD, DeGirolami U, et al. Tissue plasminogen activator: reduction of neurologic damage after experimental embolic stroke. *Arch Neurol.* 1988;45:387-391.

CHAPTER 14

Clinical Trials In Cerebrovascular Surgery

Marc R. Mayberg, MD

Clinical trials have achieved a growing role in the contemporary practice of medicine. The impetus for this trend originated from a variety of sources, including the newer methodology for multicenter studies, increasing public awareness of health-care decision-making, the role of clinical trials in determining reimbursement policies, and a general consensus in the medical community that any treatment administered should be proven effective according to rigorous scientific criteria. More recently, emphasis has been placed upon the need to document the efficacy of surgical procedures by clinical trials.

Perhaps nowhere has the impact of clinical trials upon clinical practice been more profound than in the field of cerebrovascular surgery. A single publication regarding a clinical trial[13] essentially eliminated from neurosurgical practice the extracranial-intracranial (EC-IC) bypass, which had been relatively common. Widespread recognition of this trial and its consequences led in part to the development of several studies designed to test the efficacy of carotid endarterectomy.

With the growing emphasis upon clinical trials in cerebrovascular disease, it becomes imperative for the practicing physician to become familiar with the general methodology of clinical research as well as the specific design of individual trials. Clinical decisions based upon these data will thus be based upon a better understanding of their derivation. This chapter describes the methodology employed in designing a clinical trial according to contemporary standards. In this context, all previous and current prospective, randomized trials for cerebrovascular surgery are reviewed and contrasted.

Volumes of data from retrospective and prospective nonrandomized studies in cerebrovascular disease have been published; the focus of this chapter upon prospective randomized trials does not discount the validity of these prior studies. Nevertheless, as discussed below, prospective randomized trials have several distinct methodologic advantages in demonstrating causality, or the cause-and-effect relationship between treatment (e.g. surgery) and outcome (e.g. stroke). In addition, such trials have become (whether or not appropriately) the standard by which surgical procedures are judged and ultimately applied in clinical practice.

Methodology of Clinical Trials

The design of clinical trials is important in determining their validity, applicability to broader populations, and ultimate clinical usefulness. A successful trial should be designed to provide internal validity—i.e. conclusions which are not due to erroneous observations—and external validity—i.e. inferences which relate observations in the study sample to broader populations. To accomplish this, the methodology should be constructed to minimize random error (due to chance occurrences) and systematic error (due to bias of some type). In addition, the study must pose a research question which is novel, relevant to clinical practice, feasible, ethical, and important. Failure to encompass one or more of these criteria can seriously limit the extent to which findings from a clinical trial may be applied to clinical decision-making.

Defining the Study Population

External validity for any clinical trial is determined in large part by the parameters used to define the population being studied. Inclusion criteria set forth parameters which determine the essential predictive variables to be studied—e.g. carotid stenosis and transient ischemic attacks as risk factors for subsequent cerebral infarction. Exclusion criteria, on the other hand, define a set of variables which might otherwise confound the analysis—e.g. atrial fibrillation in patients with carotid stenosis and transient ischemic attacks. These criteria define a cohort or subset of patients to be followed over time to analyze risk factors and/or describe the natural history of the condition being studied.

A delicate balance between inclusionary and exclusionary criteria must be determined to provide a cohort which is selective and relatively uniform, yet large enough to provide adequate sample size (see below) and general enough to be applicable to larger populations. Extreme care must be taken to insure that the study population is not biased by undefined selection criteria. As discussed below, the EC-IC Bypass Trial[13] was widely criticized[1,2,11,15,22] for including only a portion of all qualified patients at participating centers. In this study, referral bias may have produced a subset of patients with a stroke risk which was different from that of the general population. To assess this issue, subsequent clinical trials in cerebrovascular surgery incorporated follow-up of nonrandomized qualified patients to insure against this potential deficit.

Data Acquisition

The means by which data are collected in any clinical trial contributes to its accuracy and ultimate validity. The precision of observations is defined as the consistency of replicate measurements, which in turn are determined by random errors from the observer, the subject, and the instrument used to gather data. Precision can be enhanced by several methods, including training the observer, blinding the observer to the treatment group, and standardizing the data collection instrument (a questionnaire in most clinical trials). The sensitivity of an instrument is defined as the [number of positive observations/total number of true positive occurrences]; conversely, specificity is defined as the [number of negative observations/total number of true negative occurrences]. Variables can be continuous (e.g. serum glucose), discrete (e.g. number of prior transient ischemic attacks [TIAs] or categorical (e.g. stroke). The precision of categorical variables can be enhanced by using pre-established scales (e.g. stroke disability ratings).

Incidence and Prevalence

In contrast to cohort studies which follow a group of patients over time, cross-sectional studies measure a set of variables in a given population at one point in time. Cross-sectional studies are usually derived from general populations or data banks and define disease prevalence as the [number of patients with disease at one point in time/total number of patients at risk at that time]. Although prevalence provides important demographic information, cross-sectional studies provide less evidence for causality between any variable and outcome. For example, the prevalence of myocardial infarction is high in patients with carotid bruits; nevertheless, it is unlikely that carotid stenosis is the cause of heart attack or that carotid endarterectomy will effectively prevent it. By following patients over time, cohort trials determine disease incidence, or the [number of new cases over a period of time/total number of individuals at risk during that time]. In addition to inferring causality, cohort studies can avoid bias in measuring predictive variables, examine several outcomes over time, and determine the relative risk reduction provided by a specific therapy.

Types of Cohort Trials

Retrospective cohort trials identify a given population and analyze the existence of potential predictive variables at a prior time. For example, Sundt[23] used retrospective analysis to define perioperative risk factors in patients undergoing carotid endarterectomy. The advantage of retrospective trials is their relative simplicity, short duration, and low cost. The major disadvantages are uncontrolled patient selection, potential bias in determining predictors, and the lack of evidence for sequential cause-and-effect. Although retrospective trials may compare outcome data to that derived from other trials or cross-sectional studies, conclusions are weakened by potential differences in populations studied.

Prospective cohort trials, on the other hand, define one or more predictive variables (or treatments) in a given population and measure outcome over time. By reducing bias and controlling subject selection, true causality can be inferred with a much greater level of confidence compared to retrospective trials. The disadvantages of prospective trials include complexity, duration, cost, and potential ethical concerns. The validity of prospective trials can be further enhanced by randomization, stratification, and blinding.

Randomization eliminates bias from confounding variables by ensuring treatment groups are comparable in every regard. In most contemporary studies, treatment group is assigned by computer-generated or random number lists. Although certain variables may be analyzed retrospectively in prospective trials, additional validity can be obtained by stratification of subgroups—e.g. TIA vs. amaurosis fugax vs. completed stroke—in which separate randomization occurs for each group. Blinding of treatment to observer (single-blind) or to both patient and observer (double-blind) can reduce bias from unintended treatment or inaccurate outcome determination. In certain settings (e.g. surgical procedures) blinding is impossible.

The validity of outcome analysis is enhanced by maximizing the follow-up of patients entered into a prospective trial. Considerable effort must be made to follow as many patients as possible for the entire duration of the trial, and to minimize crossover from one treatment group to another. Intent-to-treat analysis follows outcome in all randomized patients regardless of whether they receive the intended treatment. This technique minimizes variability from unexpected occurrences such as cross-over between groups, but can produce seemingly inaccurate outcome determinations (e.g. a patient randomized to carotid endarterectomy who has a stroke prior to surgery).

Statistical Analysis

In any experiment, the null hypothesis predicts that there will be no association between the predictive variable (or treatment) and outcome. Statistical measures of outcome analyze the possibility that any observed association might have occurred by chance (alpha or p-value). A 1-tailed analysis assumes the association occurs in only one direction (e.g. fewer strokes after carotid endarterectomy), whereas 2-tailed analysis assumes the association might occur in either direction (e.g. fewer or more strokes after carotid endarterectomy). Type I errors occur when a positive association is falsely demonstrated. Type II errors occur when a falsely negative association is shown. The likelihood

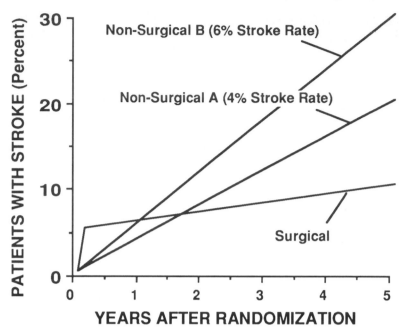

Figure 1: Schematic representation of estimated stroke rates used to calculate sample size for a prospective study of carotid endarterectomy. In each case, a perioperative stroke and death rate of 5% and subsequent annual stroke rate of 1% are used for the surgical group. If the annual stroke rate in the nonsurgical group is 4% (**A**), at 5 years there will be a 50% reduction in strokes for surgery patients. Assuming an annual 6.0% stroke rate for nonsurgical patients (**B**) provides a 67% reduction in stroke for surgery at 5 years.

of Type I or Type II errors are determined by the magnitude of the difference in expected outcome between groups and the sample size. Fewer patients may be necessary to demonstrate a valid association when outcome events are much more frequent in one group.

Statistical power is defined as the value (percentage likelihood of a Type II error). In most clinical trials, a p-value of 0.5 (i.e. < 5% chance of Type I error) and a statistical power of 0.9 (i.e. a < 10% chance of Type II error) are used to calculate sample size in the design of the study. These values are arbitrary. Calculation of sample size is critical in preventing either type of error and thereby producing misleading results.

In many cases, the outcome incidence is not known prior to the study and sample size estimates must be based upon limited data. For example, if perioperative morbidity/ mortality from carotid endarterectomy is estimated at 5% with a subsequent 1% annual stroke risk, a total of 10% of surgical patients would experience an endpoint (stroke) at 5 years. If the annual stroke rate in unoperated patients is 4%, total strokes at 5 years would equal 20% (Figure 1). Based upon these figures, approximately 600 patients would be required to demonstrate a statistically significant difference between groups at p = 0.5 and power = 0.9. However, 6% stroke rate in the nonsurgical group (n = 30%) would require a sample size of only 350 patients to demonstrate a difference with the same degree of confidence.[24]

Prospective Randomized Trials for Cerebrovascular Surgery

The EC-IC Bypass Trial

The EC-IC Bypass Trial[13] represented the first major study of cerebrovascular surgery in the era of modern clinical trials. The conclusion that surgery provided no benefit in protection against subsequent stroke in this group of patients was controversial[15,17] and has had a profound impact upon clinical practice in North America. In addition to influencing practice patterns, this study had far-reaching implications in medicolegal and reimbursement issues. Finally, the EC-IC Bypass Trial initiated an era of intense scrutiny of cerebrovascular surgery, including the development of several rigorous clinical trials for carotid endarterectomy (see below).

The EC-IC Bypass Trial was initiated in 1977 at 71 centers in the United States, Canada, Japan, and in Europe. A total of 1,377 patients with anterior circulation strokes, retinal infarction, or TIA within 3 months were randomized to surgical (N = 663) or nonsurgical (714) treatment. Qualifying lesions included middle cerebral artery (MCA) stenosis or occlusion, cervical internal carotid artery (ICA) stenosis above the C2 vertebral body, or ICA occlusion. Patients were followed for 5 years and primary endpoints were designated as fatal or nonfatal stroke (including all vascular distributions).

At an average follow-up of 55.8 months, EC-IC bypass provided no significant protection against stroke in any distribution, ipsilateral stroke, or stroke and death. Technical results of surgery were excellent with 96% of anastomoses patent on postoperative angiogram. Perioperative major stroke and death was 4.5%; however, one-third (10 of 30) of these strokes occurred prior to surgery and were included in an intent-to-treat analysis. In the equivalent time period, 1.3% of non-

surgical patients had major strokes. By 60 months, there was no significant difference in stroke rate between surgical (20%) and nonsurgical (18%) groups. Subgroup analysis showed no benefit for surgery based upon site or severity of arteriographic lesions, presence of ICA occlusion, temporal pattern of presenting symptoms, or size and location of participating center. Outcome appeared to be worse after surgery in patients with MCA stenosis or those with persistent symptoms after ICA occlusion. Analysis excluding patients with preoperative stroke did not affect outcome. There was no benefit in terms of functional status for patients receiving EC-IC bypass. The authors concluded that EC-IC bypass surgery was ineffective in preventing cerebral ischemia in patients with atherosclerotic disease in the carotid and middle cerebral arteries.

The EC-IC Bypass Trial was widely criticized on several grounds.[1,2,11,15,22] The ratio of persistently symptomatic versus asymptomatic patients studied was relatively low, and fewer than one symptomatic patient per center per year was entered into the trial. A telephone survey[22] of 57 participating centers revealed that during the period of the trial, for 1,255 patients analyzed for the study, more than twice as many (2,572) patients received surgery outside of the trial. In the U.S. and Japan, 1,014 of 1,831 nonrandomized patients receiving surgery were believed to have been eligible candidates.

These data contradicted those in the published report,[13] which described only 115 patients refusing entry and 52 patients with surgery outside of the trial. An ad hoc committee of the American Association of Neurological Surgeons (AANS)[15] examined the EC-IC Bypass Trial on several aspects and concluded that analysis for patients entered into the trial (internal validity) was appropriate. However, significant discrepancies were noted regarding the recognition and tabulation of data concerning eligible nonrandomized patients; these patients may have exceeded the reported number by 10-fold.

These findings seriously limit the external validity of the study—i.e. whether the observed results can be applied to the overall population. The ultimate fate of eligible nonrandomized patients and the possibility that randomized patients represented a distinct subgroup (perhaps at lower risk) raise significant questions about the validity of the conclusions for this study.

In addition to methodologic concerns, the EC-IC Bypass Trial did not study this procedure in a variety of other conditions including fibromuscular dysplasia, moyamoya disease, aneurysm, or tumor surgery. Despite the criticisms listed above, the study has been widely interpreted as demonstrating that surgery was not beneficial in any setting. Data suggesting a surgical benefit in patients with demonstrable cerebral hemodynamic insufficiency have been largely ignored, and at present the operation is uncommonly performed for occlusive cerebrovascular disease. At this time it appears unlikely that a second prospective randomized trial can be mounted to demonstrate efficacy for EC-IC bypass.

Trials for Carotid Endarterectomy

Early Trials

Results from three randomized trials for carotid endarterectomy were published prior to 1991. The Joint Study of Extracranial Arterial Occlusion[14] involved 24 centers in the United States. From 1962 to 1968, 316 patients with TIA and carotid stenosis were randomized to surgical or nonsurgical therapy. At a mean follow-up of 42 months, stroke occurred in 19 of 167 surgical patients (11%) compared to 18 of 145 nonsurgical patients (12%). In the endarterectomy groups, the majority of strokes (13 of 19) occurred in the perioperative period with a relatively low subsequent

stroke rate (approximately 1.5% per year). This study was flawed by a number of significant methodologic errors, including limited sample size, lack of follow-up for eligible nonrandomized patients, variability in stroke diagnosis, and inconsistency of adjunctive therapies.

Shaw et al[21] published a limited trial involving 41 symptomatic patients in Great Britain. This trial was terminated due to an excessive perioperative stroke rate (25%) among participating surgeons. A limited randomized trial for asymptomatic stenosis[10] involved only 29 patients. In summary, perhaps the only meaningful data from early prospective randomized trials for carotid endarterectomy concerned the relatively low (1% to 2% annual) risk of subsequent stroke in those patients surviving surgery. Due to serious methodologic flaws, other data regarding comparison between surgical and nonsurgical therapy in these studies must be discounted.

Current Trials for Carotid Endarterectomy

In late 1984, a series of articles appeared in the scientific[3,4,12,26] and popular literature expressing the need for prospective randomized trials to determine the efficacy of carotid endarterectomy in preventing stroke. These papers were based upon several premises: (1) that frequency of carotid endarterectomy in North America was increasing to levels approximating 100,000 cases annually;[12] (2) that wide individual variations existed in perioperative morbidity and mortality after carotid endarterectomy, with total complication rates ranging from 1% to 20%;[27] (3) that the natural history of untreated carotid stenosis was not well defined, with annual stroke incidence estimated for asymptomatic stenosis from 1% to 4%[16] and for symptomatic stenosis from 4% to 10%;[26] (4) that wide geographical variations in the frequency of carotid endarterectomy existed within the United States[17] and between countries[26];

TABLE 1
Prospective Randomized Trials for Carotid Endarterectomy—Asymptomatic Stenosis

Trial	Principal Investigator	Stenosis Criteria	Aspirin	CT	Follow-up	Sample Size	Primary Endpoints	Estimated Completion Date
Veterans Administration CSP #167	R.R. Hobson	>50% (All angio)	1300 mg/day	No	5 years	500 (444 actual)	TIA or stroke in distribution of randomized artery; death <30 days after randomization	1991
CASANOVA	H.C. Diener H. Homann	50%-90% Noninvasive	1000 mg/day +Dipyridi-mole 225 mg/day	Yes	3 years	400	TIA, stroke or death	1991
ACAS	J. Toole	>60% (Angiosurgery only)	325 mg/day	Yes	5 years	1,500	TIA or stroke in distribution of randomized artery; death <30 days after randomization	1996
MACE	D. Wiebers	>50% (Noninvasive)	80 mg/day (Nonsurgical group only)	Option	2 years	900	TIA, RIND, stroke or death	

TABLE 2
Prospective Randomized Trials for Carotid Endarterectomy—Symptomatic Stenosis

Trial	Principal Investigator	Stenosis Criteria	Aspirin	CT	Follow-up	Projected Size	Primary Endpoints	Estimated Completion Date
ECST	C. Warlow	0%-99% (All angio)	Discretion	Yes	5 years	400	Ipsilateral stroke	1991
NASCET	H.J.M. Barnett	30%-99% (All angio)	Discretion	Yes	5 years	3000 (659 actual for >70% stenosis)	Ipsilateral stroke; stroke-related death; death <30 days after randomization	1991 (>70%) ~1996 (30%-69%)
Veterans Administration CSP #309	M. Mayberg S.E. Wilson F. Yatsu	50%-99% (All angio)	325 mg/day	Yes	3 years	500 (192 actual)	Ipsilateral stroke or crescendo TIA; death <30 days	1991

(5) that the indications for carotid endarterectomy varied widely, with as few as 35% of operations being performed for "appropriate" reasons;[30] (6) that prior randomized trials for carotid endarterectomy were flawed (see above) and did not provide a scientific basis for determining the efficacy of the operation; and (7) that the EC-IC Bypass Trial demonstrated the feasibility of similar multicenter prospective trials for carotid endarterectomy.[4]

These expressions of concern were shortly followed by several trends which profoundly affected the nature of clinical practice in cerebrovascular disease. First, policy statements regarding these indica-tions for carotid endarterectomy were issued by several organizations, including the American Neurologic Association,[28] the American Heart Association,[5] and various ad hoc committees.[7,9] Second, there was a dramatic reduction in the number of endarterectomies performed in the United States overall (35%)[20] and in the Veterans Administration health care system (32%) (unpublished data). Finally, a number of prospective, randomized trials for carotid endarterectomy were undertaken.

In January, 1991, seven carotid endarterectomy trials were in progress (Tables 1 and 2). Four trials involve patients with asymptomatic carotid stenosis: Veterans

Administration Cooperative Studies Program #167 (CSP #167); the Carotid Artery Surgery Asymptomatic Narrowing Operation Versus Aspirin (CASANOVA); the Asymptomatic Carotid Atherosclerosis Study (ACAS); and, the Mayo Asymptomatic Carotid Endarterectomy Trial (MACE). Three trials deal with symptomatic patients: European Carotid Surgery Trial (ECST); North American Symptomatic Carotid Endarterectomy Trial (NASCET); and, Veterans Administration Cooperative Studies Program #309 (CSP #309).

All seven studies are prospective, randomized, nonblinded, multicenter trials. Although these studies have certain features in common, various important differences may influence their generalizability to wider populations and complicate intertrial comparisons. In this regard, the most significant differences relate to the population from which respective study patients were drawn, especially in relationship to the exclusion and ultimate fate of eligible, nonrandomized patients.

Trials for Asymptomatic Carotid Stenosis

CSP #167 is funded by the Veterans Administration Cooperative Studies Program and completed patient entry in November, 1988. A cohort of 444 patients completed follow-up in April, 1991. CASANOVA is funded by the Federal Republic of Germany and entered 400 patients by 1988. ACAS is funded by the National Institute of Neurologic Disorders and Stroke (NINDS) and projects a total sample size of 1,500 patients. MACE[29] is funded by NINDS and estimated a sample size of 900 patients.

Follow-up with regular visits is 5 years for CSP #167 and ACAS, 3 years for CASANOVA, and 2 years for MACE. ACAS and MACE will follow nonrandomized eligible patients for the duration of the study. All four trials set a probability level of 0.05 to indicate statistical significance. ACAS and CSP #167 screened participating centers for perioperative morbidity and mor-

tality $<3.0\%$. Anesthesia and surgical technique are not standardized among centers for any trial.

Patients must have no symptoms of cerebral ischemia ipsilateral to carotid stenosis in all four trials, although contralateral symptoms are permitted in ACAS and CSP #167. Criteria for carotid stenosis are comparable at 60% for ACAS and 50% for the other trials. CSP #167 requires angiographic documentation for all patients, whereas ACAS requires angiography only in surgical patients, and CASANOVA and MACE use noninvasive assessment. ACAS and CASANOVA patients are drawn from general populations at multiple centers, MACE enrolls Mayo Clinic patients, and CSP #167 utilizes men only from participating Veterans Administration medical centers. In all studies, randomization within each strata occurs at each center to minimize differences between centers. CASANOVA employs a complicated randomization procedure for patients with bilateral carotid stenosis in which one or both carotid arteries may be operated upon, and surgeons may arbitrarily exclude certain eligible patients.

Exclusion criteria are relatively consistent among the four asymptomatic trials. In general, patients who would otherwise not be considered for surgery are excluded according to a variety of neurologic, cardiovascular, and general medical (e.g. renal failure, diabetes, etc.) criteria. Confounding neurologic (e.g. seizures, dementia, etc.) and cardiac (e.g. atrial fibrillation, severe valvular disease) conditions which might affect evaluation of stroke outcome are generally grounds for exclusion.

All asymptomatic trials apply best medical management including risk-factor reduction and aspirin therapy to both medical and surgical groups, with the exception of MACE in which the surgery group does not receive aspirin. The aspirin dose varies: MACE = 80 mg/day, ACAS = 325 mg/day, CSP #167 = 1,300 mg/day, CASANOVA = 1,000 mg/day + 225 mg dipyridamole/day.

Computed tomography (CT) scans are required in ACAS and CASANOVA and are optional in MACE.

Results from Asymptomatic Trials

Results from the four asymptomatic trials are forthcoming. CSP #167 completed patient follow-up in April, 1991, and publication is in progress. A preliminary report[25] described perioperative stroke morbidity (2.4%) and mortality (1.9%) for the surgical group in this trial. CASANOVA ended patient entry in 1988 and followup was completed early in 1991. ACAS has entered slightly more than 50% of a projected sample of 1,500 patients. MACE has suspended patient entry at this time for undisclosed reasons.

Trials for Symptomatic Carotid Stenosis

ECST is funded by multiple sources and estimated a sample size of 400 patients. NASCET is funded by NINDS and has entered approximately 1,500 patients of a projected 3,000. CSP #309 was terminated after entering 192 patients of a projected 500 (see below). Follow-up is 5 years for ECST and NASCET and 3 years for CSP #309. NASCET and CSP #309 will follow eligible nonrandomized patients outside of the study. All three studies determined sample size based upon p = 0.05 and power = 0.9. NASCET and CSP #309 screened participating centers for surgical morbidity/mortality < 6.0%. Anesthesia and surgical technique are not standardized among centers for any trial.

Inclusion criteria are relatively standard among the symptomatic trials and include transient cerebral or retinal ischemia or minor completed stroke in the distribution of a stenotic carotid artery within 120 days of randomization. ECST and NASCET enter men and women from general referral populations at multiple centers, whereas CSP #309 enrolls only men at Veterans Administration centers. Angiography is mandatory in all three trials, although entry criteria vary: 0%-99% in ECST, 30%-99% for NASCET and 50%-99% for CSP #309. All three studies randomize by center according to various stratification schemes, although ECST randomizes 60% of patients to surgery. As per the asymptomatic trials, exclusionary criteria are relatively standard for NASCET and CSP #309, and seek to exclude patients who would not otherwise be candidates for surgery. ECST, on the other hand, employs nondefined (discretionary) guidelines for patient exclusion.

Among symptomatic trials, only CSP #309 defines best medical management as risk reduction plus aspirin 325 mg/day; ECST and NASCET allow discretionary administration of aspirin or other medications. CT scans are required in all studies at entry and at endpoint occurrence.

Primary endpoints in all three trials are defined as clinical infarction ipsilateral to the randomized carotid artery; ECST and CSP #309 also include death within 30 days of randomization. CSP #309 regards crescendo TIAs in the appropriate vascular distribution as a primary endpoint. Secondary endpoints for all studies include death from causes other than stroke, stroke in other vascular distributions, or myocardial infarction.

Results from Symptomatic Trials

The ECST study reported that carotid endarterectomy significantly reduced ipsilateral stroke in symptomatic patients with carotid stenosis > 70%, whereas surgery provided no benefit for stenosis < 30%.[13a] Among 778 patients with stenosis > 70%, the cumulative ipsilateral stroke rate over three years was 12.3% in the surgery group versus 21.9% in the unoperated group. Fatal or disabling ipsilateral stroke was similarly less in the surgery group (6% versus 11%). The efficacy of surgery for stenosis of 30% to 69% was not reported.

In February, 1991, NASCET prematurely stopped randomizing patients with carotid stenosis > 70% due to the overwhelming stroke risk reduction observed in the surgical group.[19] A total of 659 patients in this category of stenosis were randomized to surgical (N = 331) or nonsurgical (N = 328) therapy. At a mean follow-up of 24 months, ipsilateral stroke was noted in 26% of nonsurgical patients, compared to 9% of patients with endarterectomy, for an overall risk reduction of 17% (relative risk reduction = 71%).

The benefit for surgical patients was highly significant ($p < 0.001$) for a variety of outcomes, including stroke in any territory, major strokes, and major stroke or death from any cause. A perioperative morbidity/mortality of 5.8% was rapidly surpassed in the nonsurgical group, such that surgical benefit was apparent by 3 months. In addition, the protective effect of surgery was durable over time, with few strokes noted in the endarterectomy group beyond the perioperative period. Functional disability (assessed by a standardized disability scale) was significantly less in the surgery group over time ($p < 0.001$). Multivariate analysis demonstrated that surgical benefit was independent of a variety of concurrent demographic variables. There was a direct correlation between surgical benefit and the degree of angiographic stenosis. NASCET continues to randomize symptomatic patients with carotid stenosis of 30% to 69%; the benefit of carotid endarterectomy in this group of patients remains indeterminate.

Enrollment in CSP #309 was discontinued in February, 1991, based upon preliminary data consistent with the NASCET findings. Subsequent analysis demonstrated a statistically-significant reduction in ipsilateral stroke or crescendo TIA for patients with carotid stenosis > 50%.[18] A total of 193 men aged 35 to 82 years (mean = 64.2 years) were randomized to surgical (N = 91) or nonsurgical (N = 98) treatment. The complication rate of cerebral angiography was low, with no permanent residual deficits and transient complications in 5% (2% local vascular; 2% transient neurologic; 1%

minor allergic). Two-thirds of randomized patients demonstrated angiographic internal carotid artery stenosis greater than 70%. Duplex examination was performed in 152 patients who subsequently underwent cerebral angiography. There was poor accuracy in the lower ranges of stenoses, especially underestimating the degree of stenosis between 30% to 49%. Non-endpoint complications of surgery were relatively infrequent, including respiratory insufficiency requiring extended intensive care monitoring (5%), minor to moderate wound hematoma (5%), cranial nerve deficit (5%), myocardial infarction (2%), and pulmonary embolism (1%).

At a mean follow-up of 11.9 months there was a significant reduction in stroke or crescendo TIA in patients receiving carotid endarterectomy (7.7%) compared to nonsurgical patients (19.4%), or a risk reduction of 11.7% (relative risk reduction=60%; p=0.028). Among subgroups, the benefit of surgery was most prominent in TIA patients compared to TMB or stroke, although these differences were not statistically significant. There was a positive correlation between the degree of carotid stenosis and the subsequent risk of stroke.

For patients with carotid stenosis greater than 70%, surgery provided a risk reduction for stroke or crescendo TIA of 14.8% (p = 0.01). The benefit for surgery was apparent as early as 2 months after randomization, and persisted over the entire period of follow-up. The efficacy of carotid endarterectomy was durable with only one ipsilateral stroke beyond the 30-day perioperative period. Discounting one preoperative stroke, a perioperative morbidity of 2.2% and mortality of 3.3% (total = 5.5%) was achieved over multiple centers among relatively high-risk patients.

Symptomatic Trials — Conclusions

Several notable features are common to the three symptomatic trials. First, carotid endarterectomy provided a profound protection against subsequent ipsilateral stroke or crescendo TIA in patients with high-grade symptomatic stenosis. The stroke risk reduction was realized early after surgery, persisted over extended periods of time, and was independent of other risk factors. Second, stroke in the nonsurgical group considerably exceeded those reported from prior prospective and retrospective studies. Symptomatic patients receiving aspirin in prior prospective multicenter trials had annual stroke rates ranging from 3% to 7%,[3,6,8] compared to rates between 15% to 20% in unoperated patients from NASCET and CSP #309. Third, the inaccuracy of carotid Duplex ultrasonography noted in CSP #309 suggests that symptomatic patients with intermediate degrees of stenosis by Duplex should have definitive assessment by angiography prior to determination of therapy. Finally, efficacy of carotid endarterectomy depends in part upon an acceptable level of perioperative morbidity and mortality.

Summary

It has been stated that "if carotid endarterectomy was a drug its efficacy would require scrutiny and licensure....by the Food and Drug Administration."[26] Although this contention has widespread proponents,[3,12] surgical procedures are in fact not drugs and cannot necessarily be studied according to the same criteria. Clinical decision-making in surgery is a multifactorial process involving both subjective and objective evaluations which are difficult to quantitate and standardize. A variety of factors can otherwise confound the best clinical trial design, including referral patterns, fiscal concerns, and local variations in treatment. Most importantly, there remains the profound ethical concern regarding witholding previously accepted therapy from one group of patients in a randomized trial of a surgical procedure.

Nevertheless, the clinical trial has become the means by which existing and new surgical procedures may be judged in the near future, and the results of such trials may dictate surgical practice to some extent. For these reasons it is important that surgeons become familiar with the methodology of clinical trials and examine these studies in a critical light.

Editorial Comment: The Impact of Clinical Trials on Medical Practice

The chapter by Mayberg elegantly illustrates the technical and statistical complexities of clinical trials, potential problems of bias and internal and external validity (despite rigorous design and execution), and their profound impact on clinical practice. Rightfully or wrongfully, these trials are likely to affect referral, surgical indications, and reimbursement patterns.

Yet, trials are designed and patients are selected and stratified based on current knowledge about the disease, which is ever changing and expanding. Newer technologies may alter patient evaluation protocols and the surgical procedures themselves during the trial. Trials are rarely designed to address issues of technical performance of the procedure—which may have more than a trivial impact on surgical outcome in clinical practice. Rarely are trials sensitive to issues of combined disease, timing of surgical intervention, and highly individual contraindications. These factors may have a profound impact on individual outcomes. Clinical trials risk trivializing such issues which interact in a complex fashion in the mind of every surgeon, and clearly affect and impact upon decision-making in daily surgical practice.

Clinicians and scientists should both be aware of these factors, which are not very amenable to statistical modeling. Clinical trials should be interpreted in light of all other valid scientific information, and should supplement and not replace other lines of evidence. Clinical trials should not be extrapolated to answer questions about populations not studied in the trials, nor should secondary subgroup analyses be allowed to replace statistically valid prospective strat-ification.

The EC-IC Bypass Trial was used to condemn the procedure in subgroups of patients with peculiar angiographic and clinical features—i.e. failures of medical therapy, clear evidence of hemodynamic compromise, etc.—despite inadequate strat-ification and insufficient numbers of such patients. The EC-IC Bypass Trial was even used to determine reimbursement policy in cases of moyamoya disease, which were not even included in the trial.

Early results from trials on carotid endar-terectomy in symptomatic patients are hav-ing the opposite effect of endorsing carotid endarterectomy in all subgroups of patients. Surgeons are noticing a marked increase of referrals for this operation, and an inclina-tion by medical colleagues to urge operative intervention. Many, but not all, such pa-tients need or will likely benefit from carotid endarterectomy. In some cases, associated medical risks should prohibit surgery—despite the results of recent trials. In other patients, timing of surgery after a recent stroke, or technical and/or anesthetic fac-tors, may have a determining impact on the success or failure of surgery.

In summary, clinical trials should and will affect clinical and surgical decision-making. Yet, they should be interpreted in light of all other scientific evidence, and should not be used to replace multiple other considerations involved in surgical judgment.

Issam A. Awad, MD, MS, FACS

References

1. Ausman JI, Diaz FG. Critique of the extracranial-intracranial bypass study. *Surg Neurol.* 1986;26: 218-221.

2. Awad IA, Spetzler RF. Extracranial-intracranial bypass surgery: A critical analysis in light of the international cooperative study. *Neurosurgery.* 1986; 19:655-664.

3. Barnett HJM. Canadian Cooperative Study Group. A randomized trial of aspirin and sulfinpyrazone in threatened stroke. *N Engl J Med.* 1978;299: 53-59.

4. Barnett HJM, Plum F, Walton JN. Carotid endar-terectomy — An expression of concern. *Stroke.* 1984; 15:941-943.

5. Beebe HG, Clagett GP, DeWeese JA, et al. Assess-ing risk associated with carotid endarterectomy. A statement for health professionals by an ad hoc committee on carotid surgery standards of the stroke council, American Heart Association. *Cir-culation.* 1989;79: 472-473.

6. Bousser MG, Eschwege E, Haguenau M, et al. "AICLA" controlled trial of aspirin and dipyrida mole in the secondary prevention of athero-throm-botic cerebral ischemia. *Stroke.* 1983;14: 5-14.

7. Callow AD, Caplan LR, Correll JW, et al. Carotid endarterectomy: What is its current status? *Am J Med.* 1988;85: 835-838.

8. Candelise L, Landi G, Perrone P, et al. A random-ized trial of aspirin and sulfinpyrazone in patients with TIA. *Stroke.* 1982;13:175-179.

9. Cebul RD, Whisnant JP. American Coallege of Physicians. Indications for carotid endarterec-tomy. *Ann Int Med.* 1989;111:675-677.

10. Clagett GP, Youkey JR, Brigham RA, et al. Asymp-tomatic cervical bruit and abnormal ocular pneumo-plethysmography: a prospective study comparing two approaches to management. *Surgery.* 1984; 96:823-830.

11. Day AL, Rhoton AL, Jr., Little JR. The extracranial-intracranial bypass study. *Surg Neurol.* 1986;26: 222-226.

12. Dyken ML, Pokras R. The performance of endar-terectomy for disease of the extracranial arteries of the head. *Stroke.* 1984;15:948-950.

13. The EC/IC Bypass Study Group. Failure of extra-cranial-intracranial arterial bypass to reduce the risk of ischemic stroke: Results of an international randomized trial. *N Engl J Med.* 1985;313:1191-1200.

13a. European Carotid Surgery Trialists' Collaborative Group: MRC European carotid surgery trial: inte-rim results for symptomatic patients with severe (70-99%) or with mild (0-29%) carotid stenosis. *Lancet.* 1991;337:1235-1243.

14. Fields WS, Maslenikov V, Meyer JS, et al. Joint study of extracranial arterial occlusion, V: Progress report of prognosis following surgery or nonsurgi-cal treatment for transient cerebral ischemic attacks and cervical carotid artery lesions. *JAMA.* 1970;211: 1993-2003.

15. Goldring S, Zervas N, Langfitt T. The extracranial-intracranial bypass study. A report of the commit-tee appointed by the American Association of Neurological Surgeons to examine the study. *N Engl J Med.* 1987;316:817-820.

16. Hertzer NR. Presidential address: Carotid endar-terectomy — a crisis in confidence. *J Vasc Surg.* 1988;7:611-619.

17. Leape LL, Park RE, Solomon DH, et al. Relation between surgeons' practice volumes and geogra-phic variation in the rate of carotid endarterec-tomy. *N Engl J Med.* 1989;321:653-657.

18. Mayberg MR, Wilson SE, Yatsu F, et al. Carotid endarterectomy and prevention of cerebral ische-mia in symptomatic carotid stenosis. *JAMA.*1991; 266:3289-3294.

19. North American Symptomatic Carotid Endarter-ectomy Trial Collaborators: Beneficial effect of carotid endarterectomy in symptomatic patients with high-grade carotid stenosis. *New Engl J Med.* 1991;325:445-453.

20. Pokras R, Dyken ML. Dramatic changes in the performance of endarterectomy for diseases of the extracranial arteries of the head. *Stroke.* 1988;19: 1289-1290.

21. Shaw DA, Venables GS, Cartilidge NEF, et al. Carotid endarterectomy in patients with transient cerebral ischemia. *J Neurol Sci.* 1984;64:45-53.

22. Sundt TM, Jr. Was the international randomized trial of extracranial-intracranial arterial bypass representative of the population at risk? *N Engl J Med.* 1987;316:814-816.

23. Sundt TM Jr, Sandok BA, Whisnant JP. Carotid endarterectomy: complications and preoperative assessment of risk. *Mayo Clin Proc.* 1975;50: 301-306.

24. Taylor DW, Sackett DL, Haynes RB. Sample size for randomized trial in stroke prevention. How many patients do we need? *Stroke.* 1984;15:968-971.

25. Towne JB, Weiss DG, Hobson RW. First phase report of cooperative Veterans Administration asymtomatic carotid stenosis study — Operative morbidity and mortality. *J Vasc Surg.* 1990;11: 252-259.

26. Warlow C. Carotid endarterectomy: Does it work? *Stroke.* 1984;15:1068-1076.

27. West H, Burton R, Roon AJ, et al. Comparative risk of operation and expectant management for carotid artery disease. *Stroke.* 1979;10:117-121.

28. Whisnant JP, Fisher L, Robertson JT, et al. Committee on Health Care Issues, American Neurological Association. Does carotid endarterectomy decrease stroke and death in patients with transient ischemic attacks? *Ann Neurol.* 1987;22:72-76.

29. Wiebers DO. Mayo Asymptomatic Carotid Endarterectomy Study Group. Effectiveness of carotid endarterectomy for asymptomatic carotid stenosis: design of a clinical trial. *Mayo Clin Proc.* 1989; 64:897-904.

30. Winslow CM, Solomon DH, Chassin MR, et al. The appropriateness of carotid endarterectomy. *N Engl J Med.* 1988;318:721-727.

CHAPTER 15

Outcome and Rehabilitation in Ischemic Stroke

Bruce M. Coull, MD, and Dennis P. Briley, MD

At the onset of brain infarction, the goals of immediate management are to stabilize the patient medically, to minimize the neurologic deficit, and to begin the evaluation of rehabilitation needs. Despite promising basic and clinical research, current treatments are limited and no intervention strategies are proven effective for reducing infarction size. Thus, active rehabilitation to ameliorate the existing neurologic functional deficit is currently emphasized, as is tailoring medical and surgical management to prevent stroke recurrence.

In a broad sense, stroke rehabilitation encompasses both the pathophysiology underlying the stroke, and neurological, physical, and social conditions which ultimately impact upon the degree of recovery and return of the patient to a vigorous lifestyle. The unfortunate outcome of a more myopic view, which focuses solely on the physical needs of the patient in "rehabilitation," is often subsequent recurrent stroke which worsens the neurologic deficit, increases disability, and sometimes produces multi-infarction dementia or death.

A multiplicity of biological, environmental, and sociological factors influence stroke outcome. Within the context of stroke rehabilitation, two major aspects of these factors are addressed in this chapter.

First, short- and long-term outcome following a stroke are reviewed. Particular emphasis is given to factors that influence long-term outcome, and are potentially treatable or are predictive of patients who may benefit from a rehabilitation program. In this regard, several of the standard measures for evaluation of outcome and follow-up of patients with stroke are discussed.

The second major aspect addressed is physical rehabilitation after a stroke. Use of devices to aid rehabilitation and restoration of function are briefly reviewed, and cognitive and psychologic impairments and their rehabilitation management are discussed. The promising new advances in the pharmacologic support of physical rehabilitation, including the treatment of depression, are briefly summarized.

This review, therefore, is limited in space and scope and highlights only a few important effective components of stroke rehabilitation. Several important aspects of rehabilitative care, including diagnosis and management of speech and language disorders, neuropsychological assessment, and the role of occupational therapy, are omitted from discussion. For a detailed review of standard stroke rehabilitation practices, the texts edited by Duncan and by Kaplan and Cerullo are recommended.[23,52]

Natural History: Stroke Outcome and Stroke Recurrence

The marked variability of acute-phase stroke[20] confounds the assessment of early long-term prognosis. Roughly 15% of persons admitted to hospital with ischemic stroke die within 30 days.[18,50] A modest clinical deterioration in neurologic functions after hemispheric stroke is a typical course for 3 or 4 days after onset, but infarctions within the vertebro-basilar system sometimes progress over a week or more. The mechanisms that underlie progression are multiple, and include brain edema, disturbed function of projection pathways, and recurrent thrombosis or thromboembolism.

Relatively few factors influence short-term survival. Most of these reflect comorbidities that affect survival, such as age, heart disease, and prior stroke.[12] As might be anticipated, the volume of brain infarction is among the most important factors. In a careful study by Chambers et al of both short-term and long-term mortality, clinical findings that correlate with large infarctions indicated a poor prognosis.[12] Among these, decreased level of consciousness had the greatest correlation with early mortality.

Similar observations are reported by others.[18,50] In a study of patients admitted to hospital within 8 hours of stroke onset, a high mortality rate followed deterioration in the level of consciousness within the initial 48 hours.[20] The volume of infarct measured on computed tomography (CT) scans was largest in the group with early deterioration. Hyperglycemia and systolic hypertension at admission, and carotid artery distribution of infarction, were additional indicators of early deterioration in these patients. Of stroke survivors, the patients with neurologic deterioration within the first 48 hours after stroke onset had a worse functional outcome at 90 days.[20]

Other acute neurologic signs associated with large hemispheric infarcts and a poor prognosis include gaze palsy and bilateral leg weakness. Tijssen et al emphasized that conjugate eye deviation often heralds large infarction and a poor prognosis. Of note, eye deviation to the left had a particular poor prognosis.[100] In patients with this finding, long-term impairment was very likely, and 80% of the patients were severely disabled. Increased disability with large left-hemisphere stroke is ascribed in part to the importance of language function and the effect of aphasia upon rehabilitation and return of functional recovery.

Unfortunately, these subjective observations have limited usefulness for the clinician in deciding whether or not to advise stroke rehabilitation. One study from Sweden reported the proportionate first-year outcome of 258 patients with stroke (Figure 1).[98] Although patients with "major" stroke had persistent or severe deficits, 45% were living at home 1 year after stroke; of these, about 70% could walk independently indoors and manage personal hygiene.

A precise method for early prediction of long-term outcomes such as these, and thereby rehabilitative benefit, is not available. Thus, since the clinical status at 3 days after stroke does not accurately predict outcome,[65] evaluation for stroke rehabilitation should usually be uniformly instituted in the management of patients with acute stroke. This holds even for patients with large strokes. Although large brain infarctions as measured by either imaging or clinical means usually imply greater long-term disability, patients with large strokes may demonstrate a greater degree of improvement between days 3 and 30 following ictus than patients wth lesser deficits. Improvement thereafter usually parallels that of persons with lesser impairment for up to 90 days.

Among the best predictors of a poor long-term recovery is a low functional ability at time of discharge from the acute-care hospital. Most studies that address this problem examine the relationship between functional ability at time of admission to rehabilitation, and outcome disposition.[46,63,70,99,103]

In a landmark study using the Barthel index, a measure of independence in activi-

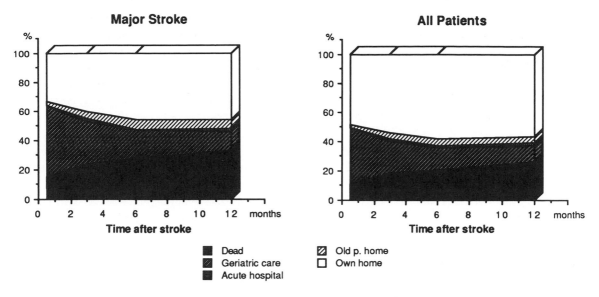

Figure 1. *Residence distribution during the first year after acute stroke in (a) all patients (total n = 258), (b) in patients with major stroke (n = 195). Geriatric care = Geriatric rehabilitation clinics and nursing homes. Old p. home = Old people's home. (From Thorngren M and Westling B., with permission[98])*

ties of daily living (ADLs), Granger and colleagues found that of patients admitted to rehabilitation with a Barthel score of 40 or less, 36% were discharged to another hospital or nursing home and fully 94% required more than 6 weeks of rehabilitation therapy.[34,35,36] In contrast, 96% of subjects with a Barthel score of more than 65 were discharged to home. At 6 months postdischarge, 70% of patients with a Barthel score of 40 or less had either died or were living in a long-term care facility. In general, a Barthel score of 61 or more directly correlates with increased independence in ADLs and better psychosocial adjustment. Patients with Barthel scores between 40 and 80 were most likely to benefit from standard rehabilitation programs.[89,90]

Whether a patient is able to go home or not is more often determined by cognition and social status than by motor-related ADL impairments on the Barthel index.[55,62] Heinemann et al confirmed that, while poor functional ADL at admission for stroke rehabilitation program was associated with poor outcome,[46] these accounted for only 30% of the variability of outcome; nonmeasured factors such as cognition and social status pre-

sumably accounted for the remainder. In this study, improvement during rehabilitation was not related to age, side of hemiparesis, or functional level at time of admission. After completing rehabilitation, approximately 85% of the patients were able to return home.[46]

The anatomic region of brain infarction has an important influence on outcome. In general, patients with hemispheric stroke usually have a worse outcome compared to brain stem infarctions.[12] In contrast to carotid territory stroke, a worse long-term survival may not be heralded by brain stem strokes in which impaired consciousness and other signs typical of a poor short-term prognosis are present.[12] The worst long-term prognosis of hemispheric infarctions is likely due to effects on cognition, language, and other higher cortical functions that are often spared in brain stem strokes. Right hemispheric infarction may impair arousal, and reduce global cerebral activation and decrease attention span.[16]

Even exquisite lesions in critical locations such as the septal region may produce diffuse derangements in cognitive function.[67] Other specific hemispheric deficits following stroke usually correlate with larger infarctions within locations such as the parietal lobes or related projection pathways. Cortical or subcortical lesions may produce either diffuse or very specific deficits that result in considerable but likewise modality-specific impediments to rehabilitation efforts.[60] In general, infarction location within the brain is less specific for degree of disability but more specific for type of disability.

Imaging studies support these concepts of lesion-specific disability. In one study, large infarct size and sulcal width (i.e. atrophy) on CT scans accounted for about 50% of the variability of outcome. Furthermore, many patients with apparent first stroke have CT or magnetic resonance imaging (MRI) evidence of a prior silent stroke. One large multi-center study found that approximately 11% of patients with "first" stroke had CT evidence for a prior silent stroke.[14]

These "silent" infarctions may add to the burden of disability to be overcome after a new symptomatic stroke. Positron emission tomography (PET) studies suggest that preserved metabolic function in ipsilateral cortex immediately surrounding infarcted brain may be critical for good recovery of function.[15] Like other indicators of outcome, however, anatomic lesions are imprecise predictors, except that the infarction location usually correlates with persistence of a given deficit.

This is particularly well documented for stroke affecting the visual and motor systems, where lesions of the primary motor or visual areas are likely to be associated with persistent, easily demonstrable deficits. For example, Bosley et al demonstrated that the presence of CT abnormalities in the primary visual cortex was associated with poor prognosis for visual recovery, compared with homonymous hemianopias produced by lesions elsewhere in the visual pathway.[8] Even cortical atrophy and severe neglect may not, however, prevent patients from showing significant recovery during stroke rehabilitation.[60] Further studies are needed to more tightly link acute or chronic abnormalities found in brain imaging after stroke to preserved functional abilities and rehabilitative outcomes.

Impaired cognition after stroke probably impedes rehabilitation more frequently than recognized. Depression often presents with cognitive decline and should be suspected in all stroke patients who demonstrate apathy, abulia, or social withdrawal or irritability.[79] A general consensus holds that poststroke depressions are most often the direct result of disturbed neurochemical functions after brain injury rather than a psychologic response to disability. These views are critically reviewed by Primeau.[75] The same clinical features of depression may signify more serious underlying cognitive pathologies.

This concept of multi-infarction dementia (MID) or vascular dementia remains controversial. In a review of stroke-related dementia, Tatemichi highlighted four characteristic aspects that were linked to cognitive dysfunction.[97] Most important was location of the infarction. This interesting finding is congruent with reports by others in which infarctions of the thalamus, the temporal lobes, and basal forebrain have been associated with marked cognitive changes.[10,67]

Of additional importance were both the "volume" of brain infarcted and the number of infarcts, which may be additive or multiplicative or produce location-specific effects. These observations bolster the classic view of Tomlinson.[101] Tatemichi cautioned that cognitive decline following infarction may reflect another underlying dementing illness such as Alzheimer's disease. At least 20% of patients with dementia coming to autopsy demonstrate findings of both cerebral infarction and Alzheimer's disease.[102]

Babikian and colleagues performed a systematic study of cognitive changes after multiple infarctions in which patients with aphasia were excluded.[2] Subjects were examined at least 1 month after their most recent infarction. Detailed neuropsychologic assessment yielded significant deficits in cognition in most patients, including those with lacunar infarctions. Using a Mini-Mental Status (MMS) score of less than 24 as a criterion, 42% of subjects with cortical or subcortical strokes were classified as demented. Such studies as these suggest that in the face of more obvious motor deficits, postinfarction cognitive changes and impaired arousal are common but neglected. Underscoring the need for a more detailed investigation of cognitive impairments is the contribution of cognitive decline as a determinator of placement in a long-term care facility.[63]

Besides an appreciation of factors that influence rehabilitation potential, and of greater importance than predictors of survival, are treatment of factors that predispose to stroke recurrence.[30,110] The high frequency of stroke recurrence is a major contributor to morbidity, and in the extreme causes multi-infarction dementia (MID), which is the second leading cause of dementia and cognitive disability in the elderly.

Brain infarctions of every type predispose to recurrent events. During the first 2 weeks after cardioembolism, recurrent brain infarction is observed with a variable frequency of 2% to 20%.[44,45,56,84,86] Studies from the Stroke Data Base Registry indicate that 30-day cumulative stroke risk of slightly over 3% is dependent upon the underlying etiology.[85] Atherothrombotic stroke recurrence approaches 8% ± 2%, whereas lacunar infarction recurrence is only about 2% ± 1% at 30 days. Other studies that have examined the early recurrence of brain infarction report recurrence rates of 1% to 4.8%, from 1 to 3 months after brain infarction.[22,93] Viitanen and colleagues report longer-term stroke recurrence rates of 14% after the first year, rising to a total of 37% at 5 years after stroke.[104] These and many other reports, emphasize that both myocardial infarction and vascular death are necessary cofactors in stroke outcome. If one considers the summation of such interrelated ("hard") endpoints, recurrence rates are frightfully high. Gent et al report a recurrence rate of 25% over 2 years for "major vascular events."[29]

A comparison of reported clinical studies suggests that both stroke recurrence rates and the rates of related major vascular events vary greatly depending upon the population studied. Nevertheless, several consistent themes emerge from these data: (1) the event rates are highest during the first year after stroke,[93] (2) this pattern holds true for stroke, myocardial infarction, and vascular death,[62] and (3) certain treatable risk factors are directly related to recurrent events, especially hyperglycemia at the onset of initial stroke, continued tobacco abuse, elevated systolic or diastolic blood pressure, or a history of either diabetes mellitus or hypertension.

Quantitative Measures for Neurologic Impairment, Dysfunction, or Handicaps

As outlined by Willoughby, three ways to assess outcome after a stroke[109] are (1) measurements of neurologic impairment that characterize the physical signs produced by the stroke, (2) functional disability that characterizes the limitations to the ADL, and (3) handicap which includes the interaction of the first two with the social and environmental limitations that follow stroke. In general, neurologic impairment is directly related to the region and extent of brain infarction, whereas functional disability and handicap depend in part upon outside influences such as family support. Thus, the patient who has a significant neurologic impairment such as a persistent flaccid hemiplegia may have relatively little functional disability by adapting the nonparalyzed arm and leg to achieve ADL.[80] Nevertheless, such a patient may remain significantly handicapped, and require nursing home placement because spouse, family, or community resources to provide assistance with day-to-day needs such as transportation and food shopping are lacking.[55] In order to evaluate disability accurately, this view of "function" must be expanded to include both nervous system and societal abilities.

As discussed above, a low functional ability at time of discharge from the acute-care hospital is predictive of a poor prognosis after stroke. The assessment of the stroke patient during hospitalization, therefore, should specifically explore physical disability as well as mood, memory, language, attention, and visual-spatial abilities since difficulties in these areas influence rehabilitation outcome. A large array of "function" scales have been developed for such applications. Many were developed for use in clinical trials, but most scales are clinically useful for either the more precise identification of disabilities or for following specific difficulties over time. A discussion of the panoply of neuropsychologic tests available for cognitive testing is beyond the scope of this review.[61] Rather, several widely used scales are briefly outlined below. For most research programs and many clinical applications these instruments are used in combinations or given as a "battery" of studies.

More than 16 stroke scales have been developed for quantifying neurologic impairment but few have been validated.[31] One exception outlined in Table 1[31] is the National Institutes of Health (NIH) stroke scale, a sensitive meaure of neurologic deficit that is both brief and highly reproducible. This scale has the particular advantage that it evaluates clinically important deficits such as neglect that simple motor stroke scales often ignore. The 13 items queried by the NIH stroke scale are listed in Table 2[31] along with comparisons and interrater reliability for several other stroke scales. From this table it is apparent that the NIH stroke scale is more comprehensive than other intruments in frequent use.[17,68,91] The NIH stroke scale is usually administered with the Supplemental Motor Examination,[1] which rates muscle strength in both the proximal and distal upper and lower extremities. Other tests of motor function such as the Fugl-Meyer scale and the Motor Assessment Scale for stroke patients are simple to perform and have also been validated.[24,28,74]

Several instruments are available for application to the functional assessment of stroke patients. These instruments probe[91] Activities of Daily Living,[73] Instrumental Activities of Daily Living (IADLs) such as shopping, meal preparation, and use of telephone, and[62] problems in thinking or behavior that result from neuropsychologic dysfunction and are socially disruptive. In most cases, evaluations are completed with the assistance of the patient and spouse or other reliable informant who can describe the patient's daily functional status.

ADLs such as bathing, dressing, feeding, transferring (mobility), toileting, and continence, are assessed in a large number of scales such as the PULSES Profile,[69] the Katz ADL Scale,[53,54] the Barthel index,[66] or the Kenney Self-Care Evaluation.[88] When applied to stroke patients, the scores achieved by the latter three scales are highly correlated, but the Barthel index is most comprehensive, sensitive to change, and statistically useful.[37] The Barthel index, which scores ADLs up to a total of 100 points for normal function, has received widespread clinical and research application among rehabilitation centers in many countries.[13,47] Modifying the Barthel index based on the amount of assistance a patient requires for a given activity may further increase the sensitivity of this scale to clinical change.[89]

A similarly designed and useful measure for the assessment of IADLs is the Multilevel Assessment Instrument developed by Lawton and colleagues.[58] These assessment tools have demonstrated satisfactory psychometric properties for reliability and validity. Alternative ADL and IADL measures exist, such as the Functional Assessment Inventory,[73] but there does not appear to be any specific advantage offered by one over the other for application to stroke patients. Upon recovery from stroke, many patients who achieved perfect ADL or IADL scores exhibit significant deficits on the NIH stroke scale or other instruments that measure behavior, mood, or cognitive functions. Thus, rather than a single scale, a combination of instruments usually best characterizes the difficulties experienced by a given stroke patient.

The MMS examination was developed by Folstein and colleagues[27] for rapid and efficient assessment of dementia and delirium. This test is now widely used for cognitive assessment. Orientation, registration, attention, simple calculation, recall, brief language

TABLE 1
NIH Stroke Scale

Test	Scale
Level of Consciousness	0 (alert, keenly responsive); 1 (drowsy, but arousable by minor stimulation to obey, answer, or respond); 2 (requires repeated stimulation to attend, or lethargic or obtunded requiring strong or painful stimulation to make movement [not stereotyped]); 3 (responds only with reflex motor or autonomic effects, or totally unresponsive, flaccid, reflexless)
Level of consciousness questions (the patient is asked the month and his or her age; only the initial answer is graded)	0 (answers both correctly); 1 (answers one correctly); 2 (answers both incorrectly or unable to speak)
Level of consciousness commands (the patient is instructed to open or close his or her hand or eyes; only initial responses are graded; credit is given if an unequivocal attempt is made but not completed)	0 (obeys both correctly); 1 (obeys one correctly); 2 (incorrect)
Extraocular movements	0 (normal); 1 (partial gaze palsy; score is given when gaze is abnormal in one or both eyes, but where forced deviation or total gaze paresis is not present); 2 (forced deviation or total gaze paresis is not overcome by the oculocephalic maneuver)
Visual fields (test for hemianopia using moving fingers on confrontation with both of patient's eyes open; double simultaneous stimulation is also performed; use visual threat where level of consciousness or comprehension limit testing, but score 1 only if clear-cut asymmetry is found; complete hemianopia [score of 2] is recorded for dense loss extending to within 5 to 10 degrees of fixation)	0 (no visual loss); 1 (partial hemianopia); 2 (complete hemianopia)
Facial palsy	0 (normal); 1 (minor); 2 (partial); 3 (complete)
Motor arm (patient is examined with arms outstretched at 90° if sitting, or at 45° if supine; request full effort for 10 s; if consciousness or comprehension are abnormal, cue the patient by actively lifting his or her arms into position as request for effort is orally given; only the weaker limb is graded)	0 (limb holds 90° for full 10 s); 1 (limb holds 90° position but drifts before full 10 s); 2 (limb cannot hold 90° position for full 10 s. but there is some effort against gravity); 3 (limb falls, no effort against gravity)
Motor leg (while supine, patient is asked to maintain weaker leg at 30° for 5 s; if consciousness or comprehension are abnormal, cue the patient by actively lifting the leg into position as the request for effort is orally given)	0 (leg holds 30° position for a 5-s period); 1 (leg falls to intermediate position by the end of the 5-s period); 2 (leg falls to bed by 5 s, but there is some effort against gravity); 3 (leg falls to bed immediately with no effort against gravity)
Limb ataxia (finger to nose and heel-to-shin tests are performed, ataxis is scored only if clearly out of proportion to weakness; limb ataxia would be "absent" in the hemiplegic, not untestable)	0 (absent); 1 (ataxia is present in one limb); 2 (ataxia is present in two limbs)

(Table 1 is continued on the next page)

TABLE 1
NIH Stroke Scale (continued)

Test	Scale
Sensory (test with pin; when consciousness or comprehension are abnormal, score sensory normal unless deficit is clearly recognized [e.g. by clear-cut grimace asymmetry, withdrawal asymmetry]; only hemisensory losses are counted as abnormal)	0 (normal, no sensation loss); 1 (mild to moderate; patient feels pinprick is less sharp or is dull on the affected side, or there is a loss of superficial pain with pinprick but patient is aware of being touched); 2 (severe-to-total sensation loss, the patient is not aware of being touched)
Neglect	0 (no neglect); 1 (visual, tactile, or auditory hemi-inattention); 2 (profound hemi-inattention to more than one modality)
Dysarthria	0 (normal); 1 (mild to moderate; patient slurs at least some words, and, at worst, can be understood with some difficulty); 2 (patient's speech is so slurred as to be unintelligible [in absence of, or out of proportion to, any dysphasia])
Language (the patient is asked to name the items on the naming sheet and is then asked to read from the reading sheet; comprehension is judged from responses to all of the commands in the preceeding general neurologic examination)	0 (normal); 1 (mild to moderate, as follows: naming errors, word-finding errors, paraphasias, and/or impairment of comprehension or expression disability); 2 (severe: fully developed Broca's or Wernicke's aphasia [or variant]); 3 (mute or global aphasia)

Each item may also be coded as "Untestable." In addition, "Impression From Previous Examination" and "Impression from Baseline" are coded as "same," "better," or "worse." These assessments were not addressed in the present study.

tests, reading, and a single block design are screened. The testing procedure is straightforward, uses routinely available clinical information, and is reliable across examiners. Upon completion, the patient receives a single score up to the total achievable normal of 30 points.

Since the cognitive function of many patients with stroke improves during recovery, application of the MMS early in the course must be interpreted with caution, lest patients be mistakenly labelled as having permanent cognitive impairment or vascular dementia. As a further drawback, this scale cannot be reliably used in aphasic patients, and isolated cognitive problems may produce inaccurate results.

Other useful instruments for measuring various aspects of cognitive function include the Wechsler Adult Intelligence Scales,[107,108] the Raven's Matrices,[76] and the Halstead-Reitan test battery[3,111] These are more exhaustive tools than the MMS, but require lengthy testing times and administration by specifically trained professionals.

Several scales are useful for detecting depression. These include the Beck Depression Inventory,[3] Multiple Affect Adjective Checklist Depression Scales,[111] and the Hamilton Psychiatric Rating Scale for Depression (HRS-D).[42,43] The former two scales are self-report measures. The HRS-D is a 21-item rating scale, completed on the basis of information derived in a psychiatric interview; as a measurement for treatment outcome, it is sensitive to clinical change. The items on the HRS-D cover both physical and psychological symptoms customarily associated with severe depression. These tests have been used in a variety of settings that include the detection and follow-up of depression and cognitive defects and right and left hemispheric infarctions.[25]

In patients where cognitive deficits are detected in the absence of depression, differentiation from Alzheimer's disease is some-

TABLE 2
Inter-rater Agreement: Stroke Rating Scales

Item	NIH Scale	Mathew et al (68)	Canadian Neurological Scale (17)	Stroke Data Bank (91)
Language	Substantial	Substantial	Almost Perfect	Moderate
Motor Leg	Substantial	Fair-Moderate	Substantial - Almost Perfect	Moderate
Motor Arm	Substantial	Moderate - Almost Perfect	Substantial - Almost Perfect	Fair - Moderate
Level of consciousness questions	Substantial	—	—	—
Neglect	Substantial	—	—	—
Visual fields	Moderate	Poor	—	Fair
Level of consciousness	Moderate	—	—	Fair
Sensory	Moderate	Fair	—	Fair
Level of consciousness commands	Moderate	—	—	—
Extraocular movements	Fair	—	—	Substantial
Dysarthria	Fair	—	—	Moderate
Facial palsy	Chance	—	Moderate - Almost Perfect	Substantial
Limb ataxia	Chance	—	—	Moderate

Levels of agreement are based on the published K statistics and are interpreted as described in the "Subjects and Methods" section. Only statistically significant items to those of the NIH Stroke Scale are included.

times difficult. The Hachinski Ischemia Scale (HIS)[40] is a 13-item list of clinical findings that are useful for distinguishing patients with MID from those with dementias of other etiologies such as Alzheimer's disease (DAT). A total derived of the items on the Hachinski scale above 7 is strongly suggestive of MID, whereas less than 4 is suggestive of DAT. A subset of the Hachinski, the modified Hachinski scale[83] contains the factors best at discriminating DAT from MID. Since the Hachinski scale was developed before the advent of modern scanning devices such as the MRI, further modification to incorporate newer evaluation technologies will likely prove to be useful.

The above scales have great utility when applied to screen patients for either unrecognized deficits or for quantification of recog-

nized difficulties. So doing helps alert the rehabilitation team to particular deficits, and may assist in focusing therapies. Following changes in scores over time may provide evidence of continuing progress or achievement of maximal benefit from rehabilitation. Patients with intermediate Barthel scores in particular appear to benefit most from standard rehabilitation efforts.[51,89,90] Patients with very low scores may require placement in a chronic-care facility rather than a rehabilitation facility. Such a patient should be followed and considered for intensive rehabilitation if there is improvement to a Barthel of 40 or more. One useful approach for using these instruments is the assessment of each patient with a stroke-specific scale such as the NIH stroke scale for neurologic impairments, a functional scale such as the Barthel index to evaluate for ADL, additional specific investigations of IADLs, and an assessment of cognitive status with the MMS and HRS-D for depression.

A recent Task Force on Stroke Impairment, Disability, and Handicap made broad recommendations for stroke outcome research and evaluation.[96] Recommendations include classification of stroke impairment by stroke type and lesion location, and categorization of impairments by psychological and physiologic subcategories. Careful documentation of complications and comorbidities such as seizures, fractures, and urinary tract infections is necessary since these may contribute to disability. Disability evaluations should be performed at stroke onset and at 3, 6, and 12 months after ictus.

By applying these guidelines, specific impairments can be identified throughout the course of recovery from stroke. This will assure a continuous, focused rehabilitation as well as coordinated effort. Management of comorbidities such as hypertension, diabetes, heart disease, obesity, and other medical conditions predisposing to stroke recurrence should be coincident with these efforts.

Rehabilitation

Although it is widely accepted that rehabilitation lessens disability following a stroke, proving that rehabilitation is useful has been more difficult. Debate continues as to whether or not focused stroke rehabilitation improves outcome.[21,80] This is due in part to disagreements regarding what to measure as a valid indicator of rehabilitation outcome.[90,103] While there is no evidence that stroke rehabilitation influences neurologic impairment, rehabilitation may be beneficial in overcoming disability.[26,80] From this perspective, rehabilitation, even when provided 1 year or more after the infarction, may produce critical improvements in the abilities needed to meet ADL and IADL.[95]

Most patients with a residual deficit after stroke benefit from rehabilitation, and many severely affected patients may receive benefit by prevention of complications. Conversely, depending upon the population studied, roughly 20% of stroke victims may not benefit from a focused rehabilitation program.[71] Typically, patients who lack benefit have severe deficits and have little functional recovery during the first month after stroke. In patients with severe residual deficits as demonstrated by a Barthel index < 40, active rehabilitation may best be delayed until the patient has regained sufficient function and awareness to participate with the rehabilitation efforts.

Most studies of stroke outcome from rehabilitation place emphasis on impairment of motor function only, with relatively little attention to the cognitive and psychological aspects of recovery. However, since these functions are critical in determining outcome, a rehabilitation program should incorporate cognitive and psychosocial evaluations.[87] Besides mood and memory, evaluations should include praxis, perceptual problems, and sexuality.[5] The most effective rehabilitation techniques for stroke patients are yet to be fully defined, and more effective techniques are needed not only for overcoming certain motor problems such as spasticity,[21,26,39,80] but also for management of neglect and impulsivity. Whether techniques such as cognitive retraining after stroke are useful for treatment of those impaired higher cortical functions is unproved and remains quite controversial.[4,59,105]

Rehabilitation should be started as soon as possible after onset of stroke, but overvigorous early rehabilitation should be avoided lest the patient fall or sustain serious joint injuries because of muscular weakness and inability to stabilize his legs. At this stage, swallowing, speech and language functions, as well as pulmonary, cognitive, and psychosocial evaluations should be conducted. Problems with neglect and apraxias should be identified early in the course of treatment.

During the acute phase of stroke, the initial goals are to prevent complications such as aspiration, contracture, and pressure sores. Intravenous lines should not be placed in a paretic extremity. Each joint in a paralyzed or paretic extremity should be moved through a full range of motion several times daily. Splints are a useful adjunct for prevention of contracture;[3] in particular, a posterior foot splint to prevent plantar contracture is helpful.

Despite their utility, splints are not an adequate substitute for range-of-motion procedures. If the patient will likely be bed bound for a prolonged period, prophylaxis against deep venous thrombosis and pulmonary embolus should be instituted. Intermittent subcutaneous heparin in a dose of 5000 units every 8 hours is effective prophylaxis.[41] In patients where heparin is contraindicated, leg pneumatic devices are suitable alternatives. Frequent turning and appropriate cushioning are effective for preventing pressure sores.

Nutritional status is another important management consideration in which early attention should be directed to the patient's ability to maintain caloric or fluid needs by oral feeding. A catabolic state develops as early as 12 hours after stroke, even in obese patients. Patients with good nutritional status improve faster and have fewer medical complications such as infections and decubiti. If swallowing is impaired or the patient is lethargic, a danger with early oral feeding is aspiration. Aspiration is especially common after bilateral hemispheric strokes or brain stem infarctions, but may even occur with unilateral hemispheric infarction.[49] A diminished cough and the presence of dysphonia are good clinical clues that aspiration will be a problem. The presence or absence of a gag reflex is of little use for assessment of swallowing. If difficulties with glutition are present or suspected, the patient should initially receive intravenous fluids and undergo a formal evaluation for dysphagia.

Speech pathologists often assist in the evaluation and treatment of dysphagia, and assessment usually includes a videofluoroscopic barium swallow. Many patients with dysphagia may be aided by comparatively simple maneuvers such as sitting upright for meals, using a semisolid texture, eating one small bolus of food at a time, and avoiding thin liquids or the use of straws. When these techniques are insufficient, nasogastric feeding is needed.

In the short term, a small nasogastric feeding (Dobhoff) tube may be placed with caution. Infrequent but serious complications that accompany Dobhoff tube use include sinusitis; nasal, pharyngeal, and esophageal erosions; and the potential for displacement. In patients with altered consciousness the tubes are sometimes misguided into the lung, causing complications such as pneumothorax or diaphragmatic perforation. A chest x-ray should be obtained whenever a Dobhoff tube is placed or replaced. When enteric feeding of about 1 month or more is necessary, a feeding gastrostomy should be constructed by the percutaneous route. With appropriate management of dysphagia, the prognosis for eventual return of oral feeding appears to be fairly good.[48,49]

Lethargy and confusion states frequently accompany the acute phase of stroke. This may be manifest as impulsiveness, agitation, and impaired communication. Communication difficulties during this time are often further exacerbated by lack of eyeglasses, hearing aids, and dentures. Neglect of a body side, with consequent lack of awareness of neurologic deficit, may also be a major problem; in the short term, because of agitation, passive restraints are sometimes necessary to prevent falls. Certain patients, such as those with acute Wernicke's aphasia, are frequently bewildered and agitated because of the sudden loss of receptive language and a related gnostic deficit. Having a family member at the bedside for reassurance is often useful in this setting.

Active rehabilitation should begin once the patient is medically stable and out of the acute phase. In particular, metabolic, respiratory, and cardiovascular functions should be optimal and the patient should have sufficient awareness to cooperate with active rehabilitation. Rehabilitation efforts are first directed at improving each significant physical impairment. Goals include increasing strength and coordination of paretic extremities, and stabilizing sitting and standing posture and eventually gait. The longer-term goals usually involve occupational therapy directed at overcoming IADL disabilities.

The usual causes of physical impairments are loss of strength, spasticity, and problems with order and timing of movement. The consequences of these difficulties are loss of range of motion, and loss of joint alignment. With continued paralysis, range-of-motion exercises should remain as a daily exercise routine. Splinting, particularly of the lower extremity, may assume greater importance in this phase of rehabilitation as a mechanism to allow resumption of walking. The ankle-foot orthosis (AFO) assists ankle dorsiflexion, aids efficient ambulation, and helps to prevent tripping.

When the quadriceps is weak, knee hyperextension may occur. This can be partially assisted by knee bracing, which may be linked to an AFO. For minor degrees of impairment, particularly if the deficit involves sensory modalities, a cane provides some added support and sensory input. The use and misuse of braces is discussed by Redford.[78] All braces require patient training to assure proper use, and often physical reconditioning, as an integral part of the rehabilitation process. Physical therapists provide assistance in such management, and guide the retraining process. Most patients with stroke do not require bracing.

Spasticity is a common and sometimes a disabling problem following stroke. Muscle-stretching exercises which may help control mild degrees of spasticity are, when effective, the preferred management option. A brief massage with ice or moist heating may be a useful adjunct to the stretching exercises. Current drug treatments for severe or refractory spasticity are disappointing. Most drugs such as benzodiazepines, baclofen, and dantrolene impede recovery from stroke by clouding consciousness, promoting depression, or producing other untoward side effects.[32,33,57] There is also an increased risk of falls with these medications; as much as possible, their use should be avoided.[77] One exception is the occasional patient who experiences severe generalized spasticity in episodic or nocturnal spasms or when significant weakness is absent. If a single muscle group is problematic, local techniques such as motor point blocks or surgical release of contracture may be considered.[9,78]

A variety of rehabilitation and occupational therapies are useful for patients with upper extremity impairments. With arm paresis, shoulder subluxation is frequent and often painful. When this happens, attempts to move the arm become painful and disuse ensues, which further increases impairment. Simple shoulder slings are helpful. A wrist splint may improve hand function in some patients. Occupational rehabilitation is directed toward the use of adaptive techniques such as learning to dress with the aid of Velcro straps instead of shoelaces, and zippers and snaps instead of buttons. Occupational therapists provide guidance for the selection of specific therapies, and retraining that is needed to achieve IADLs such as relearning how to cook.

Major depression is perhaps the most overlooked treatable cause of failure to achieve or to maintain maximal gains in rehabilitation. Several studies suggest that depression is more likely with infarctions of the left anterior hemisphere,[7] but stroke of every type and location may cause depression.[75] Patients who are depressed have more functional impairment, and do less well in rehabilitation.[92] With depression prevalence between 30% and 50%, at one time or another most patients experience poststroke depression.[72,94,106] In a study of subjects followed at 3 weeks, 6 months, and 12 months following infarction, Wade et al found that approximately one-third of patients were depressed at any given time, and half of those depressed at 3 weeks remained depressed at 1 year.[106] Despite symptoms of major depression, treating physicians failed to diagnose depression in most cases and only rarely prescribed antidepressant therapy. This failure to recognize depression is particularly grievous since treatment of stroke patients with antidepressants is efficacious.[64,81] The use of a screening scale such as the HRS-D for Depression to detect occult depression is recommended.

Cognitive impairment in the convalescing stroke patient is a theoretical contraindication to antidepressant therapy, since antidepressant drugs may impair cognition. This is a less relevant consideration, however, since depression and cognition are clinically linked— i.e. depression may present as cognitive decline.[79] As reported by Lipsey, cognition improved after treatment with antidepressants, even in depressed patients with lower initial mental status scores.[64]

Thus, strong clinical evidence indicates that treatment of depression is useful, even if cognition appears impaired. Depression should be suspected in all patients after stroke, and, if detected, aggressively treated. Re-evaluation of cognitively impaired patients may be assisted by detailed neuropsychological evaluation to provide management guidelines, especially when only one domain of cognition is affected.

The influence of drug treatments upon stroke outcome has received relatively little study. Most patients enrolled in rehabilitation programs are receiving one or more medications, either to treat medical conditions such as hypertension, or to ameliorate behavioral difficulties such as agitation or insomnia. Certain of these drugs may impair recovery. Some drugs not only impair mood and alertness as mentioned previously, but may actually impede brain healing. This latter effect is currently somewhat speculative, but benzodiazepines, neuroleptics, and alpha agonists such as clonidine all have been shown to impair recovery from stroke in experimental animals.[32,33] The medications that patients are receiving during rehabilitation should be carefully reviewed, and the putative benefits of drugs known to affect the sensorium weighed against the adverse effects.

Even less well studied than drugs that cause adverse effects are medications that may aid recovery. There has been one anecdotal report that treatment with bromocriptine benefits recovery from aphasia.[11] Other studies indicate that amphetamine treatment after stroke may aid recovery. In animal experiments of brain injury, amphetamine accelerated motor recovery but did not affect outcome. One small pilot study in man reported that the combination of amphetamine and physical therapy leads to a better outcome. The authors speculate that the improvement results from augmented release of norepinephrine from the diffuse projections of locus ceruleus neurons.[19,33] Although studies to date hold but meager promise, the recent recognition that nervous system growth and other trophic factors have major influences upon neuronal plasticity and brain healing will undoubtedly have increasing importance for research and therapeutic developments in stroke rehabilitation during the next decade.

Summary

Rehabilitation after stroke is an ongoing and recurring process that requires periodic monitoring and review so that patients can maintain or gain functions. This process requires teamwork. The best results are obtained by a multidisciplinary coordinated approach[26] which should include risk-factor management. The use of scales to help assess deficits and monitor progress is recommended. No single measure, scale, or clinical finding is sufficiently accurate early in the course of stroke to predict outcome. Application of a variety of scales is useful for identifying particular problems, focusing rehabilitation efforts, and plotting recovery.

As documentation of improved cognition or neurologic status is obtained, the patient may further benefit from brief courses of focused rehabilitation efforts.[95] The chronic maintenance of functional abilities is a critical need of many elderly patients who require community and social supports to maintain independent living.[82,87]

Most patients with stroke are deconditioned or quickly become so as a consequence of stroke. An individually tailored exercise program is an excellent strategy for building

muscle strength, trimming weight, and helping to improve certain medical conditions
such as hypertension and diabetes. A rehabilitation program for both evaluation and
therapy is most useful. The majority of
patients are able to return home to independent living after stroke, but up to a third
will remain dependent in ADL.[38] In younger
patients, roughly 50% return to work,[6] but
many remain significantly disabled. These
impaired or disabled patients, young and old,
remain the ongoing challenge for better stroke
treatments and rehabilitation.

References

1. Asplund K. Clinimetries in stroke research. *Stroke.* 1987;18:528-530.
2. Babikian VL, Wolfe N, Linn R, et al. Cognitive changes in patients with multiple cerebral infarcts. *Stroke.* 1990;21:1013-1018.
3. Beck AT, Ward CH, Mendelson M, et al. An inventory for measuring depression. *Arch Gen Psychiatry.* 1961;4:561-571.
4. Berrol S. Issues in cognitive rehabilitation. *Arch Neurol.* 1990;47:219-220.
5. Binder LM, Howieson D, Coull BM. Stroke: causes, consequences and treatment. In: Caplan B, ed. *Rehabilitation Psychology Desk Reference.* Rockville, Md: Aspen Publishing Company; 1987:65-100.
6. Black-Schaffer RM, Osberg JS. Return to work after stroke: development of a predictive model. *Arch Phys Med Rehabil.* 1990;71:285-290.
7. Bolla-Wilson K, Robinson RG, Starkstein SE, et al. Lateralization of dementia of depression in stroke patients. *Am J Psychiatry.* 1989;146:627-634.
8. Bosley TM, Dann R, Silver FL, et al. Recovery of vision after ischemic lesions: positron emission tomography. *Ann Neurol.* 1987;21:444-450.
9. Braun RM, West F, Mooney V, et al. Surgical treatment of the painful shoulder contracture in the stroke patient. *J Bone Joint Surg.* [Am] 1971; 53-A:1307-1312.
10. Caplan LR. Top of the basilar syndrome. *Neurology.* 1980;30:72-79.
11. Catsman-Berrevoets CE, von Harskamp F. Compulsive pre-sleep behavior and apathy due to bilateral thalamic stroke: response to bromocriptine. *Neurology.* 1988;38:647-649.
12. Chambers BR, Norris JW, Shurvell BL, et al. Prognosis of acute stroke. *Neurology.* 1987; 37:221-225.
13. Chino N. Efficacy of Barthel index in evaluating activities of daily living in Japan, the United States and United Kingdom. *Stroke.* 1990;21(suppl II): II-64-II-65.
14. Chodosh EH, Foulkes MA, Kase CS, et al. Silent stroke in the NINCDS Stroke Data Bank. *Neurology.* 1988;38:1674-1679.
15. Chollet F, DiPiero V, Wise RJS, et al. The functional anatomy of motor recovery after stroke in humans: a study with positron emission tomography. *Ann Neurol.* 1991;29:63-71.

16. Coslett HB, Bowers D, Heilman KM. Reduction in cerebral activation after right hemisphere stroke. *Neurology.* 1987;37:957-962.
17. Côté R, Hachinski VC, Shurvell BL, et al. The Canadian neurological scale: a preliminary study in acute stroke. *Stroke.* 1986;17:731-737.
18. Coull BM, Brockschmidt JK, Howard G, et al. stroke diagnosis and its relationship to demographics, risk factors, and clinical status after stroke. *Stroke.* 1990;21:867-873.
19. Crisostomo EA, Duncan PW, Propst M, et al. Evidence that amphetamine with physical therapy promotes recovery of motor function in stroke patients. *Ann Neurol.* 1988;23:94-97.
20. Dávalos A, Cendra E, Teruel J, et al. Deteriorating ischemic stroke: risk factors and prognosis. *Neurology.* 1990;40:1865-1869.
21. Dobkin BH. Focused stroke rehabilitation programs do not improve outcome. *Arch Neurol.* 1989;46: 701-703.
22. Donnan GA. In: Donnan GA, Vajda FJE, eds. *Perspectives in Stroke.* Victoria, Australia: York Press; 1986.
23. Duncan PW, Badke MB, eds. *Stroke Rehabilitation: the Recovery of Motor Control.* Chicago, Illinois: Year Book Medical Publishers; 1987.
24. Duncan PW, Propst M, Nelson SG. Reliability of Fugl-Meyer assessment of sensorimotor recovery following cerebrovascular accident. *J Am Assoc Phys Ther.* 1983;63:1606-1610.
25. Egelko S, Simon D, Riley E, et al. First year after stroke: tracking cognitive and affective deficits. *Arch Phys Med Rehabil.* 1989;70:297-302
26. Ernst E. A review of stroke rehabilitation and physiotherapy. *Stroke.* 1990;21:1081-1085.
27. Folstein MF, Folstein SE, McHugh PR. "Minimental state." A practical method for grading the cognitive state of patients for the clinician. *J Psychiat Res.* 1975;12:189-198.
28. Fugl-Meyer AR, Jääskö L, Leyman I, et al. The post-stroke hemiplegic patient, I: A method for evaluation of physical performance. *Scand J Rehabil Med.* 1975;7:13-31.
29. Gent M, Blakely JA, Easton JD, et al. The Canadian-American ticlopidine study (CATS) in thromboembolic stroke. *Lancet.* 1989;1:1215-1220.
30. Goldberg G, Berger GG. Secondary prevention in stroke: a primary rehabilitation concern. *Arch Phys Med Rehabil.* 1988;69:32-40.
31. Goldstein LB, Bertels C, Davis JN. Interrater reliability of the NIH stroke scale. *Arch Neurol.* 1989;46: 660-662.
32. Goldstein LB, Davis JN. Physician prescribing patterns following hospital admission for ischemic cerebrovascular disease. *Neurology.* 1988;38:1806-1809.
33. Goldstein LB, Davis JN. Restorative neurology: drugs and recovery following stroke. *Stroke.* 1990; 21:1636-1640.
34. Granger CV, Dewis LS, Peters NC, et al. Stroke rehabilitation: analysis of repeated Barthel index measures. *Arch Phys Med Rehabil.* 1979;60:14-17.
35. Granger CV, Hamilton BB, Gresham GE. Stroke rehabilitation outcome study, I: general description. *Arch Phys Med Rehabil.* 1988;69:506-509.
36. Granger CV, Hamilton BB, Gresham GE, et al. The stroke rehabilitation outcome study, II: relative merits of the total Barthel index score and a four-item subscore in predicting patient outcomes. *Arch Phys Med Rehabil.* 1989;70:100-103.

37. Gresham GE, Phillips TF, Labi MLC. ADL status in stroke: relative merits of three standard indexes. *Arch Phys Med Rehabil.* 1980;61:355-358.

38. Gresham GE, Phillips TF, Wolf PA, et al. Epidemiologic profile of long-term stroke disability: the Framingham study. *Arch Phys Med Rehabil.* 1979;60:487-491.

39. Hachinski V. Stroke rehabilitation. *Arch Neurol.* 1989;46:703.

40. Hachinski VC, Lassen NA, Marshall J. Multi-infarct dementia: a cause of mental deterioration in the elderly. *Lancet.* 1974;2:207-210.

41. Halkin H, Goldberg J, Modan M, et al. Reduction of mortality in general medical in-patients by low-dose heparin prophylaxis. *Ann Intern Med.* 1982;96:561-565.

42. Hamilton M. A rating scale for depression. *J Neurol Neurosurg Psychiatry.* 1960;23:56-62.

43. Hamilton M. Development of a rating scale for primary depressive illness. *Brit J Soc Clin Psychol.* 1967;6:278-296.

44. Hart RG, Coull BM, Miller VT. Anticoagulation and embolic infarction. *Neurology.* 1983;33:252-253.

45. Hart RG, Miller VT, Coull BM, et al. Cerebral infarction associated with lupus anticoagulants—preliminary report. *Stroke.* 1984;15:114-118.

46. Heinemann AW, Roth EJ, Cichowski K, et al. Multivariate analysis of improvement and outcome following stroke rehabilitation. *Arch Neurol.* 1987;44:1167-1172.

47. Hewer RL. Outcome measures in stroke. a British view. *Stroke.* 1990;21(suppl II):II-52-II-55.

48. Horner J, Massey EW, Brazer SR. Aspiration in bilateral stroke patients. *Neurology.* 1990;40:1686-1688.

49. Horner J, Massey EW, Riski JE, et al. Aspiration following stroke: clinical correlates and outcome. *Neurology.* 1988;38:1359-1362.

50. Howard G, Walker MD, Becker C, et al. Community hospital-based stroke programs: North Carolina, Oregon and New York, III: factors influencing survival after stroke: proportional hazards analysis of 4219 patients. *Stroke.* 1986;17:294-299.

51. Jongbloed L. Prediction of function after stroke: a critical review. *Stroke.* 1986;17:765-776.

52. Kaplan PE, Cerullo CJ, eds. *Stroke Rehabilitation.* Boston, Mass: Butterworths; 1986.

53. Katz S, Downs TD, Cash HR, et al. Progress in development of the index of ADL. *Gerontologist.* 1970;10:20-30.

54. Katz S, Ford AB, Moskowitz RW, et al. Studies of illness in the aged. The index of ADL: a standardized measure of biological and psychosocial function. *JAMA.* 1963;185:914-919.

55. Kelly-Hayes M, Wolf PA, Kannel WB, et al. Factors influencing survival and need for institutionalization following stroke: the Framingham study. *Arch Phys Med Rehabil.* 1988;69:415-418.

56. Koller RL. Recurrent embolic cerebral infarction and anticoagulation. *Neurology.* 1982;32:283-285.

57. Larson EB, Kukull WA, Buchner D, et al. Adverse drug reactions associated with global cognitive impairment in elderly persons. *Ann Intern Med.* 1987;107:169-173.

58. Lawton MP, Moss M, Fulcomer M, et al. A research and service oriented multilevel assessment instrument. *J Gerontol.* 1982;37:91-99.

59. Levin HS. Cognitive rehabilitation: unproved but promising. *Arch Neurol.* 1990;47:223-224.

60. Levine DN, Warach JD, Benowitz L, et al. Left spatial neglect: effects of lesion size and premorbid brain atrophy on severity and recovery following right cerebral infarction. *Neurology.* 1986; 36:362-366.

61. Lezak MD. *Neuropsychological Assessment.* New York, NY: Oxford University Press; 1983.

62. Lincoln NB, Blackburn M, Ellis S, et al. An investigation of factors affecting progress of patients on a stroke unit. *J Neurol Neurosurg Psychiatry.* 1989;52:493-496.

63. Lincoln NB, Jackson JM, Edmans JA, et al. The accuracy of predictions about progress of patients on a stroke unit. *J Neurol Neurosurg Psychiatry.* 1990;53:972-975.

64. Lipsey JR, Robinson RG, Pearlson GD, et al. Nortriptyline treatment of post-stroke depression: a double-blind study. *Lancet.* 1984:1:297-300.

65. Loewen SC, Anderson BA. Predictors of stroke outcome using objective measurement scales. *Stroke.* 1990;21:78-81.

66. Mahoney FI, Barthel DW. Functional evaluation: the Barthel index. *Maryland State Med J.* 1965;14:61-65.

67. Mann DMA, Yates PO, Marcyniuk B. The nucleus basalis of Meynert in multi-infarct (vascular) dementia. *Acta Neuropathol (Berl).* 1986;71:332-337.

68. Mathew NT, Meyer JS, Rivera VM, et al. Double-blind evaluation of glycerol therapy in acute cerebral infarction. *Lancet.* 1972;2:1327-1329.

69. Moskowitz E, McCann CB. Classification of disability in the chronically ill and aging. *J Chronic Dis.* 1957;5:342-346.

70. Olsen TS. Arm and leg paresis as outcome predictors in stroke rehabilitation. *Stroke.* 1990;21:247-251.

71. Osberg JS, Haley SM, McGinnis GE, et al. Characteristics of cost outliers who did not benefit from stroke rehabilitation. *Am J Phys Med Rehabil.* 1990;69(3):117-125.

72. Parikh RM, Lipsey JR, Robinson RG, et al. Two-year longitudinal study of post-stroke mood disorders: dynamic changes in correlates of depression at one and two years. *Stroke.* 1987;18:579-584.

73. Pfeiffer E., ed. *Multidimensional functional assessment; the OARS methodology: a manual.* Durham, NC: Center for the Study of Aging and Human Development, Duke University; 1975.

74. Poole JL, Whitney SL. Motor assessment scale for stroke patients: concurrent validity and interrater reliability. *Arch Phys Med Rehabil.* 1988;69:195-197.

75. Primeau F. Post-stroke depression: a critical review of the literature. *Can J Psychiatry.* 1988;33:757-765.

76. Raven JC. Guide to using the coloured progressive matrices. London, England: Lewis; 1965.

77. Ray WA, Griffin MR, Schaffner W, et al. Psychotropic drug use and the risk of fracture. *N Engl J Med.* 1987;316:363-369.

78. Redford JB. Orthotics, State of the Art Reviews. *Phys Med Rehab.* 1987;1:1-175

79. Reding M, Haycox J, Blass J. Depression in patients referred to a dementia clinic: a three-year prospective study. *Arch Neurol.* 1985;42:894-896.

80. Reding MJ, McDowell FH. Focused stroke rehabilitation programs improve outcome. *Arch Neurol.* 1989;46:700-701.

81. Reding MJ, Orto LA, Winter SW, et al. Antidepressant therapy after stroke: a double-blind trial. *Arch Neurol.* 1986;43:763-765.

82. Reed RL, Gerety MB, Winograd CH. Expanded access to rehabilitation services for older people: an

urgent need. *J Am Geriatr Soc.* 1990;38:1055-1056.

83. Rosen WG, Terry RD, Fuld PA, et al. Pathological verification of ischemic score in differentiation of dementias. *Ann Neurol.* 1980;7:486-488.

84. Rothrock JF, Dittrich HC, McAllen S, et al. Acute anticoagulation following cardioembolic stroke. *Stroke.* 1989;20:730-734.

85. Sacco RL, Foulkes MA, Mohr JP, et al. Determinants of early recurrence of cerebral infarction: the Stroke Data Bank. *Stroke.* 1989;20:983-989.

86. Sage JI, Van Uitert RL. Risk of recurrent stroke in patients with atrial fibrillation and non-valvular heart disease. *Stroke.* 1983;14:537-540.

87. Santus G, Ranzenigo A, Caregnato R, et al. Social and family integration of hemiplegic elderly patients 1 year after stroke. *Stroke.* 1990;21:1019-1022.

88. Schoening HA, Anderegg L, Bergstrom D, et al. Numerical scoring of self-care status of patients. *Arch Phys Med Rehabil.* 1965;46:689-697.

89. Shah S, Vanclay F, Cooper B. Predicting discharge status at commencement of stroke rehabilitation. *Stroke.* 1989;20:766-769.

90. Shah S, Vanclay F, Cooper B. Efficiency, effectiveness, and duration of stroke rehabilitation. *Stroke.* 1990;21:241-246.

91. Shinar D, Gross CR, Mohr JP, et al. Interobserver variability in the assessment of neurologic history and examination in the Stroke Data Bank. *Arch Neurol.* 1985;42:557-565.

92. Sinyor D, Amato P, Kaloupek DG, et al. Post-stroke depression: relationships to functional impairment, coping strategies, and rehabilitation outcome. *Stroke.* 1986;17:1102-1107.

93. Sobel E, Alter M, Davanipour Z, et al. Stroke in the Lehigh Valley: combined risk factors for recurrent ischemic stroke. *Neurology.* 1989;39:669-672.

94. Starkstein SE, Robinson RG. Affective disorders and cerebral vascular disease. *Br J Psych.* 1989;154:170-182.

95. Tangeman PT, Banaitis DA, Williams AK. Rehabilitation of chronic stroke patients: changes in functional performance. *Arch Phys Med Rehabil.* 1990;71:876-880.

96. Task Force on Stroke Impairment, Task Force on Stroke Disability, and Task Force on Stroke Handicap. Symposium recommendations for methodology in stroke outcome research. *Stroke.* 1990;21 (suppl II):II-68-II-73).

97. Tatemichi TK. How acute brain failure becomes chronic: a view of the mechanisms of dementia related to stroke. *Neurology.* 1990;40:1652-1659.

98. Thorngren M, Westling B. Rehabilitation and achieved health quality after stroke. A population-based study of 258 hospitalized cases followed for one year. *Acta Neurol Scand.* 1990;82:374-380.

99. Thorngren M, Westling B, Norrving B. Outcome after stroke in patients discharged to independent living. *Stroke.* 1990;21:236-240.

100. Tijssen CC, Schulte BPM, Leyten ACM. Prognostic significance of conjugate eye deviation in stroke patients. *Stroke.* 1991;22:200-202.

101. Tomlinson BE, Blessed G, Roth M. Observations on the brains of demented old people. *J Neurol Sci.* 1970;11:205-242.

102. Ulrich J, Probst A, Wüest M. The brain diseases causing senile dementia. *J Neurol.* 1986;233:118-122.

103. Vanclay F. Functional outcome measures in stroke rehabilitation. *Stroke.* 1991;22:105-108.

104. Viitanen M, Eriksson S, Asplund K. Risk of recurrent stroke, myocardial infarction and epilepsy during long-term follow-up after stroke. *Eur Neurol.* 1988;28:227-231.

105. Volpe BT, McDowell FH. The efficacy of cognitive rehabilitation in patients with traumatic brain injury. *Arch Neurol.* 1990;47:220-222.

106. Wade DT, Legh-Smith J, Hewer RA. Depressed mood after stroke: a community study of its frequency. *Br J Psych.* 1987;151:200-205.

107. Wechsler D. *Manual for the Wechsler Adult Intelligence Scale.* New York, NY: Psychological Corporation; 1955.

108. Wechsler D. *Wechsler Adult Intelligence Scale.* Revised manual. New York, NY: Psychological Corporation, 1981.

109. Willoughby EW, Paty DW. Scales for rating impairment in multiple sclerosis: a critique. *Neurology.* 1988;38:1793-1798.

110. Wolf PA, D'Agostino RB, Belanger AJ, et al. Probability of stroke: a risk profile from the Framingham Study. *Stroke.* 1991;22:312-318.

111. Zuckerman M, Lubin B. *Manual for multiple affect adjective checklist.* San Diego, Calif: Educational and Industrial Testing Services; 1965.

CHAPTER 16

A Unified Concept of Cerebrovascular Occlusive Disease and Brain Ischemia

Issam A. Awad, MD, MS, FACS

Cerebrovascular occlusive disease is a complex multifocal disease affecting the heart, great vessels, cerebral arteries of all sizes, brain parenchyma, and/or blood. Complex interactions between these entities result in one or more of the clinical manifestations of brain ischemia. Preceding chapters in this book have addressed a wide spectrum of issues related to the basic and clinical aspects of this disease. In this final chapter, we present a conceptual synthesis of many of these issues, aiming toward a consensus perspective that is useful to clinicians. Each of the aspects summarized below has been well covered in other chapters of the book. The reader is referred to these individual chapters for additional detail, including a more exhaustive survey of controversial points and references to the literature. It is hoped that this editorial overview will highlight a unified concept of cerebrovascular occlusive disease and brain ischemia, without wrongly oversimplifying its many complex facets.

Epidemiology and Natural History

Asymptomatic Cerebrovascular Disease

Clinically silent cerebrovascular occlusive disease is difficult to define, follow, and "treat." Uncertainty about the natural history and individual variability of clinical courses make it difficult to justify recommending any treatment modalities that may be associated with any significant risk. Yet, asymptomatic cerebrovascular occlusive disease cannot be ignored. Of major disabling strokes, more than half are not preceded by clearly recognized warning spells or minor strokes. The most common unwarned major stroke is massive hemispheric infarction with internal carotid artery (ICA) occlusion or cardiogenic embolism. Both entities represent an end stage of large-vessel disease and cardiac disease, respectively, which may have remained asymptomatic for many years.

It is extremely important to recognize that warning spells or minor strokes may be ignored or missed, or both, by the patient or physicians despite the most aggressive preparation and education. Many zones of the brain may sustain ischemia and infarction without clinically evident symptoms. Other ischemic spells may occur during sleep and go totally undetected. Still other spells may be misinterpreted by the most astute patient or physician.

Prevalence and Significance of Cervical Bruits

The incidence of cervical bruits detectable on clinical examination increases with age and with risk factors of systemic atherosclerosis. The presence of a cervical bruit more than doubles the risk of subsequent stroke and myocardial infarction; however, a cervical bruit is neither a sensitive nor a specific predictor of "significant" carotid stenosis (see below). Only 60% of subsequent strokes are ipsilateral to the bruit, and many strokes are lacunar infarctions secondary to small-vessel parenchymal disease.

Cervical bruits represent an index of generalized atherosclerotic vasculopathy but are neither a necessary nor sufficient indicator of clinically significant large-vessel atherosclerotic occlusive disease.

Risk Factors of Stroke

The most significant risk factor of stroke is previous symptomatic brain ischemia. Patients with a transient or permanent ischemic insult are under a nearly 30% risk of subsequent major stroke within 3 years when followed prospectively. The risk is not uniform, and some subgroups of patients have a more or less severe prognosis, depending on the specific pathophysiology of their initial ischemic insult. Patients with a lacunar-type infarction and no significant large-vessel disease have a more benign risk of subsequent major stroke, whereas patients with pre-occlusive ICA stenosis have a more critical risk. Subsequent risk of brain ischemia is weakly related to the severity of symptoms and more strongly related to the underlying pathophysiology of ischemic symptoms.

Other significant and independent risk factors of ischemic stroke include age, hypertension, coronary artery disease, and diabetes mellitus. Other risk factors in special groups of patients include the use of birth control pills, sickle-cell disease, and so on. Other secondary or indirect risks include the presence of cervical bruit and peripheral atherosclerotic occlusive disease. Cigarette smoking used to be thought of as a secondary or indirect risk; it has recently been shown to be an independent and significant risk factor for progression of large-vessel and small-vessel

cerebrovascular occlusive disease, regardless of other accompanying risks, and an independent predictor of subsequent stroke.

High-Risk Angiographic Lesions

Certain vascular lesions carry a significant risk of subsequent stroke in their respective distribution. These include the "tight" (pre-occlusive) ICA stenosis, which has been shown in several studies to carry at least a 7% to 10% per year risk of ipsilateral major stroke. The risk of subsequent stroke is even greater if there have been previous symptoms related to the lesion.

Deep, shaggy ulcerated lesions have been shown to carry a similar risk of major ipsilateral stroke. In this setting, the majority of subsequent strokes appear to be preceded by recognizable transient or minor ischemic spells. The presence of a "string sign" or luminal thrombus within the ICA signals a serious (greater than 50%) risk of impending major stroke. This risk may be substantially lessened by anticoagulant therapy.

In any of these so-called high-risk angiographic lesions, the risk of subsequent stroke might be magnified by prior symptoms or an unfavorable risk factor profile. The risk of subsequent stroke may be modified by medical or surgical strategies for stroke prevention (see below).

Special Case of ICA Occlusion

The greatest risk of stroke in ICA occlusion is at the time of occlusion and/or in the period just preceding or immediately following documented occlusion.

The greatest risk of stroke in ICA occlusion is not hemodynamic. Most patients harbor physiologic collateral pathways that would make ICA occlusion well tolerated; however, propagating thrombosis and thromboembolism from the fresh thrombus within the lumen of the acutely occluded artery may compromise collateral pathways and/or occlude other cerebral arteries downstream, resulting in massive brain infarction.

Subsequent stroke risk following a previously documented ICA occlusion is 6% to 8% per year, but the risk of major subsequent ipsilateral stroke is less than 2% per year. Subsequent strokes following a documented ICA occlusion have multiple etiologies and do not always coincide with the territory of the occluded artery. Small-vessel disease, occlusion of collateral pathways, and disease in other vascular territories, as well as cardiopathy can all result in subsequent stroke in the setting of known ICA occlusion.

Special Case of Intracranial Stenoses

Intracranial stenotic lesions of cerebral arteries are significant markers of generalized atherosclerotic disease. They are associated with a greater than 5% subsequent yearly risk of myocardial infarction. Subsequent risk of stroke is also high, estimated at 10% to 12% per year; however, nearly half of subsequent strokes occur in territories other than those of the stenosed arteries.

Intracranial arterial stenoses represent a serious index of advanced generalized vasculopathy, including cerebrovascular disease. Intracranial stenoses are dynamic lesions and have been well documented to progress in severity to occlude or to resolve altogether. Hemodynamic compromise and artery-to-artery embolism have been shown to occur from such lesions, although in many instances they may be asymptomatic and incidental to other cerebrovascular or systemic vascular occlusive disease.

New Concepts in Pathophysiology
Uniformity of Ischemic Thresholds

The brain is endowed with a rich source of blood supply and with several levels of potential physiologic collateral pathways to ensure appropriate blood flow in situations of vascular occlusion. In addition, cerebral blood flow (CBF) is closely controlled by tight autoregulatory mechanisms in the face of variations in perfusion pressure or substrate and oxygen availability.

Studies in animals and in humans have demonstrated a consistent threshold of CBF (18-22 ml/100 g/min) below which there is disturbance of electrophysiologic cellular function (e.g. electroencephalographic slowing, abolition of evoked responses) and corresponding clinical manifestations of dysfunction in respective brain regions. Despite such electrophysiologic disturbance, no disruption of cellular structural integrity occurs at such levels of CBF.

When regional CBF falls below the range of 8-10 ml/100 g/min, cellular structural integrity is threatened, with tissue damage more likely with increasing duration of time at which regional CBF remains so impaired.

Therefore, the likelihood of tissue damage from brain ischemia is related to both the depth and duration of ischemia. Reversible clinical manifestations of brain ischemia can occur without tissue damage as long as CBF does not fall for any length of time below the threshold of structural integrity, with clinical symptoms resolving whenever CBF is restored to levels above the threshold of cellular dysfunction. The concept of ischemic thresholds has implications with regard to the possibility of cellular dysfunction in the absence of cell death. Such a concept of "idling neurons" has been demonstrated in the laboratory and in selected clinical scenarios.

Other implications of the concept of ischemic thresholds involve the situation of temporary arterial occlusions in the operating room. In carotid endarterectomy or temporary arterial occlusion for aneurysm repair, electroencephalographic or evoked potential monitoring, or both, may be used to ensure that regional CBF does not drop below levels of cellular dysfunction. There may be hemodynamic and pharmacologic manipulations

Mechanisms of Focal Ischemia

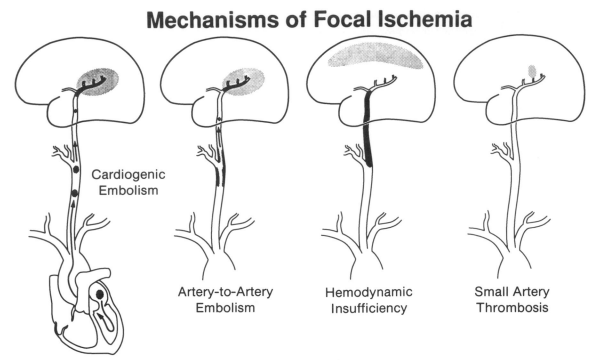

Figure 1. *Pathophysiologic mechanisms of brain ischemia. One or more of these mechanisms is operating in the majority of clinical situations. Other less frequent mechanisms include hematologic abnormalities and arterial dissections (not illustrated in this figure).*

that temporarily enhance the tolerance of brain tissue to lower levels of CBF.

Multifactorial Mechanisms of Tissue Damage

In the experimental setting, several factors have been shown to independently contribute to tissue damage from ischemia. In the clinical situation, it is likely that all these factors operate simultaneously. There is no evidence that a single "final common pathway" is solely responsible for cell death. Consequently, it is not likely that any single agent will ever be found that can solely protect against cell damage; however, several mechanisms may contribute in a cumulative fashion to final ischemic damage, and the manipulation of these mechanisms may limit the extent of ischemic injury.

Mechanisms of ischemic tissue damage include microcirculatory impairment that results in further deterioration of local CBF and aggravation of focal brain ischemia. Ischemic cellular edema (cytotoxic edema) may result in the swelling of astrocytes, which will further infringe on local microcirculation. Ischemic disruption of the blood-brain barrier (vasogenic edema) causes gross disruption of endothelial tight junctions, and spillage of fluid and proteins into the extracellular space. Oncotic and osmotic factors might aggravate this edema and result in focal tissue pressure elevations and further perfusion compromise. Ischemic edema may result in further neurologic dysfunction and tissue damage.

Cellular membrane disruption causes the release of arachidonic acid and the activation of multiple cascades, including the bradykinin-kallikrein system and thromboxane generation, which may result in further microcirculatory compromise and magnification of focal ischemia. In individual studies, a multitude of molecules have been shown to play important roles in these mechanisms. Recent attention has been focused on endothelium-mediated factors, including the peptide endothelin, which is the most potent vasoconstrictor known.

The concept of excitotoxicity, or cell death by excitation, has been shown to be operative in certain regions of the brain during ischemia. Ischemic tissue may result in the activation of certain synaptic pathways, including the release of certain amino acids, which results in receptor-mediated ischemic cell damage even in the absence of exhaustion of cellular energy reserves. Such excitotoxicity has been linked to focal seizure activity that may increase metabolic demands within the ischemic brain, at a time when CBF is already impaired.

Several of the above pathways have been implicated at the cellular level with activation of specific calcium channels, allowing drastic compartmental changes in intracellular calcium. These have been linked directly to irreversible cell death.

It is likely that additional research on the molecular mechanisms of ischemic cell damage will further uncover the complexities and multifactorial aspects of this process.

Pathophysiologic Heterogeneity

At another level, there is considerable etiologic heterogeneity (Figure 1), which may result in brain ischemia. Cardiac pathology may result in brain ischemia via a variety of mechanisms, including cerebral hypoperfusion from cardiac arrhythmia, and more importantly from cardiogenic cerebral embolism via

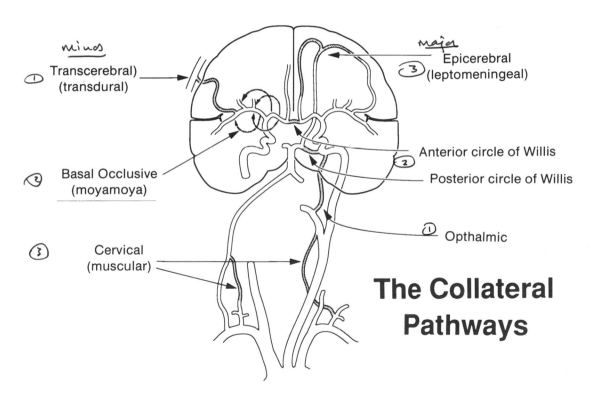

The Collateral Pathways

Figure 2. Cerebral collateral pathways. Major collateral pathways include leptomeningeal (epicerebral) collaterals, anterior and posterior circle of Willis collaterals, and opthalmic artery collaterals. Other collateral pathways operating in situations of more profound and chronic ischemia (pathologic collateral pathways) include transdural transcerebral collaterals, cervical muscular collaterals, and basal occlusive (moyamoya) collaterals.

a patent atrial foramen ovale, atrial or ventricular mural thrombi, or valvular vegetations.

Large vessels may result in artery-to-artery embolism or in progressive hemodynamic compromise. Small end-vessel disease within the brain parenchyma may also result in focal brain ischemia within the territory of the respective vessels.

Major physiologic collateral pathways provide significant protection against brain ischemia in the face of vascular occlusions (Figure 2). These include leptomeningeal epicerebral collaterals, anterior and posterior circle of Willis collaterals, and ophthalmic artery collaterals. Other collateral pathways imply more profound hemodynamic compromise and are less likely to totally prevent brain ischemia. These include cervical muscular collaterals, transdural transcerebral collaterals, and proliferative collaterals of penetrating vessels in basal occlusive disease (moyamoya collaterals). The presence of one or more of these pathologic collateral patterns is typically indicative of more pronounced and chronic hemodynamic compromise.

In the face of such etiologic heterogeneity and variability of collateral pathways, the clinical spectrum of cerebrovascular occlusive disease and brain ischemia is highly diverse. Significant cerebrovascular occlusive disease may occur in totally asymptomatic patients. In other patients, symptoms of brain ischemia may be brief and reversible, depending on the particular pathoetiologic mechanism and collateralization to the affected brain region. Paucity of symptoms does not necessarily imply a favorable prognosis. In other situations, brain ischemia is manifested as an ischemic stroke with varying degrees of clinical severity, depending once again on the extent of parenchymal damage and eloquence of brain regions affected. Patients with minor brain ischemia have much to lose from further clinical manifestations in the same vascular territory. Patients with devastating ischemic insults suffer from the consequences of brain damage and from potential consequences of further ischemia in other vascular territories.

Cerebrovascular occlusive disease is a mul-

tisystem disease with simultaneous progression of pathology in the heart, large vessels, small vessels, and brain parenchyma. Hematologic factors may interact with vascular pathology with further clinical consequences. Cerebrovascular occlusive disease is subject to uniform risk factors that have been shown to aggravate the extent of pathology at all levels.

New Concepts in Diagnosis
High-Resolution Computed Tomography

The pattern of ischemic damage on computed tomographic (CT) scanning can be closely related to the mechanism of infarction. Thromboembolic infarctions have an appearance distinct from those resulting from hemodynamic compromise or small end-vessel disease. CT scanning may also reveal occult infarctions that are clinically silent, but that may represent an index of the extent of cerebrovascular occlusive disease. Chronic cerebrovascular disease also may be related to brain atrophy with sulcal dilatation or to periventricular leukoaraiosis, which may represent subcortical arteriosclerotic encephalomalacia.

Limitations of CT scanning include the inability of this modality to visualize acute brain ischemia (within the first 24 hours of tissue damage) or symptomatic ischemic zones without tissue damage.

Angiogenic Techniques

Cerebral angiography remains the gold standard of angiogenic diagnosis in cerebrovascular occlusive disease. The safety of this modality has been greatly enhanced by newer catheter designs and technical experience. Digital subtraction imaging has enhanced the practicality, precision, and safety of angiography. Cerebral angiography can reveal the nature and extent of occlusive vascular lesions at all levels, possible embolic sources, and physiologic and pathologic patterns of collateral supply.

Noninvasive vascular techniques have evolved into reliable methods of screening for significant vascular occlusive disease and certain patterns of collateral supply. Limitations of precision and accuracy have prevented their universal or exclusive application in all clinical scenarios.

The recent introduction of magnetic resonance angiography (MRA) has vastly improved the reliability of noninvasive techniques. In its current form, this technique remains an excellent tool for screening and follow-up, but it does not provide sufficient spacial resolution and dynamic flow information to guide invasive therapeutic decisions.

Magnetic Resonance Imaging (MRI)

MRI has provided exquisite sensitivity in the delineation of parenchymal regions of previous ischemic brain damage. Such exquisite sensitivity paradoxically has somewhat limited clinical usefulness in that MRI does not reliably distinguish recent and remote lesions and symptomatic and asymptomatic lesions. MRI abnormalities that are also visualized by CT scan tend to be the most relevant clinically; however, the extent of parenchymal abnormalities on MRI may represent an overall index of parenchymal "wear and tear" associated with chronic cerebrovascular disease and the brunt of vascular risk factors. These have been correlated significantly with age and cerebrovascular risk factors and with overall risk of subsequent stroke.

Recent innovations of MR diffusion and perfusion imaging may allow the delineation of zones of ongoing ischemic damage in the first minutes of infarction, in time to allow meaningful therapeutic manipulations to limit infarction size. MR spectroscopy provides unique opportunities for functional imaging of metabolic disturbances associated with brain ischemia.

More Sophisticated Diagnostic Modalities

Numerous techniques of regional CBF assessment have been developed that are practical and reliable. These include xenon CT and single photon emission CT. In selected clinical scenarios, they may provide complementary information to other diagnostic studies, adding insights to the hemodynamic and functional impact of cerebrovascular occlusive disease.

Other functional modalities including positron emission tomography (PET) have limited availability and may or may not provide reliable and useful clinical information. They represent powerful research tools into the mechanisms and therapeutic modification of brain ischemia.

New Therapeutic Concepts
Treatment of Acute Stroke

The management of acute brain ischemia includes measures designed to minimize infarction size. If instituted in the critical early hours of evolving ischemic damage, such modalities may limit the extent and functional impact of ischemic stroke. General medical measures contribute much in this regard, including optimization of oxygenation, electrolyte balance, hemodynamic function, hemostatic function, blood viscosity, and nutrition. Deep vein thromboembolic prophylaxis, gastrointestinal bleeding prophylaxis, respiratory therapy, and physical therapy are all applied early to prevent secondary systemic complications that may further the functional impact of stroke.

More specific measures including hypervolemic hemodilution, anticoagulation, vigorous prevention and treatment of brain edema, and avoidance of extremes of hyperglycemia and hypoglycemia may all contribute to the limitation of infarction size. Other measures in the setting of acute stroke are designed to prevent recurrent stroke.

Stroke Prevention

Stroke prevention includes specific measures aimed at avoiding the consequences of existing vascular pathology and more general measures aimed at modifying the progression of cerebrovascular occlusive disease.

Specific measures are aimed at particular occlusive lesions and pathophysiologic mechanisms operating in the individual patient. Antiplatelet therapy has been shown to decrease the risk of subsequent stroke in several clinical settings, including previous transient ischemic attack, minor stroke, and atrial fibrillation. Antiplatelet therapy is not the universal answer to stroke prevention and is not effective in hemodynamically significant lesions, nor is it capable of totally eliminating macroembolism. Antiplatelet therapy provides excellent stroke prophylaxis in patients with multifocal low-risk lesions, in patients with platelet microembolism, in patients awaiting diagnostic evaluation, and in asymptomatic patients with multiple risk factors.

Anticoagulation therapy may be useful in situations of active propagating thrombosis, impending occlusion, or stroke in evolution where propagating thromboembolism is operative. Anticoagulation is a useful temporizing measure in dynamic lesions such as arterial dissections and intracranial stenoses. It has been shown to decrease the risk of subsequent stroke from cardiogenic thromboembolism in atrial fibrillation. Anticoagulation is not totally effective in hemodynamic lesions, but it may delay thrombotic occlusion of high-grade stenoses. Anticoagulation is associated with significant hemorrhagic risk that is cumulative over time and may be prohibitive in elderly and noncompliant patients.

Surgical intervention is effective for specific lesions and in the setting of specific symptoms. The risk of surgery must be balanced against the natural risk of the disease; both factors are quite variable among patients. Surgical intervention must be performed by surgeons who have training and expertise in cerebrovascular surgery because a surgeon's performance may be critical to the effective-

ness or lack of effectiveness of the procedure in an individual clinical scenario. Recent clinical trials have demonstrated the effectiveness of carotid endarterectomy in severe ICA stenosis with previous ischemic symptoms in the same distribution.

More general measures of stroke prevention include risk factor management. This is essential in all patients and provides the greatest epidemiologic impact on stroke prevention. Education about cerebrovascular disease and likely symptoms of brain ischemia is important to risk factor modification (e.g. diet, exercise, compliance with antihypertensive therapy) and to the recognition of subsequent transient and minor ischemic symptoms that may precede more devastating strokes. Risk factor modification and education about ischemic symptoms should complement more specific medical measures of stroke prevention, but they are not to be used as a substitute for such specific measures.

Toward a Unified Concept of Ischemic Cerebrovascular Disease
Limitations of Classic Concepts and Terminology

Classic teaching about cerebrovascular disease has been heavily influenced by concepts and terminology without clear and unifying clinical relevance. Concepts such as transient ischemic attack, carotid bruit, amaurosis fugax, reversible ischemic neurologic deficit, and stroke with minor residuum are all illustrative of symptoms of the overall disease that often have been misinterpreted as individual disease entities. Clinical diagnosis of the symptomatology of the disease has often been confused with the underlying lesion diagnosis and pathophysiologic events. There has been much confusion about asymptomatic disease, tending to minimize its individual and epidemiologic impact, and about advanced cerebrovascular disease, tending to emphasize nihilistic therapeutic attitudes.

CLINICAL AND PATHOLOGIC SPECTRUM OF BRAIN ISCHEMIA

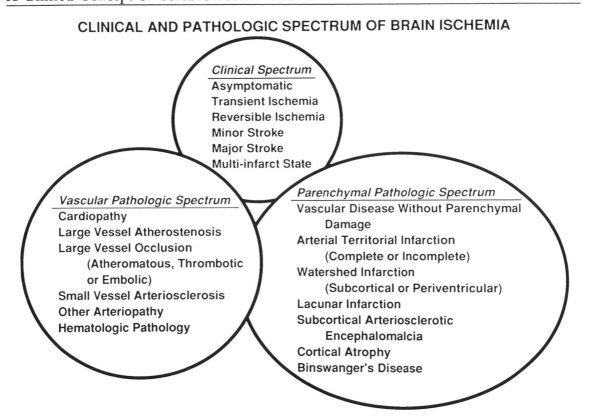

Clinical Spectrum
Asymptomatic
Transient Ischemia
Reversible Ischemia
Minor Stroke
Major Stroke
Multi-infarct State

Vascular Pathologic Spectrum
Cardiopathy
Large Vessel Atherostenosis
Large Vessel Occlusion
    (Atheromatous, Thrombotic
    or Embolic)
Small Vessel Arteriosclerosis
Other Arteriopathy
Hematologic Pathology

Parenchymal Pathologic Spectrum
Vascular Disease Without Parenchymal
    Damage
Arterial Territorial Infarction
    (Complete or Incomplete)
Watershed Infarction
    (Subcortical or Periventricular)
Lacunar Infarction
Subcortical Arteriosclerotic
    Encephalomalcia
Cortical Atrophy
Binswanger's Disease

Figure 3. Clinical and pathologic spectrum of brain ischemia. Minimal criteria of definition of the disease should include clinical information and definition of the extent of cardiac, vascular, and parenchymal disease.

Such ill-focused and imprecise concepts are no longer permissible in light of recent advances in the understanding of pathophysiology and novel concepts of diagnosis and treatment. The past decade has witnessed numerous clinical trials that have demonstrated scientifically the value of specific medical and surgical treatment modalities in individual clinical scenarios. These advances demonstrate the importance of continued basic and clinical research on this subject and speak strongly against nihilistic therapeutic attitudes.

Minimal Criteria for Accurate Definition of the Disease

Cerebrovascular occlusive disease cannot be defined by its clinical symptomatology alone nor solely by the presence of a specific vascular or parenchymal lesion. Minimal criteria for accurate definition of the disease (Figure 3) should include the following:

1. Clinical manifestations.
2. Occult and clinically symptomatic vascular lesions.
3. Occult and clinically symptomatic parenchymal lesions.

Complementary information about each of these three aspects of cerebrovascular occlusive disease and brain ischemia is necessary in individual cases and forms the basis of rational management strategies for each particular patient.

Multifaceted Therapeutic Strategy

The clinician faced with a patient with cerebrovascular occlusive disease and brain

MANAGEMENT OF ACUTE BRAIN ISCHEMIA

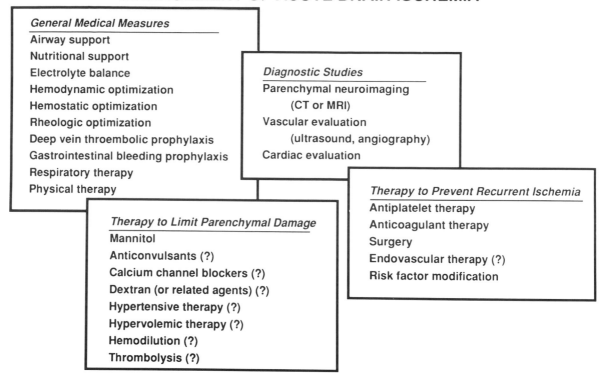

General Medical Measures

Airway support
Nutritional support
Electrolyte balance
Hemodynamic optimization
Hemostatic optimization
Rheologic optimization
Deep vein throembolic prophylaxis
Gastrointestinal bleeding prophylaxis
Respiratory therapy
Physical therapy

Diagnostic Studies

Parenchymal neuroimaging
(CT or MRI)
Vascular evaluation
(ultrasound, angiography)
Cardiac evaluation

Therapy to Prevent Recurrent Ischemia

Antiplatelet therapy
Anticoagulant therapy
Surgery
Endovascular therapy (?)
Risk factor modification

Therapy to Limit Parenchymal Damage

Mannitol
Anticonvulsants (?)
Calcium channel blockers (?)
Dextran (or related agents) (?)
Hypertensive therapy (?)
Hypervolemic therapy (?)
Hemodilution (?)
Thrombolysis (?)

Figure 4. Multifaceted approach to the management of acute brain ischemia. In every case, diagnostic measures are designed to define the extent of the disease. General and specific therapies are instituted to limit extent of ongoing parenchymal damage and to prevent recurrent ischemia. Specific therapeutic measures are individualized according to pathophysiologic mechanisms and the extent of the disease in individual patients.

ischemia should adopt a multifaceted management strategy (Figure 4). This should include diagnostic studies aimed at defining the extent of the disease as highlighted above. In addition, general medical measures to limit parenchymal damage are instituted as per the requirements of the individual case. General therapy to prevent recurrent ischemia is indicated in every case and consists of risk factor modification and patient and family education about the disease. More specific interventions to prevent recurrent ischemia may include medical and surgical therapy as indicated by the specific extent of the disease and risk/benefit considerations in individual cases.

Index

Page numbers for tables, figures, and illustrations are in *boldface italics.*

A

ACAS (Clinical trial), *257,* 258-260
Acetazolamide, *93,* 93-94
Acidosis
 extracellular, 2, 5
 intracellular, 13
 metabolic cascades, 9
Acylated plasminogen-streptokinase activated complex
 comparison of thrombolytic agents, *232,* 232-234
 intracranial hemorrhage, 238
 major thrombolytic trials, *237*
Adenosine, 6, *6*
Adenosine diphosphate, 2
Adenosine triphosphate (ATP)
 decline and ischemia, 14-15
 levels and arterial occlusion, *8*
 MR spectroscopy, 83
 parenchymal, *3*
 phosphorylation, 2
Adenylate cyclase, 7
ADP, 2
Adventitial rupture
 intracranial vertebral artery dissection, 199
Age
 arterial occlusion risk factors, 120-121
 carotid endarterectomy risks, 168
 vascular risk factors, 60
Agraphia, 63
Albumin, 30, 51
Alcohol consumption, 123-124
Alexia, 63
Allergies, 88
Alpha agonists, 277
Alpha-tocopherol, 21
Amaurosis fugax, 73, 77, 85
Amino acids
 excitatory, 11-12, 20, 22
 MR spectroscopy, 83
Amphetamines, 277
Anemia, 43, 54
Anesthesia
 barbiturate, 180
 carotid endarterectomy, 169

Aneurysms
 angiography, 74
 concurrent carotid disease, 162
 dangerous rupture, 191-192
 dissecting, 191, 192, *192,* 194, 195, 199, 200
 dissecting (vertebrobasilar), 204
 extracranial, 194, 195, 200
 extradural, *198*
 false, 181, 187, 188, 191-192
 formation (dissecting intramural hematoma), 196
 giant, 224
 intracranial, 200
 pseudoaneurysms, 86, 196, 204
 rupture, 200
 spontaneous resolution, 195
 surgical obliteration, *21*
Angina pectoris, 167
Angiography
 aneurysm obliteration, *21*
 anticoagulation follow-up, 200
 basilar artery stenosis, *204*
 carotid ulceration, 81, *82*
 circle of Willis, *223*
 common carotid artery, *191*
 completed stroke, 74
 definitive test, 84
 dissecting aneurysm (internal carotid), *192*
 extracranial carotid artery, 84-86
 extracranial carotid artery dissection, 194, 195, *195*
 extracranial vertebral artery dissection, *198*
 focal web, *191*
 general description and uses, 84-88
 gold standard of evaluation techniques, 96, 287
 internal carotid artery, *190*
 internal carotid occlusion, *223*
 internal carotid stenosis, bifurcation, *84*
 internal carotid traumatic dissection, *76*
 intracranial vertebral artery dissection, 199
 intracranial vessels, 86-87
 intraoperative, 180-181
 neck, skull base trauma, 188
 neurologic deficits, 74
 preoperative evaluation for endarterectomy, 90
 risks, 87-88
 speedy evaluations, 74, 235-236
 spontaneous healing, *190*
 surgical candidate evaluation, 74

transient ischemic attacks (TIAs), 87
  vertebral artery, *206*
  vertebrobasilar disease, 207
Angioplasty
  complications, 212
  delayed, 238
  percutaneous transluminal, 243-245
  venous patch, 177-178
  vertebral artery, 208-209
Animals
  hemodilutional research, 45-46
  models of focal ischemia, 238-239
Ankle-foot orthosis, 276
Anticoagulation therapy
  angiographic evaluation, 74
  arterial dissections, 194, 200
  atherosclerotic occlusive disease, 223
  contraindications, 200
  controversial role, 150
  heart disease patients, 129
  infarction management, 142-143
  intracranial hemorrhage risk, 158
  moyamoya disease, 224
  thromboembolism, thrombosis protection, 200
  traumatic arterial injuries, 191
  uses, 288
  vertebrobasilar disease, 207-208, 213
Antiphospholipid antibody syndrome, 60
Antiplatelet therapy
  carotid bruit, stenosis, 156
  EC-IC bypass alternatives, 223
  stroke risk reduction, 129-130
  transient ischemic attacks (TIAs), 158-159
  uses, 288
AP-7, *11*, 20
Aphasia, 63, 67, 277
Apoplexy, 118, 119
APSAC, see Acylated plasminogen-streptokinase
  activated complex
Arm
  exercise, 276
  hemiparesis, 67
  movement, *271, 273*
Arterial blood pressure, see Blood pressure
Arterial carbon dioxide ($PaCO_2$), *3*, 7
Arterial dissection, see also names of arteries,
  e.g. Carotid artery dissection
  angiography, *86*
  anticoagulant therapy, 194
  extracranial, 147
  extracranial carotid, 193-197
  extracranial vertebral, 197-199
  intracranial carotid, 197
  intracranial vertebral, 199
  spontaneous healing, *190,* 191
  surgical indications, 189, 191

traumatic injury versus, 192-193
  ultrasonography, 113
  underlying vasculopathy, 193
  vertebral, 204, *206*
Arterial injuries, see Trauma
Arterial occlusion, see Occlusive diseases; names of
  specific arteries, e.g., Carotid artery occlusion
Arterial oxygen (PaO_2), 2, 7
Arteries, see names of specific arteries
Arterioles, see also Microcirculation
  delayed hypoperfusion, *16*
  dilatation, 49
  penetrating, 5
  role in cerebral blood flow, 3-4, *4*
Arteriovenous malformations, 74, 182
Ascorbate, 21
Asia, 223
Aspartate, 12
Aspiration, 275
Aspirin
  adjunct in hemodilution, 50
  asymptomatic carotid stenosis, 156-157
  carotid endarterectomy preoperative care, 169
  stroke, death reduction, 159
Asymptomatic Carotid Atherosclerosis Study, *257*, 258-260
Ataxia, 206, *271, 273*
Ataxic hemiparesis, 67
Atherosclerotic large-artery disease
  B-scanning of plaque, 108-109
  dissection, 193
  EC-IC bypass surgery, 228
  extracranial vessels, 106-110, 143-144
  headache, 64
  medical management, 143-144
  microembolism, 62
  natural history, 68-69
  occlusive disease classification, 60
  revascularization surgery criteria, 222-223
  risks, 118
  stenosis as defining characteristic, 60
  stroke risk, 68-69
  transient ischemic attacks (TIAs), 61
  ultrasound imaging, 106-110
  ultrasound screening, 128
  vascular risk factors, 60-61
ATP, see Adenosine triphosphate
Atrial fibrillation, 61, 69
Auricular nerve, 182
Axial cellular flow, 26, *26,* 31-35

B

B-mode ultrasound
  arterial dissection, 113
  description, 89-90, 105
  intraoperative monitoring, 91

plaque, 107-109
Balis effect, 5
Balloon angioplasty, 210
Barbiturates
    anesthesia, 180
    carotid endarterectomy, 173
    ischemia during surgical carotid occlusion, 182
    neuronal energy requirements, 17
Barthel index, 266-267, 273-274
Basal occlusive disease, *285*
Basilar artery, see also Vertebrobasilar arteries
    anatomy, 203
    angioplasty, *245*
    atherosclerosis, *204*
    circumferential, 203
    posterior cerebral arteries and, 204
    stenosis, *204*
    transcranial Doppler, 106, 108
Basilar artery occlusion
    streptokinase and urokinase therapy, 208
Basilar artery stenosis
    angioplasty, *245*
    poor prognosis, 69
    transient ischemic attacks (TIAs), 61
Basophils, 40
Benzodiazepines, 277
Binswanger's disease, 67, *80,* 81
Blacks (stroke risk factors), 61
Blindness, Transient monocular, 61
Blood-brain barrier, 2, 5, 54
Blood cells, see Erythrocytes; Leukocytes; Platelets
Blood coagulation disorders, 148, 149
Blood flow, Cerebral, 1-24, see also Blood viscosity;
    Macro circulation; Microcirculation
    axial cellular flow, 26, *26,* 31-35
    brain metabolic relationships, *3*
    complexity of regulation, 5
    coupled to metabolism, 2
    coupling agents, 5-7
    decreases, 18
    diagnostic assessment, 287
    hematocrit, viscosityand, 42-43
    hemodilutional therapy, 45-48
    inverse relationship with viscosity, 27
    ischemia thresholds, 7-9, *7*
    ischemic vasoconstriction, 14
    leukocytes and, 52-53
    luminal narrowing, velocity and, 104-105
    metabolism coupling agents, *6*
    microanatomy, 3-5
    modulation, 19-20
    optimal hematocrit for oxygen delivery, 47-50, 54
    PET imaging, 95, 96
    plasma viscosity and plasma proteins, 50-52
    reduction with intracellular acidosis, 13
    reduction and tissue damage, 150

regulation, 4, 5-7
resting, 1
role of hematocrit and viscosity, 42-45, 49-50
secondary vasospasm, 14
sedimentation, 39-40
SPECT imaging, *94*
    limitations, 236
surgical monitoring, 92
therapeutic increase, 16, 18-20, 22
ultrasound measurement, 104-105
vasodilators, vasoconstrictors, *6*
viscosity in microcirculation, 49
xenon-enhanced, 92-94, *93*
Blood flow velocity
    blood cell axial distribution, 32, 33, *33*
    diastolic and systolic, 104, 108
    intraoperative monitoring, 112-113
    leukocyte and erythrocyte, 41
    luminal narrowing, blood flow and, 104-105
    plasma and sedimented erythrocytes, 40
    thixotropy, macrocirculation and microcirculation, 28-30
    transcranial Doppler imaging, 112-113, *114*
    ultrasound measurement, 104-105
    viscosity and shear, 26
Blood glucose, 151
Blood plasma, see Plasma
Blood pressure, see also Hypertension
    arterial, 5
    carotid endarterectomy postoperative care, 177
    control, vertebrobasilar disease, 208
    infarction risk factor, 43
    vertebrobasilar disease, 208
Blood sedimentation, 39-40
Blood viscosity
    apparent, in macrocirculation and microcirculation, 28-30
    determination with viscometer, *28*
    erythrocyte aggregation and shear rate, 31
    erythrocyte influence in microcirculation, 50
    fibrinogen and globulins, 31
    hematocrit and, 35-36, *36*
    hematocrit, blood flow and, 42-43
    hematocrit, cerebral ischemia and, 43-45, 49-50
    hematocrit less important in microcirculation, 50
    hematocrit, shear rate and, *29*
    importance in ischemia, 54
    importance in microcirculation, 27
    microcirculation and blood cell aggregation,
        axial flow, 34, *35*
    macrocirculation, microcirculation and, 31, 42
    optimal hematocrit for oxygen delivery, 47-49, 50, 54
    plasma viscosity, 50-52
    postischemic hypoperfusion, 16
    relative, and shear rate, *35*
    shear and, 25-27
    thixotropy (shaken, disturbed liquids), 27
    vessel diameter and, *32,* 35

Brain
    biochemical changes, 149
    blood flow coupling agents, *6*
    dependency on oxidative phosphorylation, 1
    energy requirements, 2-3
    metabolism and blood flow described, 1-24
    neoplasms, 207
    neuronal damage and energy failure, *10*
    oxygen consumption decrease, 18
    reperfusion, 234-238, 240
    tissue damage mechanisms, 284-285
    tissue rescue, 150-153
    vasodilators, vasoconstrictors, *6*
Brain stem, 177, 267
Bromocriptine, 277
Bruit
    arterial dissection sign, 194
    arterial occlusion risk factors, 128
    asymptomatic, 74, 155-158, 167
    cervical, prevalence and significance, 281-282
    classification of occlusive diseases, 64-65
    preoperative patients, 158
    surgery, 167
Bypass (revascularization) surgery, see Surgery
Bypass surgery, Extracranial-Intracranial, see
    Extracranial-Intracranial bypass surgery

C

Calcitonin-gene-related peptide, 6, *6*
Calcium
    hypothesis of cell injury, 11
    influx, 13, 15
Calcium antagonists
    cerebral blood flow, 18-20, 22
    metabolic cascades, 20
    role in normal cellular events, 10
    tissue rescue, 152-153
Calcium-ATPase, 11, 12
Calcium-binding proteins, 13
Calcium channel blockers, 18
Calcium channels, 12, 14, 20
Calcium ions, 11-13
Canadian Neurological Scale, *273*
Capillaries, see also Microcirculation
    cerebral blood flow, 4, *4*
    delayed hypoperfusion, *16*
    diameter and relative hematocrit, *39*
    occlusion by leukocytes, 41, 42, 43
Carbon dioxide, *3*, 7
Cardiac output, 1
Cardioembolism
    headache, 64
    heart disease and, 120
    medical management, 144-145
    myocardial infarction and, 61

natural history, 69
occlusive disease classification, 60
recurrent stroke, 69
stroke of undetermined cause, 68
stroke risk, 69
transient ischemic attacks (TIAs), 61
vascular risk factors, 60-61
Cardiopulmonary bypass, 244-245
Carotid arteries
    asymptomatic disease, 155-158
    bifurcation, 105
    blood flow velocity, 82
    bruits, 155-156
    collateral circulation, 158
    common, *171, 172*
    concurrent intracranial aneurysm, 162
    CT imaging, 78
    embolic disease and surgery, 159
    endarterectomy, 167-185
    extracranial, 106
    internal, 203
    internal, recanalization, 194
    luminal irregularities, *196*
    luminal thrombosis, 161-162
    neurologic deficits, 159-160
    recent stroke, 160-161
    silent disease and risks in general surgical
        patients 157-158
    stump syndromes, 160
    symptomatic disease, 158
    transient ischemic attacks (TIAs), 141, 158-159
    ulceration, 68, 81, *82,* 85-86, 167
    webs, *191*
Carotid artery dissection
    carotid endarterectomy risks, 168
    cervical aneurysms, 191
    internal, 197
    intramural hematoma, 196
    magnetic resonance uses, *196*
    multiple, 195
    recurrent, 195
    spontaneous, 195
    vertebral dissections simultaneously, 198-199
Carotid artery occlusion
    angiography, 85
    bruit, 64
    carotid endarterectomy risks, 168
    common configurations, *84,* 85, *85,* 86
    complete, 160
    CT imaging, *66*
    delayed surgery, 160
    Doppler techniques, 107-108
    duration, 160
    emergency carotid endarterectomy, 163
    external, *189*
    extracranial, 194

general characteristics, 67
internal, 194
recanalization, 112
STA-MCA bypass, 216
stroke risk, 68, 282-283
stump syndrome, 160
surgical, 182
transient ischemic attacks (TIAs), 67
Carotid artery stenosis
angiography, 85, 195
angioplasty, *245*
asymptomatic, 64, 68, 163, 258-259
asymptomatic and preoperative patients, 158
asymptomatic (medical and surgical treatment
   compared), 156-157
atrial fibrillation and, 61
bruit and hypertension, 64
carotid endarterectomy benefits, 244
carotid endarterectomy indications, 167
carotid endarterectomy risks, 168
carotid endarterectomy trials, 258-261
critical (80% or more), 161, 163
EC-IC bypass lack of benefits, 219
extracranial *107*
fifty-percent, 157
high-percentage, 156, 158, 159, 163
hypoperfusion, 182
intracranial, 86
lesions, 282
Magnetic resonance angiography (MRA), 82
perioperative stroke risk, 158
"pseudo-tandem," 162
recurrrent, 162-163
severe, and surgery, 167
STA-MCA bypass, 216
stroke risk, 68
surgical considerations, 161
surgical treatment for 70% or more stenosis, 159
symptomatic, 259-261
transcranial Doppler ultrasound, 196
transient ischemic attacks (TIAs), 61, 163
transient monocular blindness and, 61
ultrasound screening for endarterectomy, 115
Carotid artery surgery asymptomatic
   narrowing operation versus aspirin, *257,* 258-260
Carotid artery, Common
angioplasty, *245*
continuous-wave Doppler, 105
Doppler techniques, 108
ultrasonography, 113
Carotid artery, External (Extracranial)
angiography, 84-86
carotid endarterectomy procedure, *171*
continuous-wave Doppler, 105
dissection, 193-197
occlusion, *189*

stump, 218
surgical indications, 155-165
ultrasound imaging, 106-110
ultrasound screening, 128
Carotid artery, Internal (Intracranial)
angiography, 86-87
angioplasty, 243, *245*
carotid endarterectomy procedure, *171,* 171, *174*
continuous-wave Doppler, 105
dissecting aneurysm, *192*
dissection, 197
Doppler techniques, 108
extracranial, 61, 105, 106
lesions, stenosis, 282
magnetic resonance angiography (MRA), 81, *82*
recanalization, 112
stenosis and STA-MCA bypass, 216
stenosis, bifurcation, *84*
stroke risk, 68
stump, 218
surgical treatment of stenosis, 159
transcranial Doppler imaging, 91-92, 106, 108, *109*
traumatic dissection, *76*
Carotid artery, Internal (Intracranial—Occlusion)
angiogram, *223*
angiography, *85, 86*
angioplasty for stenosis, *245*
EC-IC bypass study, 218, 220
neurologic deficits and, 218
recanalization, 242
siphon, 106
special case (time and risks of stroke), 282-283
STA-MCA bypass, 216
stenosis, 86
surgical risk, 158
transcranial Doppler, 91
ultrasonongraphy, 110-113
Carotid endarterectomy, 167-185
alternative techniques, 177-181
anesthesia, positioning, 169-170
angiography preoperative evaluation, 90
candidate screening by ultrasound, 115
carotid occlusion and, 163
complications, 181-183
condemnation and endorsement, 262
elective, 169
emergency, 159, 160, 163
fibrostenosis, 244
mortality, 155, 163, 167, 181
myocardial infarction, 181
neurologic deficits and, 163
operative procedures, 170-176
perioperative stroke, 167
postoperative care, 176-177
procedures illustrated, *169-176*
prophylactic, 155, 157, 158, 163, 260-261

proven indications, 163
recent stroke, 160-161
recurrent stenosis, 162
risk and preoperative assessment, 158, 167-169
siphon disease resolution, 162
stroke rates, *254*
surgical positioning, *169*
surgical risk grading system, 168
transient ischemic attacks (TIAs), 260-261
trials, 256-261, *257*
Carotid sheath, *170,* 171
Carotid siphon disease, 86, 162, 168
CASANOVA (Clinical trial), *257,* 258-260
Cerebellar arteries
anterior, 203
diaschisis, 95
posterior, 203-204
superior, 203
transcranial Doppler, 91, 106, 108
ultrasonography, 110-112
Cerebral arteries, see subject headings beginning with
"Arteries; "Arterial..;" names of specific arteries,
e.g. Carotid arteries
Cerebral artery occlusion, see Occlusive diseases; names
of specific arteries, e.g., Carotid artery occlusion
Cerebral artery, Middle
angioplasty, 243, *245*
CT imaging, *75, 76,* 77
decreased perfusion pressures, 215-216
infarction, *189*
internal carotid artery dissection, 197
recanalization, 112
SPECT imaging, *94*
STA-MCA bypass, 216
stroke risk factors, 61
transcranial Doppler, 91, 106, *109*
ultrasonography, 110-112
velocity, 91, 92
Cerebral artery, Middle—Occlusion
ATP and lactate levels, *8*
delayed hypoperfusion, *16*
ischemic vasoconstriction and reperfusion, *15*
MR spectroscopy, 83
recanalization, 242
Cerebral artery, Middle—Stenosis
imaging, 85, *87*
transcranial Doppler, *111*
Cerebral artery occlusion, see Occlusive diseases;
names of specific arteries, e.g. Carotid artery occlusion
Cerebral blood flow, see Blood flow, Cerebral
Cerebral ischemia, see Ischemia
Cerebral vasculitis, 147
Cerebral venous thrombosis, 149, 150
Cerebrovascular occlusive diseases, see Occlusive diseases;
names of specific cerebrovascular arteries
Cervical vertebrae, 206

Chinese, 61
Chiropractic manipulation, 206
Cholecystokinin, 6, *6*
Cholesterol, 123
Chronic obstructive pulmonary disease, 168
Cigarette Smoking, see Tobacco
Circle of Willis
angiography, *223*
collateral pathways, *285,* 286
Doppler ultrasonography, 106, *114*
Circumferential arteries, 203
Clinical trials, see also Surgery; Thrombolysis
impact on medical practice, 261-262
Clonidine, 277
Clot formation, 231-232
Coagulation disorders, 148, 149, 207
Cognition, 267
Cognitive impairment, 270-272, 274, 277
Cohort trials, 253
Collateral pathways, *285,* 286
Color Doppler
carotid occlusion 107-108
carotid stenosis, *107*
description, 90, 106
Comma-shaped lesions, 65
Common carotid artery, see Carotid artery, Common
Communicating arteries, 203-204
Compaction stasis, 40
Computed tomography (CT)
acute ischemia vs intracerebral hemorrhage, 73
acute stage, *75*
asymptomatic carotid bruits, 74
carotid artery, 78
carotid endarterctomy assessment, 168
completed stroke, 74
hemispheric stroke 75-78
high-resolution, 286
infarction features, 65-66, *75*
lacunar infarctions, 77-78
lacunar, vertebrobasilar and watershed
infarctions, 77-78
left hemisphere, *190*
middle cerebral artery *75, 76*
neurologic deficits, 74
parenchymal infarction, *66*
SPECT compared to, 94
speedy evaluation of stroke, 235-236
subacute stage, 77
subcortical infarction, *66*
transient ischemic attacks (TIAs), 77
vertebrobasilar disease, 207
vertebrobasilar ischemia, 78
watershed zone, 78
wedge-shaped cortical infarction, *66*
xenon, 236
Confusion, 275

Congestive heart failure, 167
Consciousness, Loss of, 2, 266, *271, 273*
Contraceptives, 207
Coronary artery disease, 69
Coronary bypass surgery, 158, 244-245
Corticosteroids, 149-150
Cranial nerves
arterial dissection symptoms, 194
injury from carotid endarterectomy, 182-183
palsies, 194, 199
Crossed cerebellar diaschisis, 95
CSP (clinical trial), @257, 258-260
CT, see Computed Tomography

D

Data acquistion, 252
Dementia, 268
Demyelinating disease, 207
Depression, 276-277
Dextran
    erythrocyte aggregation, 31
    erythrocytes, relative viscosity and shear rate, *35*
    high molecular weight, 30, 34
    low molecular weight, 19, 45-48
Dextromethorphan, *11,* 20
Diabetes
    arterial occlusion risk factors, 125-126
    stroke recurrence, 269
    stroke risk factors, 61
Diagnosis, see also specific diagnostic techniques, e.g.
    Angiography, Computed tomography; Doppler
    ultrasound; Magnetic resonance imaging (MRI)
    acute ischemia, 135-138
    angiography as gold standard, 287
    candidates and timing, 73-75
    evaluation of ischemia, 73-101
    noninvasive studies, 88-92
    speedy evaluation for thrombolytic therapy, 234-236
    vertebrobasilar disease, 207
Diamox™, *93,* 93-94
Diaschisis, 95
Diastolic velocities, 104
Diet, 124-125
Digital cerebral angiography, 207
Digital subtraction angiography, 87, 90, 107-108
Diplopia, 206
Dipyridamile, 159
Disabilities, see also Neurologic deficits and
    impairments evaluation, measurement, 269-274
    independent living, 278
    infarction location and, 268
    stroke outcome and rehabilitation, 265-280
Dobhoff tube, 275
Dolichoectasia, 113
Doppler ultrasound
    asymptomatic carotid bruits, 74
    continous-wave, 104-106, 109, 113
    description, 88, 89
    external vertebral artery dissection, 199
    extracranial carotid artery dissection, 195-196
    general principles and applications, 103-116
    intraoperative monitoring, 91
    pulsed-wave, 104, 106
Drug abuse, 123-124
Duplex ultrasound
    carotid artery evaluation, 96, 107-108
    description, 90
    extracranial arteries, 106, *107*
    inaccuracy in carotid endarterectomy trials, 261
    innominate artery, 109
    uses, 105
Dysarthria, 67, 206, *271, 273*
Dysmetria, 206
Dysphagia, 275
Dysrhythmias, 207

E

EC-IC bypass, see Extracranial-intracranial anastomosis
    (bypass)
Echocardiography, 68
ECST (Clinical trial), *257,* 258-260
Edema, 54
    exacerbation by hemodilution, 152
    hemodilution contraindications, 152
    MRI, 80
    postischemic hypoperfusion, 16
    postoperative, 182
    subacute stage, 77
EEG, see Electroencephalography
Electroencephalography (EEG)
    attenuation, *3,* 7-8
    carotid endarterectomy monitoring, 179
    intraoperative monitoring, 21
Electrolyte disorders, 149, 150
Electrons, 2, 3
Embolism
    artery-to-artery, *284,* 286
    associated neurologic deficits, 63
    hemorrhagic infarction, 65
    microemboli, 112
    ocular and cerebral, 218, 219
    recurrent, 149
    stroke classification, 59
    vertebrobasilar disease, 207
Embolization, carotid endarterectomy complications, 182
Emopamil™, 19
Encephalo-myo-synangiosis, 227
Encephalo-omental-synangiosis, 224
Encephalomyo-synangiosis, 224
Endothelial cells, 4, 5

Endothelial-releasing factor, 5
Endothelin, 5, *6*
Endothelium, 41
Endovascular thrombolysis, see Thrombolysis
Energy production, 2-3
Eosinophils, 40
Erythrocyte
   sedimentation, 29
Erythrocyte aggregation
   fibrinogen, albumin, globulin role, 51
   leukocyte displacement, 41
   mechanism in infarction, 51
   and axial flow, 33
   and cell free margin, 33, 34, *34*
   and deformability, 30-31
   and microcirculation, 31
   and pH, 31
   and shear rate, 30
   viscosity and shear rate, 31, 35
Erythrocytes
   aggregation, axial flow and viscosity, 34, *35*
   axial distribution, 32, *33*
   deformability, 30
   deformation and vessel diameter, 35
   impedance by leukocytes, 41
   influence on viscosity in microcirculation, 50
   platelet interaction, 50
   sedimentation, 39-40
   velocity, 41
Ethics, medical, EC-IC bypass surgery, 228
Etomidate
   carotid endarterectomy, 173, 180
   decreased metabolic demand, 21
   ischemia during surgical carotid occlusion, 182
   neuronal energy requirements, 18
European Carotid Surgery Trial, *257*, 258-260
Excitatory amino acid antagonists, 20
Excitotoxic theory, *11*, 11-12, 20
Excitotoxicity, 285
Exclusion effects, 36-39
Extracranial atherosclerosis, see Atherosclerotic large-artery disease
Extracranial carotid artery, see Carotid artery, External (Extracranial)
Extracranial-intracranial (EC-IC) anastomosis (bypass), 215-230
   agreement on correct procedure, 221
   Bypass Study, Trial 216-222, 252, 255-257, 262
   complications, 212
   ethical considerations, 228
   natural, 223-224
   patients who may benefit, 218
   procedures and techniques, 225-228
   prophylactic, elective, 224
   strict criteria, 228

   vertebrobasilar occlusive disease, 211-212, *211*
Eye deviation, 266
Eye movements, *271, 273*

F

Facial nerve, 182
Facial palsy, *271, 273*
Facial vein, *170, 171*, 171
Fahraeus effect, 36-39, *39*, 48, 49
   reversal (erythrocyte sedimentation), 40
Fahraeus-Lindqvist effect, 30-35, 48, 49
   inversion phenomenon, 35
Fb-Fb-CF, 238
Feeding, artificial, 275
Fentanyl, 169
Fibrin, 231-233, *232*
Fibrinogen
   blood viscosity, 31
   clot formation and thrombolytic agents, 231-233
   erythrocyte aggregation and deformability, 30, 51
   plasma viscosity, 51
   stroke risk factors, 124
Fibrinolysis, 148
Fibromuscular dysplasia, 147-148, 193, 196-197, 244
Fibromuscular hyperplasia, 204
Fibrostenosis, 244
Fistula, carotid-cavernous, 194
Foramina transversaria, 210
Free radical scavengers, 20-22
Functional ability, see stroke, and activities of daily living

G

Gadolinium-DTPA, 78, 80
Gaze palsy, 266
Globulins
   blood viscosity, 31
   erythrocyte aggregation, 51
Glucose
   brain energy requirements, 1
   brain pH and, *14*
   delivery, 2
   metabolic rate, 3
   oxidationn, 2-3
   PET imaging, 95
Glutamate, 11, 12
Glutamate antagonists, 153
Glutathione, 21
GM1 ganglioside, 153
Gosling's Index, 104
Grafting, see Venous patch angioplasty
Granulocytes, 40, 41
Gunshot wounds, 188, *189*

H

Hagen-Poiseuille equation, 27, 49
Hamilton Psychiatric Rating Scale for
    Depression, 272-274
Hand weakness, 64
Handicaps, see Disabilities
Headaches
    classification of occlusive diseases, 64-65
    extracranial vertebral artery dissection, 197-198
Heart diseases
    anticoagulant therapy, 129
    cardiogenic emboli and, 120
    ischemic, 75
    major thrombolytic trials, 237-238, *237*
    stroke cause in young adults, 146-147
    stroke complications, 150
    thrombolytic therapy, 237-238
Heart valve, Prosthetic, 61
Hematocrit
    blood flow determination, 35-36
    blood flow, viscosity and, 42-43
    decreased, and oxygen delivery, 44, 45
    discharge, 38
    elevated 43, 45, 49, 54
    feed, 38
    inverse correlation with oxygen delivery, 152
    optimal for oxygen delivery, 47-50, 54
    platelet aggregation, 50
    reduced, 48, 49
    reduction in microcirculation, 36-39
    relative, *39*
    relative, and erythrocyte sedimentation, 40
    tube, 38
    viscosity, 35-36, *36*
    viscosity, cerebral ischemia and, 43-45, 49-50
    viscosity, shear rate and, *21*
Hematoma
    dissecting arterial, 200
    dissecting, in intracranial vertebral artery
        dissection, 199
    dissecting intramural 196, *196*
    MRI, 199
    surgical wounds, 181-182
Hemianopsia, 67, 206
Hemiparesis, 62-64, 67
Hemisensory loss, 67
Hemispheres of brain
    CT imaging, 75-78, *109*
    hyperperfusion, 182
    stroke outcome prediction, 267
Hemodilution therapy
    animal research, 45-46
    aspirin adjunct, 50
    clinical trials, 46-48, 54

complexity and disappointing results, 53
    hypervolemic, 19, 45, 46-48, 152
    infarct size reduction, 19
    isovolemic, 45, 46, 152
    optimal hematocrit for oxygen delivery, 50
    questionable benefit for acute ischemia, 48
    tissue rescue, 151-152
Hemodynamic insufficiency, *284*
Hemoglobin, 43, 127
Hemorheology, 25-58
Hemorrhage
    CT imaging, 73
    differentiation from ischemia, 137
    intracranial, associated with thrombolysis, 238
    intracranial, risk after anticoagulation, 158
    intraplaque, 161
    postoperative, 183
    recurrent, 199
    reperfusion-related, 20
Hemorrhage, Subarachnoid
    arterial dissections, 199
    nimodipine treatment, 19, 20, 152
    vasospasm, 54
Hemorrhagic conversion (Thrombolysis), 239-243
Hemorrhagic shock, 42
Heparin
    arterial dissection treatment, 200
    carotid endarterectomy, 173
    carotid endarterectomy preoperative care, 168
    effectiveness examined, 150
    hemorrhagic conversion, 239
    intraluminal thrombus, 161-162
Herniation, 152
Hexamethylpropyleneamineoxime, 94
High-molecular weight-dextran, see Dextran
HMWD (High-molecular-weight dextran), see Dextran
Hypotension, 45
Hydrogen ions, 5, 13
Hyperglycemia, 13, 151, 266, 269
Hyperlipidemia, 61
Hyperperfusion, 182
Hypertension
    arterial occlusion risk factors, 122-123
    carotid endarterectomy, 177
    control, 129
    early deterioration of stroke patients, 266
    induced, 19, 22, 54
    infarction management, 142
    postoperative, 182
    stroke recurrence, 269
    stroke risk factors, 61
    surgical risk factors, 167
Hypervolemia, 54, 152
Hypoglossal artery, 204
Hypoglossal nerve, *171,* 171, 182

Hyponatremia, 150
Hypoperfusion
  delayed, postischemic, 15-16, *16*
  global, *66*
  postischemic, 18
  revascularization candidates, 222
Hypotension
  carotid endarterectomy, 173, 177
  neutrophil role, 42
Hypothermia, 17-18, 22
Hypoxia, 45, 49

I

ICA, see Carotid artery, Internal (Intracranial)
Idiopathic basal occlusive disease, see Moyamoya disease
Incidence, 252-253
Independence, see Stroke, and activities of daily living
Infarction, see also Ischemia; Stroke
  brain stem, 199
  cortical, 65, *66*
  elevated hematocrit, 43
  erythrocyte aggregation and mechanism for, 51
  established, 142
  hematocrit and atherosclerosis, 45
  hemodilution contraindications, 152
  hemoglobin concentration as risk factor, 43
  hemorrhagic, 65
  ischemic thresholds, *10*
  lacunar, 64, 77-78, 80, 145-146, *205*
  location and patient outcome, 267, 268
  MRI, early, 287
  multi-infarction dementia, 268
  multiple (surgical risks), 168
  parenchymal, 54, *66*, 222
  PET imaging, 96
  rare, 146-149
  recurrent, 143
  schematization, with ischemic penumbra, *9*
  severity and increased hematocrit, 49
  size decrease after speedy reperfusion, 234
  size and headache, 65
  size reduction in hemodilution, 19, 20
  stages (acute, subacute, chronic), 75, 77
  striatocapsular, 65, *66*
  subcortical, 60, 64, *66*
  transient, 194
  volume and prognosis for recovery, 266
  watershed, 77-78
  wedge-shaped, *66*
  young adult, 146-149
Informed consent, 228
Innominate artery, 106, 109, 110
Intensive care, 53
Internal carotid artery, see Carotid artery, Internal
  (Intracranial)

Intracranial carotid artery, see Carotid artery,
  Internal (Intracranial)
Intracranial pressure, 149
Intubation, 176
Iodine[123]-labeled propanediamine, 94
Ischemia, see also Infarction; Stroke
  acute, 135-154
  acute, and CT, 73
  acute, "therapeutic window," 153
  brain metabolic relationships, *3*
  calcium channel blockers, 18
  cardiac, 181
  carotid occlusion, 182
  cerebral, and arterial dissection, 199
  clinical and pathologic spectrum illustrated, *289*
  complete, and tissue damage, 151
  diagnostic evaluation, 73-101
  diagnostic tests summarized, 96
  differences between focal and global, 1
  differentiation from hemorrhage, 137
  elevated hematocrit, 49, 54
  focal, 15, 16, 18
  focal, and accompanying diseases, 1
  focal, and hemodilution, 46
  focal, mechanisms, *284*
  global, 16
  hematocrit, viscosity, and blood flow, 27, 43-45, 49-50
  hemodilutional therapy, 45-48
  hypoperfusion, 15-16, *16*, 18, *66*, 222
  inappropriate application of theory, 53
  incomplete, and tissue damage, 151
  mechanisms illustrated, *284*
  metabolic cascades, 9-10
  need for continuous and dynamic monitoring, 53
  occlusive disease as risk factor, 118-120
  parenchymal, 222
  penumbra, 9, *9*, 150, 151
  posterior circulation, 199
  previous, as occlusion risk factors, 128
  progression to infarction, PET imaging, 96
  recurrent (prevention), *290*
  reperfusion, *15*, 22, 41-42, 234-238, 240, 241
  retinal, and arterial dissection, 199
  rheological characteristics, 50-53
  subclass identification for better clinical trials, 54
  thresholds, 7-9, *7*, *10*
  threshold uniformity, 283-284
  transient ischemic attacks (TIAs), 194
  treatment and monitoring dynamics, 53
  unified concept, 281-291
  vasoconstriction, *6*, 14, *15*
  vertebrobasilar, 197-198, 213
  viscosity importance, 27
Ischemic penumbra, 9, *9*, 150, 151
Ischemic thresholds, 7-9, *7*, *10*, 283-284
Isoflurane, 18, 21, *21*

Isoproterenol, 19

J

Japan, 45, 223
Jugular vein, *170,* 170-171

K

Knee bracing, 276

L

L channels, 14, 20
Lactate, *8*
Lactic acid
  brain metabolic relationships, *3*
  ischemia thresholds, 8-9
Lactic acidosis, 5, 83
Lacunar hypothesis, 63-64
Lacunar infarction
  asymptomatic and symptomatic, 80
  coexistent carotid stenosis, 64
  CT imaging, 77-78
  description, 145-146
MRI, *205*
  stroke classification, 59
  syndrome, 60, 62
Language ability, 267, *271, 273*
Large-vessel hemodynamics, see Macrocirculation
Laryngeal nerves, *170,* 183
Lateral medullary syndrome, 63
Leg
  carotid occlusive disease, 67
  movement, *271, 273*
  weakness, 266
Leptomeningeal collateral pathway, *285*
Lethargy, 275
Leukocytes
  adhesion, 41
  capillary occlusion, 41, 42, 43
  flight, 41
  postischemic hypoperfusion, 16
  rheology, 40-42
  rheological characteristics of ischemia, 52-53
  velocity, 41
Leukomalacia, *80,* 81
Limb ataxia, *271, 273*
Lipids, 129
Lipohyalinosis, 63
Long-term care, *267*
Lumbar puncture, 138
Lumen
  narrowing (blood flow, velocity), 104-105
  narrowing (dissecting intramural hematoma), 196
  narrowing, in intracranial vertebral artery

dissection, 199
narrowing (quantification), 107-108
outpouching, 187, 191
stenosis, 187
thrombosis
surgical considerations, 161-162
webs, 191, *191*
Lymphocytes, 40

M

MACE (Clinical trial), *257,* 258-260
Macrocirculation
  differences from microcirculation, 25
  hematocrit and viscosity, *36*
  hematocrit reduction and elevation, 49
  plasma proteins and stroke pathogenesis, 52
  shear rate, erythrocyte aggregation and viscosity, 36, *37*
  viscosity, 28-30, 42
  viscosity, less important than in microcirculation, 27
  viscosity and shear rate in, 29, 31
Macroglobulinemias, 207
Magnetic resonance angiography (MRA)
  anticoagulation follow-up, 200
  carotid bifurcations, 81
  combination with MRI, 82
  internal carotid artery, 81, *82*
  luminal irregularities, *196*
  MRI combination, 96
  normal, *83*
  reliability, 287
  ultrasound compared to, 114
  uses, 81-82
  vertebral artery stenosis, *205*
  vertebrobasilar disease, 207
Magnetic resonance imaging (MRI)
  acute ischemia, 137
  asymptomatic carotid bruits, 74
  Binswanger's disease, 67
  brain stem and cerebellar structures, 207
  carotid artery, hematoma, *196*
  carotid blood flow velocity, 82
  carotid endarterectomy assessment, 168
  combination with MRA, 82
  combination with MR spectroscopy, 83
  current diagnostic uses, 287
  early imaging of infarction, 287
  edema, 80
  external vertebral artery dissection, 199
  extracranial carotid artery dissection, 194
  extracranial vertebral artery dissection, *198*
  general description and uses, 78-84
  infarction features, 65-66
  infarction near middle cerebral artery, *189*

intracranial vertebral artery dissection, 199
lacunar infarctions, *205*
leukomalacia (Binswanger's dementia), *80*, 81
MRA combination, 96
potential in speedy evaluations of stroke, 236
small-vessel disease, 74
transient ischemic attacks, 81
uses, limitation, 78-84
vertebral artery dissection, *206*
watershed zone, *79*, 81
Mannitol, 150
Marfan's syndrome, 193
Mass effect, 77, 78, 199
Mayo Asymptomatic Carotid Endarterectomy Trial, *257*, 258-260
MCA, see Cerebral artery, Middle
Metabolic cascades
    blocking, 22
    decreasing, 20-21
    ischemia, 9-10
    neuronal injury, 9-13
    therapeutic blocking, 16, 20-21
Metabolism, Brain, 1-24
    neuronal damage and energy failure, *10*
    oxygen consumption decrease, 18
Methodology of clinical trials, see Research
    Microcirculation
    axial flow, aggregation and viscosity, 34, *35*
    blood cell axial distribution, 32, *33*
    blood viscosity, 28-30
    capillary diameter and relative hematocrit, *39*
    differences from macrocirculation, 25
    erythrocyte aggregation and viscosity, 31, 51
    erythrocyte impedance by leukocytes, 41
    erythrocyte influence on viscosity, 50
    hematocrit, less important in viscosity
        determination, 50
    hematocrit reduction, 36-39
    hematocrit, and viscosity, *38*
    inversion phenomenon between viscosity and vessel
        diameter, 35
    microanatomy, 3-5
    MRI, 74
    neuronal injury, 13-16
    neutrophil role in hypotension, 42
    plasma proteins and stroke pathogenesis, 52
    postischemia reperfusion, 41
    viscosity, 28-31, 33, 36-39, 42, 49
viscosity increase prevented, 30
viscosity, more important than in macrocirculation, 27
Microembolism, 112
Microscope, operating, 180
Middle cerebral artery, see Cerebral artery, middle
Migraine
    basilar, 207
    classification of strokes, 60

headache in stroke diagnosis, 65
stroke cause in young adults, 146
Mini-mental status, 268, 270, 271, 274
Misery perfusion, 96
Mitochondria, 2, 12-13
Mitral stenosis, 61
MK801, *11*, 20
Mortality   angiography, 88
    carotid endarterectomy, 155, 163, 167, 181
    coronary artery disease,69
Moyamoya disease, 148, 223-224, *285*
MRA, see Magnetic resonance angiography
MRI, see Magnetic resonance imaging
Multi-infarction dementia, 268
Myocardial infarction
    cardioembolism causes, 69
    following transient ischemic attack, 69
    postoperative, 181
    risk factor in subsequent carotid endarterectomy,
        167
    stroke-in-evolution (progressing), 149
    stroke risk factors, 61
    surgical mortality, 157
    thrombolytic trials, *237*, 237-238
Myocardial insufficiency, 207

N

N-isopropyl-123-iodoamphetamine, 94-95
NADH, Nicotinamide adenine dinucleotide
NASCET, see North American Symptomatic Carotid
    Endarterectomy Clinical Trial
Nasogastric feeding, 275
National Institutes of Health Stroke Scale,
    see NIH stroke scale
Neck movements (injuries), 193, 197
Neck wounds, 188
Neglect, *271, 273*
Nerve palsies, 194, 199
Neurokinin A, 6, *6*
Neuroleptics, 277
Neurologic deficits and impairment
    angiography risks, 88
    carotid artery disease, 159-160
    carotid endarterectomy complications, 182-183
    carotid endarterectomy indications, 167
    carotid endarterectomy risks, 168
    classification of occlusive diseases, 63-64
    early deterioration of stroke patients, 266
    emergency carotid endarterectomy, 163
    ICA occlusion and, 218
    imaging, 74
    measurement, 269-274
    postoperative complications, 181
    rating scales, 270-274, *271-273*
    temporal profile, 63

thrombolysis effect, 20
Neurons
    calcium entry, 152
    damage and energy failure, *10*
    energy requirements, 17-18
    injury, 7-16
    injury and reperfusion, 22
    ischemic injury, 21
    SPECT portrayal of dysfunction, 95
    therapeutic decrease in energy requirements, 16-18
Neuropeptide Y, 5, *6*
Neuropeptides, 5
Neurotransmitters, 5, *6*, 11
Neutropenia, 52.
Neutrophils, 40, 42, 52
Nicotinamide adenine dinucleotide
    brain energy production, 2
    brain metabolic relationships, *3*
    NADH, 3, 13
NIH Stroke Scale, *271-273*, 273
Nimodipine, 18, 19, 20, 152
NMDA, 11, 20, 153
Nonatherosclerotic large-artery disease
    headache, 64
    microembolism, 62
    occlusive disease classification, 60
    revascularization (bypass) surgery, 223-224
    risks, 118
    transient ischemic attacks (TIAs), 61
    vascular risk factors, 60
Norepinephrine, 5, *6*, 15
North American Symptomatic Carotid
    Trial (NASCET), *257*, 258-260
Null hypothesis, 253
Nursing homes, *267*
Nutrition, 275

O

Obesity, 126, 168
Occipital-anterior inferior cerebellar anastomosis,
    211-212
Occipital artery, 210
Occipital-posterior-inferior cerebellar anastomosis,
    211
    safety, 212
Occlusion, planned, 224
Occlusive diseases, see also names of arteries
    asymptomatic, 281
    candidates for revascularization surgery, 222-225
    classification, 59-60
    coronary artery disease as cause of death, 69
    duration as classifying system, 59
    intracranial, 110-112
    intracranial stenosis, 283
    natural history, 68-69

recanalization, 151
revascularization surgery, 222-230
risk factor for ischemia, 118-120
risk factors, 120-128
thrombolytic therapy (reperfusion, recanalization,
    hemorrhagic conversion), 231-249
types and symptoms described, 60-71
unified concept, 281-291
vertebrobasilar, 203-214
Oculoplethysmography, 88-89
Oculosympathetic paresis, 194
Omohyoid muscle, *170*, 171
One-tailed analysis, 253
Ophthalmic artery
    carotid stump syndrome, 160
    collateral pathways, *285*, 286
    transcranial Doppler, 106, 108
Osteophytic spurs, 206
Osteotomy, 210
Otic artery, 204
Outcome, see under Stroke
Outcome analysis, 253
Oxidative phosphorylation 1, 2, 152
Oxygen
    arterial and venous tensions, 2, 7
    metabolism 1-3
Oxygen delivery
    decreased hematocrit and, 44, 45
    hemodilution therapy, 45
    inverse correlation with hematocrit, 152
    optimal hematocrit, 47-50, 54
    tissue rescue, 150
    viscosity reduction and, 46
Oxygen extraction ratio, 95, 96

P

$PaCO_2$, see Arterial carbon dioxide
Pain
    abrupt, 199
    extracranial carotid artery dissection, 194
Palsy, nerve, see Nerve palsies
Pancuronium, 169
PaO_2, see Arterial oxygen
Paralysis, *10*
Parenchyma
    ATP, *3*
    brain ischemia spectrum, *289*
    infarction, ischemia, 54, 222
    ischemic penumbra, 9, *9*
    microcirculation, 25
    MRI, 287
    oxygen transport, 45
    therapy to limit damage, *290*
Paresis, Oculosympathetic, 199
Penetrating artery disease

bruit and hypertension, 64
description, 67
features on CT, MRI, 65
hemiparesis, 64
natural history, 69
neurologic deficit, 63, 64
occlusive disease classification, 60
recurrent stroke, 69
sensory stroke, 64
transient ischemic attacks (TIAs), 61-62
vascular risk factors, 60-61
Pentobarbital, 17
Pentoxifylline, 153
Percutaneous transluminal angioplasty, 243-245
Perfusion, 150
Perfusion pressure, 7
Periventricular infarction, 80
PET, see Positron emission tomography
pH
brain, *14*
erythrocyte shape, 31
extracellular, 5
MR spectroscopy, 83
Phenobarbital, 17
Phenylalkamine, 19
Phenylephrine, 173
Phonoangiography, 89
Phosphate, 83
Phosphocreatine, 83
Physical therapy, 274-277
Plaque
B-mode imaging, 107
carotid endarterectomy risks, 168
morphology, 106-107, 161
removal (carotid endarterectomy), *173,* 173-174,
174, 175, *176*
ulceration, 161
vertebrobasilar occlusive disease, 204, 209
Plasma
cell free zone, 39, 40
erythrocytes, relative viscosity and shear rate, *35*
hemorheologic properties, 27
proteins, 50-52
proteolytic state, *232*
viscosity, 50-52
Platelets
abnormalities, 148
adhesion and aggregation, 50
aggregation, 16, 231-232
antiplatelet therapy, 129-130, 156, 158-159, 223
erythrocyte interaction, 50
Pneumonia, 149, 150
Polyarteritis nodosa, 193
Polycythemia 43-44. 127, 148
Positron emission tomography (PET)
evaluation of ischemia, 95-96

limitations and research use, 287
limits, 95
SPECT compared to, 95
use in research, 96
vertebrobasilar disease, 207
Posterior fossa, 199
Postoperative care
carotid endarterectomy, 176-177
Postoperative complications
carotid endarterectomy, 181-183
vertebral artery angioplasties, anastomoses, 212
Potassium, 8
Potts scissors, *172,* 173
Pourcelot's Resistivity Index, 104
Precapillary sphincter, 4
Preoperative care
carotid endarterectomy, 168-169
Pressure perfusion, 7
Prevalence, 252-253
Preventive techniques, 129-130
Pro-atlantal artery, 204
Procoagulant state, 60
Prospective cohort trials, 253
Prostacyclin, 7, 153
Pseudoaneurysms, 86, 196, 204
Pseudostroke, 136
Pulmonary embolism, 149, 150
Pulsatility index, 104
Pulsatility transmission index, 108
Pyruvic acid, 2, 3

Q-R

Quantitative phonoangiography, 89
Race (Occlusive disease risk factors), 126-127
Randomization, 253, 254
Recanalization
thrombolytic therapy, 151, 238-242
transcranial Doppler imaging, 112
Red blood cells, see Erythrocytes
Rehabilitation, 274
Renal failure, 88
Reoperation, see Surgery
Reperfusion
blockage (leukocyte plugging), 41
neuronal injury, 22
postischemic, and neutrophils, 42
temporary occlusion, *15*
thrombolytic therapy, 234-238, 240, 241
Research
biases, problems in trials, 221
lessons of EC-IC bypass study, 220-222
representative cases, 221
Retina, 194
Retrospective cohort trials, 253
Revascularization surgery, see

Extrancranial-intracranial EC-IC
    anastomosis (bypass)
Reversible ischemic neurologic deficit
RINDs, 59, 73, 161
RINDs, see Reversible ischemic neurologic deficits
Risk factors, 117-134
    carotid endarterectomy, 167-168
    cerebral artery occlusion, 120-128
    classification of occlusive diseases, 60-61
    stroke, summarized, 282
Rouleau, see Erythrocytes
Rummell tourniquets, *172,* 172

S

Sample size, *254*
Saphenous veins, 177-178, *178-179,* 201, *225, 226*
ScuPA, see Single chain urokinase plasminogen
    activator
Sedentary lifestyle, 125
Sedimentation, see Blood sedimentation
Seizures, 182
Seldinger technique, 87
Sensitivity (Data collection), 252
Sensory tests, *271, 273*
Serotonin, 5-6, *6*
Serotonin antagonists, 19, 22
Serum glucose, 20
Sex factors, 126
Shear rate
    blood-cell axial distribution, 32, *33*
    erythrocytes and, 31, *34, 35*
    low, 50, 51
    macrocirculation, 49
    microcirculation hematocrit and viscosity, *38,* 50
    relative viscosity, *35*
    sedimentation and, 39-40
    viscosity, hematocrit and, 25-27, *29*
Shear stress, 26
Shunts
    carotid endarterectomy, *176,* 176, 178-179
    carotid occlusion, 162
Sickle-cell disease, 60,113, 127-128, 148, 207
Single chain urokinase plasminogen activator,
232, 232-234
Single photon emission computed tomography
(SPECT)
    cerebral blood flow, *94*
    CT compared to, 94
    evaluation of ischemia, 94-95
    limitations, 236
    PET compared to, 95
    speedy evaluation of stroke, 235-236
Skull base injuries, 188
Skull base neoplasms, 224
Smoking, see Tobacco

Sodium, 8, 10
Sodium-calcium ATPase, 10
Sodium ions, 11-12
Sodium-potassium-ATPase, 8, 12
Spasticity, 276
SPECT, see Single photon emission computed
tomography
Speech pathology, 275
Statistical analysis, 253-254
Statistical power, 254
Steal syndrome, 110, 206, 208-209
Stenosis, arterial, see names of specific arteries
Streptokinase
    comparison of thrombolytic agents, *232,* 232-234
    hemorrhagic conversion, 239
    intracranial hemorrhage, 238
    intravenous thrombolytic studies, *240, 241*
    major thrombolytic trials, *237*
    recanalization 151, 238
    vertebrobasilar disease, 208
Striatocapsular infarctions, 65, *66*
String sign, 86, 187
Stroke, see also Infarction, Ischemia
    and activities of daily living, 267, 269, 270, 273,
    274, 276, 278
    angiography risks, 88
    antiphospholipid antibody syndrome, 60
    brain stem, 267
    carotid artery occlusion, 194
    completed, 59, 74
    complications, 149, 150
    distribution by type, 60
    embolic, 59
    fatal, nonfatal and EC-IC bypass, *217*
    hemispheric, 75-78, 267
    in-evolution, 59, 88, 149-150, 160
    lacunar, 59, 63-64, 77-78, 80, 145-146, *205*
    large-artery thrombotic, 59
    major, (postoperative), 181
    migraine, 60
    minor, (postoperative), 181
    miscellaneous group, 60
    occlusive disease risk factors, 120-128
    outcome, 265-274, 277-278
    percutaneous transluminal angioplasty, 243-245
    perioperative, 157, 158, 167
    postoperative mortality, 181
    prevention, 61, 117-134, 288
    procoagulant state, 60
    progressing, 149-150
    prophylactic surgery, 160
    pure sensory, 67
    rating scales (inter-rater agreement), *273*
    recent, 160-161
    recurrent, 69, 269
    rehabilitation, 265, 274-278

risk factor reduction, control, 129-130
risk factors summarized, 282
sensory, 64
sickle-cell disease, 60
static vs dynamic treatment paradigm, 53
subtypes, 117-118
survival after, 266
thrombolytic therapy, 231-243, *240*
transient ischemic attacks (TIAs) and risk of,
　　61, 168
undetermined cause, 60, *67-69*
vertebrobasilar disease, 213
Stroke Data Bank (rating scale), *273*
Stump syndromes, 160
Subarachnoid hemorrhage, see Hemorrhage,
　　Subarachnoid
Subclavian artery, 106, 110, 203
Subclavian steal syndrome, 206, 208-209
Substance abuse, 123-124
Substance P, 6, *6*
Sulfinpyrazone, 159
Superficial temporal artery
　　—AICA anastomosis, 225
　　donor vessels in revasacularization surgery, 225
　　—MCA anastomosis, 215-218, 225, *225, 226,*
　　　226-228
　　—MCA bypass compared to EC-IC bypass, 216-218
　　—PICA anastomosis, 225
　　posterior cerebral artery anastomosis, 212, 215
Superior cerebellar artery anastomosis, 212
Surgery, see also Carotid endarterectomy
　　angiographic evaluation, 74
　　angiography (intraoperative), 180-181
　　arterial dissections, 189, 191, 200
　　barbiturate anesthesia, 180
　　blood velocity monitoring, 112-113
　　carotid stenosis over 70%, 159
　　carotid stump syndrome, 160
　　clinical trials, 251-263
　　crescendo transient ischemic attacks (TIAs),
　　　159-160
　　delayed for carotid occlusion, 160
　　Doppler and B-mode ultrasound, 91
　　EEG monitoring, 21
　　general considerations, 288
　　indications for extracranial carotid disease, 155-165
　　induced hypertension, 19, 22, 54
　　microscopy, 180
　　mortality, 155, 157, 163, 213
　　noncarotid procedures and silent carotid
　　　disease, 157-158
　　prophylactic, 130, 155
　　reoperation for carotid stenosis, 163
　　revascularization, 215-230
　　shunting, 178-179
　　special cases, 161-163

stroke and occlusive disease risk reduction, 130
stroke-in-evolution, 160
stroke rates, *254*
temporary vessel occlusion, 21
transcranial Doppler monitoring of blood flow, 92
venous patch angioplasty, 177-178
vertebrobasilar occlusion, 208-213
wound closure, 176
wound hematoma, 181-182
wound infection, 181
Swallowing, 275
Swan-Ganz catheter, 168
Sweden, 266
Syangiosis, 224, 227
Syphilis, 193
Systolic velocities, 104, 108

T

Thiopental, 17, 169, 173
Thixotropy, 27-30
Thrombocytosis, 148, 207
Thromboembolism
　　arterial dissections, 187, 197-198, 200
　　arterial occlusion and, 216
　　arterial trauma, 187
　　carotid artery ulceration, 85-86
　　extracranial vertebral artery, 197-198
　　planned large-vessel occlusion, 224
　　role in transient ischemic attacks (TIAs) and minor
　　　strokes, 218
Thrombolysis
　　agents, 232-234
　　animal models, 238-239
　　bleeding complications, *232*, 238
　　cardiac trials, *237*, 237-238
　　cerebral blood flow modulation, 20
　　clot formation and lysis, 231-232
　　cost *232*
　　hemorrhagic conversion, 239-243
　　intra-arterial trials, 239-241, *240, 241*
　　recanalization, 112, 151, 238-242
　　reocclusion rate, *232*
　　reperfusion, 151, 234, 238-240, 241
　　reperfusion-related hemorrhage, 20
　　risks, 242-243
　　time factors, 151
　　tissue rescue, 151
　　trials, 239-242
　　ultra-early evaluation, 234-236
Thrombosis
　　acute ischemia management, 149
　　arterial dissections, 200
　　carotid endarterectomy complications, risks, 168,
　　　182
　　extracranial vertebral artery dissection, 197-198

large-artery stroke, 59
luminal, 161-162
propagating, 187, 200, 224
small-artery, *284*
venous, 149, 150
Thromboxane A₂, 6, 7
Thyroid artery, 171, *172*
TIAs, see Transient ischemic attacks
Tinnitus, 199
Tissue plasminogen activator
    comparison of thrombolytic agents, *232,* 232-234
    description, trials, 151
    hemorrhagic conversion, 239, 242
    infarct size reduction, 20
    intracranial hemorrhage, 238
    intravenous thrombolytic studies, *240, 241,* 241-242
    intravenous, 241-242
    major thrombolytic trials, *237*
    recanalization, 238, 242
    reperfusion, 238
    vertebrobasilar disease, 208
Tissue rescue, see Brain
Tobacco
    arterial occlusion risk factors, 121-122
    infarction, stroke risk factors, 43, 61
    smoking cessation, 128-129
    stroke recurrence, 269
Tomography, see Computed tomography (CT);
    Positron emission tomography (PET); Single photon
        emission computed tomography (SPECT)
tPA, see Tissue plasminogen activator
Transcranial Doppler
    arterial dissection, 113
    blood velocities, 112-113, *114*
    circle of Willis, *114*
collateral pathways, 108
    dolichoectasia, 113
    expanding role, 103
    extracranial carotid stenosis, *109*
    extracranial internal carotid artery, 106
    general description, 106
    innominate stenosis, 109
    intracranial occlusive disease, 110-112
    intracranial vessels, 91-92, 196
    limitations, 235
    MCA stenosis, *111*
    microemboli, 112
    recanalization, 112
    sickle-cell vasculopathy, 113
    speedy evaluation of stroke, 235-236
    subclavian artery and steal syndrome, 110
    surgical monitoring of blood flow, 92
    velocities, 108, *109*
Transient ischemic attacks (TIAs)
    angiography, 87
    angiography risks, 88

antiplatelet aggregating agents, 158-159
carotid artery disease, 67, 85, 158-159
carotid endarterectomy clinical trials, 260-261
carotid stump syndrome, 160
crescendo, 62, 159
CT imaging, 77
diagnosis, management, 138-141
etiology, 61
evaluation same as stroke, 63
frequency and timing, 61
frequent (carotid endarterectomy risks), 168
heparin, 168
MRI, 81
MRI and MRA combination, 96
myocardial infarction in following year, 69
occlusive disease classfication, 59, 61-63
postoperative (carotid endarterectomy), 181
preceding stroke, 61-62
recurrent, 158-159
SPECT imaging, 95
stroke rate after first month, 168
stroke risk following, 158
subtypes, 62
surgical indication with 70% stenosis, 163
warning before acute stroke, 156
Transient monocular blindness, 61
Transtentorial herniation, 149
Trauma
    arterial dissection, 192-193, 199-200
    nonpenetrating injuries, 188-192
    penetrating injuries, 187-188
    spontaneous arterial dissection versus, 192-193
    vertebrobasilar occlusion, 206
Trigeminal artery, 204
Two-tailed analysis, 253
Type I and II errors, 253-254

U-V

Ultrasonography, 103-116, see also B-mode
        ultrasound; Color Doppler; Doppler ultra-
        sound; Transcranial Doppler
    asymptomatic carotid bruits, 74
    MR angiography compared to, 114
    transient ischemic attacks (TIAs), 115
Uric acid, 128
Urokinase
    comparison of thrombolytic agents, *232,* 232-234
    infarct size reduction, 20
    intravenous thrombolytic studies, *240, 241*
    major thrombolytic trials, *237*
    recanalization 151, 238
    vertebrobasilar disease, 208
US National Institutes of Health
    Stroke Scale, *271-273,* 273
Vagus nerve, 182-183

Validity (Clinical trials), 253
Vascular dementia, 268
Vascular reserve assessment, 108-109
Vasculitis, Cerebral, 147
Vasoactive intestinal peptide, 6, *6*
Vasoconstriction, *6,* 14, *15*
Vasodilation, 2, 5, *6*
Vasospasm
    chronic cerebral, 224-225
    fibrous, stenotic lesions, 244
    following subarachnoid hemorrhage, 54
    secondary, 14
    subarachnoid hemorrhage-induced, 20
Vecuronium bromide, 169
Velocity, see Blood flow velocity
Venesection, 43-44
Venous thrombosis, 149, 150
Vertebral arteries, see also specific arteries
    and conditions under Vertebral artery
    and Vertebrobasilar arteries
    anatomy, sections, 203
    angioplasty, *245*
    arteriosclerotic lesions, 210
    circumferential, 203
    continuous-wave Doppler, 105
    endarterectomy, 211
    stroke risk, 68-69
    transcranial Doppler, 106
    transposition, 208, *209*
    ultrasound techniques, 109, 113
Vertebral artery dissections
    angiography, 204, *206*
    carotid dissections simultaneously, 198-199
    extracranial, 197-199, *198*
    intracranial, 199
Vertebral artery, extracranial
    anastomosis to intracranial VA, 211-212, *211*
    dissection, 197-199, *198*
    reconstructions, 208, 212
    ultrasonography, 106, 110
Vertebral artery, internal (Intracranial)
    anastomosis from extracranial VA, 211-212, *211*
    dissection, 199

Vertebral artery occlusion
    dissection leading to, 198
    extracranial-to-intracranial anastomosis,
        (EC-IC), 211-212, *211*
    neurologic deficit, 63
Vertebral artery stenosis
    angioplasty, *245*
    endarterectomy, 211
    extracranial-to-intracranial anastomosis,
        (EC-IC), 211-212, *211*
    MRA, *205*
    poor prognosis, 69
    ultrasound techniques, 109
Vertebrobasilar arteries
    angiography, 207
    insufficiency, 206, 207
    infarctions, CT imaging, 77-78
    ischemia, 197-198
    transient ischemic attacks (TIAs), 141
Vertebrobasilar occlusion, 203-214
    abnormalities, 204
    dissecting aneurysms, 204
    dolichoectatic changes, 204
    no controlled trial of therapies, 223
    plaques, 204
    recanalization, hemorrhagic conversion, 240-241
    thrombolytic therapy, *240,* 240-241
Veterans Administration Cooperative Studies
    Program, *257,* 258-260
Viscometers, *28,* 28, 29, 31, 32
Viscosity, see Blood viscosity
Visual fields, *271, 273*
Vocal cord paralysis, 183

W-X-Y

Warfarin, 200
Watershed zones, 77-78, *79,* 81
Wernicke's aphasia, 63
Women (Vertebrobasilar disease and), 207
Wounds, surgical, see under Surgery
Xenon cerebral blood flow, 92-94, *93,* 236
Young adults (infarctions in), 146-149

Previously Published Books in the *Neurosurgical Topics* Series

Management of Posttraumatic Spinal Instability
  Edited by Paul R. Cooper, MD

Malignant Cerebral Glioma
  Edited by Michael L.J. Apuzzo, MD

Intracranial Vascular Malformations
  Edited by Daniel L. Barrow, MD

Neurosurgical Treatment of Disorders of the Thoracic Spine
  Edited by Edward C. Tarlov, MD

Contemporary Diagnosis and Management of Pituitary Adenomas
  Edited by Paul R. Cooper, MD

Complications of Spinal Surgery
  Edited by Edward C. Tarlov, MD

Neurosurgical Aspects of Epilepsy
  Edited by Michael L.J. Apuzzo, MD

Complications and Sequelae of Head Injury
  Edited by Daniel L. Barrow, MD

Practical Approaches to Peripheral Nerve Surgery
  Edited by Edward C. Benzel, MD

For order information call (708) 692-9500.